Effective Functional Progressions in Sport Rehabilitation

Todd S. Ellenbecker, DPT, CSCS

Physiotherapy Associates
Scottsdale Sports Clinic, Scottsdale, AZ

Mark S. De Carlo, PT, MHA, SCS, ATC

Methodist Sports Medicine
The Orthopedic Specialists, Indianapolis, IN

Carl DeRosa, PT, PhD, FAPTA

Northern Arizona University
DeRosa Physical Therapy at Summit Center, Flagstaff, AZ

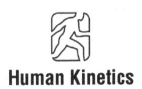

Human Kinetics

Library of Congress Cataloging-in-Publication Data

Ellenbecker, Todd S., 1962-
  Effective functional progressions in sport rehabilitation / Todd Ellenbecker, Mark De Carlo, Carl DeRosa.
    p. ; cm.
  Includes bibliographical references and index.
  ISBN-13: 978-0-7360-6381-4 (soft cover)
  ISBN-10: 0-7360-6381-1 (soft cover)
  1. Sports injuries. 2. Athletes--Rehabilitation. I. De Carlo, Mark, 1960- II. DeRosa, Carl. III. Title.
  [DNLM: 1. Athletic Injuries--rehabilitation. 2. Physical Therapy Modalities. QT 261 E45e 2009]
  RD97.E45 2009
  617.1'027--dc22
                         2008048273

ISBN-10: 0-7360-6381-1
ISBN-13: 978-0-7360-6381-4

The Web addresses cited in this text were current as of November 2008, unless otherwise noted.

Acquisitions Editor: Loarn D. Robertson, PhD; **Developmental Editor:** Amanda S. Ewing; **Assistant Editors:** Kate Maurer, Melissa J. Zavala, Nicole Gleeson, and Christine Bryant Cohen; **Copyeditor:** Patricia L. MacDonald; **Proofreader:** Joanna Hatzopoulos Portman; **Indexer:** Gerry Lynn Shipe; **Permission Manager:** Dalene Reeder; **Graphic Designer:** Fred Starbird; **Graphic Artist:** Patrick Sandberg; **Cover Designer:** Keith Blomberg; **Photographer (cover):** © kevinswan.com; **Photographer (interior):** photos on pages 9 and 185 © Human Kinetics; photos on pages 7-8, 14, 42, 46, 48, and 50-99 courtesy of Todd Ellenbecker; photos on page 137 courtesy of Gary Cook, PT, PC; photos on pages 138-147 and 154-161 © kevinswan.com; photos on pages 177-178, 181, 183, 197-207, and 209-214 courtesy of Carl DeRosa; **Photo Asset Manager:** Laura Fitch; **Photo Production Manager:** Jason Allen; **Art Manager:** Kelly Hendren; **Associate Art Manager:** Alan L. Wilborn; **Illustrator:** Jason M. McAlexander, MFA; **Printer:** Total Printing Systems

Printed in the United States of America   10 9 8 7 6 5 4 3

The paper in this book is certified under a sustainable forestry program.

Human Kinetics
Web site: www.HumanKinetics.com

United States: Human Kinetics, P.O. Box 5076, Champaign, IL 61825-5076
800-747-4457
email: info@hkusa.com

Canada: Human Kinetics, 475 Devonshire Road Unit 100, Windsor, ON N8Y 2L5
800-465-7301 (in Canada only)
email: info@hkcanada.com

Europe: Human Kinetics, 107 Bradford Road, Stanningley, Leeds LS28 6 AT, United Kingdom
+44 (0) 113 255 5665
email: hk@hkeurope.com

Australia: Human Kinetics, 57A Price Avenue, Lower Mitcham, South Australia 5062
08 8372 0999
e-mail: info@hkaustralia.com

New Zealand: Human Kinetics, P.O. Box 80, Mitcham Shopping Centre, South Australia 5062
0800 222 062
e-mail: info@hknewzealand.com

E3723

HUMAN KINETICS ONLINE RESOURCE

How to access the supplemental online resource

We are pleased to provide access to an online resource that supplements *Effective Functional Progressions in Sport Rehabilitation*. This resource offers an image bank, which contains all of the art, content photos, and tables from the book delivered via PowerPoint; a blank PowerPoint template; and a blank Word handout template. We are certain you will enjoy this unique online feature.

Accessing the online resource is easy!
Follow these steps if you purchased a new book:

1. Visit **www.HumanKinetics.com/ EffectiveFunctionalProgressionsInSportRehabilitation**.

2. Click the <u>first edition</u> link next to the book cover.

3. Click the Sign In link on the left or top of the page. If you do not have an account with Human Kinetics, you will be prompted to create one.

4. If the online product you purchased does not appear in the Ancillary Items box on the left of the page, click the Enter Key Code option in that box. Enter the key code that is printed at the right, including all hyphens. Click the Submit button to unlock your online product.

5. After you have entered your key code the first time, you will never have to enter it again to access this product. Once unlocked, a link to your product will permanently appear in the menu on the left. For future visits, all you need to do is sign in to the textbook's website and follow the link that appears in the left menu!

→ Click the Need Help? button on the textbook's website if you need assistance along the way.

For technical support, send an e-mail to:
support@hkusa.com . . . . U.S. and international customers
info@hkcanada.com . . . . Canadian customers
academic@hkeurope.com . . . . European customers
keycodesupport@hkaustralia.com . . . . . Australian and New Zealand customers

HUMAN KINETICS
The Information Leader in Physical Activity & Health

12-2015

This unique code allows you access to the online resource.

Product: Effective Functional Progressions in Sport Rehabilitation online resource

Key code: ELLENBECKER-CNMAL4-OSG

Access is provided if you have purchased a new book. Once submitted, the code may not be entered for any other user.

To my wife, Gail, for her constant love and support; and my mentors in physical therapy who have taught me the tremendous value in the progression of exercise
~ Todd Ellenbecker

To Christian and Sarah, I love you to heaven and back; and to my colleagues Patti Hunker, Debbie Carroll, Ryan McDivitt and Kathy Oneacre, for your contributions to this project
~ Mark De Carlo

To Riley and Cooper, with love forever
~ Carl DeRosa

Contents

Preface   vii

Part I
Components of Functional Progressions 1

Chapter 1   **Introduction to
Functional Progression** 3

Benefits of a Functional Progression   4
Clinical Guidelines for Functional Progression   6
Guidelines for Initiating Functional Progression   8
Summary   10

Chapter 2   **Developing Successful Functional
Progression Programs.** 11

Key Components of
Functional Progression Programs   12
Kinetic Link Principle   15
Summary   20

Part II
Regional Functional Progressions 21

Chapter 3   **Upper Extremity** **23**

Anatomy of the Upper Extremity   23
Muscular Stabilization of the Upper Extremity   26
Biomechanics of the Upper Extremity   28
Injuries   36
Functional Testing of the Upper Extremity   41
Functional Exercise Progressions   49
Summary   108

Chapter 4   **Lower Extremity** **109**

Anatomy of the Lower Extremity   109
Muscular Stabilization of the Lower Extremity   115
Biomechanics of the Lower Extremity   120
Injuries   129
Functional Testing of the Lower Extremity   134
Clinical Exercise Progressions   138
Functional Exercise Progressions   147
Summary   161

Chapter 5   **Trunk** **163**

Anatomy of the Trunk   164
Muscular Stabilization of the Trunk   175
Biomechanics of the Trunk   187
Injuries   189
Functional Testing of the Trunk   190
Functional Exercise Tests and Progressions   195
Summary   215

References   217

Index   229

About the Authors   239

Preface

One of the most challenging tasks encountered in the rehabilitation of an orthopedic and sports injury is the provision of exercise progressions that adequately simulate and prepare the individual for their return to an active lifestyle and ultimately athletic activity. The purpose of this book is to provide the clinician with an objectively based approach to the progression of functional exercise for the individuals following orthopedic injuries to the upper and lower extremities and trunk. This book is designed to provide vital information that will allow the clinician to better understand the important concepts of functional progressions as well as provide specific examples of functional progressions for the upper and lower extremity and trunk. Each individual author has many years of clinical and research experience in their regional area and is best able to provide the specific information on exercise progression, functional testing, and return to sport functional progressions.

One unique emphasis in this book is the use of referenced material and scientific basis to the material presented. While each author has presented their exercise and functional progressions, each author provided evidence for the inclusion of these exercises and activities and functional tests. This will for some readers provide the necessary justification for inclusion of these exercises and progressions in their treatment programming.

Our goal is that this book provide a unique reference for the practicing clinician and provide usable material that can be quickly and easily referenced and applied. It provides a "how to" approach with a "why to" approach integrated into one text. While the book can be read in a comprehensive front to back fashion, it is designed and organized with specific, detailed sections on the upper and lower extremities and the trunk. This organization can allow the reader to hone in on a specific area of exercise progression realizing that the core stabilization information described in chapter 5 will be ultimately applicable when progressing exercise for the extremities as well.

In part I of this book key introductory information is presented on exercise progression outlining the critical elements of exercise progression imbedded with clinically relevant examples of how the material in the subsequent chapters can be applied. Chapter 1 looks specifically at the benefits of functional progressions and the guidelines one needs to follow to initiate functional progressions. Chapter 2 outlines how exactly to design a successful functional progression program.

In part II, each of the three areas (chapter 3, upper extremity; chapter 4, lower extremity; and chapter 5, trunk) are presented comprehensively, highlighting the specific anatomical and biomechanical nuances inherent in each area while also presenting the neuromuscular basis for the specific approaches to each region. While each of these chapters does have concise and clinically relevant anatomy and biomechanical information, it is not meant to be all-encompassing in this area. Rather, the clinically most important anatomical and biomechanical concepts are developed prior to the exercise progressions themselves.

Each of the chapters in part II also includes specific functional tests for each region. Tests are reviewed with normative data provided when applicable to allow clinicians to interpret test results in their patients and use those results to objectively progress resistive and functional exercise programming. The exercise progressions themselves are presented in a consistent fashion throughout the text and provide information on how to specifically perform the exercise, illustrate how that exercise fits into the progression, and provide additional clinical insight into why that particular exercise or progression is needed and essential to rehabilitation for that region of the body. Each progression is presented using a consistent format providing specific information on the starting position of the exercise, the exercise action, and both the indications and contraindications of the exercise. Additionally, reference to the muscles or muscle groups that are targeted with each exercise are provided along with, when applicable, clinically important information termed "pearls of performance." Photos illustrate the movements required to successfully perform the progression. In addition to the regional breakdown provided, several sport specific functional progressions are provided as examples to return patients to specific sport activities such as throwing and running.

To further help clinicians use the information in this book to create functional progressions and instructors to teach classes, an image bank is provided online at www.HumanKinetics.com/EffectiveFunctionalProgressionsInSportRehabilitation/.

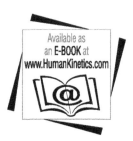

The image bank provides all of the art, tables, and photos used in the book. These images can be used by clinicians to create handouts for their clients (a blank handout template is provided) or by instructors to create a PowerPoint presentation (a blank PowerPoint template is provided) or other class handouts. The image bank is provided free to anyone who purchases the book and can be accessed by following the instructions on the key code letter at the front of the book.

Components of Functional Progressions

Functional progression is of critical importance to the rehabilitation professional. In addition to having a detailed understanding of the specific exercises that may form a functional progression, the clinician must also have an understanding of the basic components that form a progression, the factors that dictate the progression and, perhaps most important, the rate of progression of the exercises. Part I provides the basic elements needed to design a functional progression program. A brief review of functional exercise and exercise progression is provided in chapter 1, followed in chapter 2 by clinical examples of applying many of these components.

C·H·A·P·T·E·R 1

Introduction to Functional Progression

Functional progression has become increasingly more common in all sport rehabilitation programs. Using the functional progression concept in rehabilitation is not new. More than 30 years ago, Yamamoto and colleagues (1975) described a functional progression program used in the rehabilitation of injured West Point cadets. This program placed emphasis on restoring agility through dynamic exercise after knee injury, versus what the authors termed a static exercise program. Kegerreis (1983) added specific movement patterns and skills to the program and introduced the importance of addressing the psychological needs of injured athletes. He also addressed the scientific principles that play an important role in functional progression, specifically healing-time constraints and proprioception. Specificity of the functional progression program was given high priority as well. The need to break down sport-specific functions to be gradually addressed within rehabilitation was put into perspective in later publications (Kegerreis, Malone, and McCarroll 1984; Kegerreis and Wetherald 1987).

Advances in medicine have allowed clinical professionals to become much more proficient in the diagnosis and treatment of athletic injuries. However, though an athlete may have achieved clinical goals, a physician or other medical professional can be sure the athlete is able to return to his sport only by having him complete a functional assessment specific to his activity. A functional progression is a series of basic sport-specific movement patterns graduated according to the difficulty of the skill and the athlete's tolerance. The end goal of functional progression is an athlete's timely and safe return to competition.

Functional progression is a vital component of a conscientious return-to-sport program. Inclusion of a functional progression in a treatment program is a sign of a prudent rehabilitation professional. It is of utmost importance that the athlete advance one step at a time. Function within a given sport must be broken down into basic skills and movements that are progressed gradually as the athlete tolerates them. As the athlete regains the skills specific to her sport, appropriate safeguards against further injury must be taken.

Functional progression is based on a principle known as specific adaptations to imposed demands (SAID) (Kegerreis 1983). The SAID principle, which states that the body adapts to the specific demands placed on it, should guide the clinician in creating a functional progression that incorporates key movements associated

3

with the specific activity. Demands vary within sports as well as across sports. Specific positions within a sport may require speed and agility, while others may focus on strength. The functional progression for a football player will be different from one developed for a volleyball player. An effective rehabilitation program must prepare each person for the demands that will be placed on the injured area once the program has been successfully completed. A sound functional progression program needs to address each athlete's role in his sport. Once the specific activity has been broken down into required fundamental movements, the athlete stresses his injured body part progressively until function is adequate for him to return to sport-specific demands.

This chapter discusses the psychological and physiological benefits of a functional progression for the athlete and guidelines for implementation. Clinicians are given guidelines to transition from clinical rehabilitation to a functional progression that emphasizes a gradual building of intensity, movements, duration, and joint loads.

BENEFITS OF A FUNCTIONAL PROGRESSION

Both the clinician and the athlete benefit from a sound functional progression program. The athlete benefits physiologically and psychologically, while the clinician has objective measurements by which to advance the athlete safely into her sport.

Physiological Benefits for the Athlete

During the healing process, injured tissue must be stressed according to the manner in which it functions. Stress applied to the tissue must be sufficient to encourage healing, but not so stressful as to inhibit healing. Following is a discussion of the physiological principles governing the healing process, as well as the physical benefits of the functional progression program.

At the heart of the physical benefits of functional progression are Davis' law and Wolff's law. These two physiological principles state that soft tissue (Davis' law) and bone (Wolff's law) heal according to the manner in which they are stressed (Tippet and Voight 1995). Wolff's law, a theory developed by the German anatomist and surgeon Julius Wolff (1835-1902) in the 19th century, states that bone in a healthy person or animal will adapt to the loads it is placed under. If loading on a particular bone increases, the bone will remodel itself over time to become stronger to resist that sort of loading. The converse is true as well: If the loading on a bone decreases, the bone will become weaker because of turnover, as it is less metabolically costly to maintain and there is no stimulus for continued remodeling to maintain bone mass.

As Davis' law describes, healing tissue responds to stress by reacting along the lines of the given stress. For optimum healing, tissue must be stressed gradually to accept a given force. During rehabilitation, if healing tissue is not stressed in the way required of it before the injury, the tissue will not be ready to fully accept preinjury requirements. Making the soft tissue accept this stress during rehabilitation will lead to strengthening of the tissue. Wolff's law states that the same principle applies to healing bone. For example, with an inversion ankle sprain in a basketball player, if the athlete were allowed to return to basketball after completing straight-plane resisted activities only, the healing lateral ankle ligaments would not be stressed to provide for optimum healing required for basketball activities.

Tippet and Voight (1995) describe postinjury performance enhancement as another benefit for the athlete who participates in a comprehensive functional progression program. While participating in a functional progression program, the athlete proceeds from simple, safe skills to complex skills that more closely mimic competition. The differences in the performance of an athlete who has not undergone adequate functional progression training and an athlete who is prepared for a return to sport are readily apparent. Typically, performance of the person who has not taken part in the functional progression program is characterized by inadequate speed, strength, or endurance in a given sport skill. This is especially true as the degree of difficulty of a skill or the duration of participation is increased. The athlete who returns prematurely to competition usually favors the injured area and ends up either voluntarily or involuntarily being removed from competition. The athlete who has completed a functional progression program usually performs on the same level as his noninjured teammates. Normal, unencumbered postinjury performance is the goal of the functional progression program.

Psychological Benefits for the Athlete

Any health care professional who has assisted in sport rehabilitation knows that the psyche deserves as much attention as the physical body. Helping the athlete return to competition with confidence after an injury is clearly a vital concern. Sport psychologists have studied and documented the emotional reactions of athletes who have been injured (Tippet and Voight 1995; Carr 2006). At the point of injury and immediately after the injury, the athlete may demonstrate shock, emotional disorganization, and denial, while uncertainty and excessive anxiety may set in as treatment options are being considered (Carr 2006). Often, removing an athlete from a sport after an injury can be devastating. Sports may be the focal point in life for some athletes, and the inability to participate because of injury may completely disrupt their lives. The sooner they can resume normal activities, the better for their peace of mind. Questions such as "What will I be like?" and "Will I be able to function?" are normal, and through the course of functional progression, these questions are answered. This could be compounded if the injury occurs at a critical time during the season, such as just before a championship game (Carr 2006).

Functional progression drills are introduced during rehabilitation as soon as the sport participant is ready. Those involved in team sports should be encouraged to perform these drills during regular practice sessions. When appropriate (e.g., with stretching exercises), the person can perform the drills alongside noninjured teammates. When teammates are doing drills that the injured person is not ready for, she can perform appropriate functional progression drills alongside teammates.

Returning the athlete to a familiar environment as soon as possible minimizes the stress of not fitting in because of injury. Remember that the athlete must be sufficiently rehabilitated before returning to competition. Just as feelings of deprivation are normal for the injured person, feelings of uncertainty are also common. During the progression, the athlete may experience emotions of both fear and relief (Carr 2006). The athlete may be concerned as to whether or not he will be able to return to his preinjury level of competition, and the fear of reinjury may be present. Extraneous pressures may be placed on the person to recover well enough to maintain a starting position on the team, to keep a scholarship, or to continue to earn a living. As the athlete responds to rehabilitation, functional progression activities are introduced that prepare him for competition. Preparation enhances confidence. If the person tolerates a graduated series of progressively difficult drills, self-confidence improves right along with specific sport function. The functional progression program will ready the athlete for any situation he may encounter after returning to sport. The key is that the person tackles each of the steps in a controlled, supervised functional progression program before being asked to perform competitively. Therefore, the athlete enters the competitive arena confident that function will be up to playing standards.

CLINICAL GUIDELINES FOR FUNCTIONAL PROGRESSION

Functional progression drills are the activities that bridge the gap between clinic-based rehabilitation and sport function. The athlete is ready to advance from traditional rehabilitation to functional progression activities when she has met specific clinical goals.

Tissue Healing

It is beyond this book's scope to discuss sequelae of all sport injuries as they relate to healing parameters. However, it is vital during every phase of rehabilitation not to stress healing tissue beyond its tolerance. Many factors play a direct role in how the injured body part responds after a sports injury. These factors include the effects of immobilization after the injury, the natural course after surgical and nonsurgical intervention, the condition of the injured tissue, the overall general conditioning of the person before injury, and the age of the athlete (Barrack et al. 1990; Buckley, Barrack, and Alexander 1989; Elmqvist et al. 1988; Harter et al. 1988; Indelicato, Hermansdorfer, and Huegel 1990; Jokl et al. 1987; Noyes et al. 1974; Odensten, Lysholm, and Gillquist 1985; Weiss et al. 1989). The clinician must consider all these variables and implement, monitor, and modify the functional progression program accordingly.

Swelling

Swelling is an indicator of an overzealous rehabilitation program. After injury to a joint, there should be very minimal to no swelling when a functional progression is initiated. If swelling is present, activities that do not increase swelling should be stressed. Therapeutic modalities such as high-volt galvanic stimulation, intermittent or constant compression, and cryotherapy should be emphasized.

Pain

Pain is a determinant of whether or not the activity is too strenuous during rehabilitation. In a carefully advanced program, the athlete should experience minimal to no pain. If pain occurs with any rehabilitation activity, that particular activity should be avoided. Pain is counterproductive to rehabilitation exercises because of reflex muscle inhibition. If pain is present, activity should be curtailed, and analgesics, electrotherapeutic modalities, or cryotherapy can be employed before the initiation of a functional progression.

Range of Motion

Range of motion (ROM) equal to that of the noninjured side must be present before initiating a functional progression (figure 1.1). Joints have normal ROM guidelines as well as normal end feels (e.g., soft tissue approximation, bone to bone, springy). If ROM deficits are present, functional progression activities should be deemphasized and

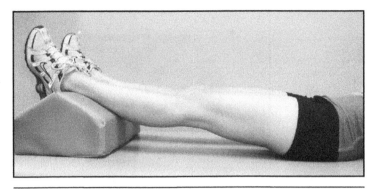

Figure 1.1 Symmetrical knee ROM.

active, active-assisted, or passive ROM exercises stressed. As soon as range of motion is sufficient to allow unimpeded performance of the simplest functional progression activities, the formal program may be initiated.

Strength

Muscle strength provides dynamic stability to any given joint and must be adequate for the rigors of functional progression. An adequate strength base is absolutely essential for any sport activity. When rehabilitating an injury of the lower extremity, therapists should look for strength to be symmetrical. After injury to the upper extremity, however, equal strength on both sides may not be satisfactory. Ideally, strength of the athlete's dominant arm in throwing activities should be 10 to 15%

greater than the nondominant arm. A stronger dominant arm is especially important to the throwing athlete or to those who play racket sports.

Strength can be assessed in a number of ways. Isokinetic dynamometers vary among different manufactures, and readings may vary (figure 1.2). The same holds true in regard to the extrapolation of agonist–antagonist ratios, torque-output–body-weight ratios, and other generally accepted data (Cook et al. 1987; Walmsley and Szybbo 1987; Wyatt and Edwards 1981). Strength may also be assessed with handheld dynamometers (figure 1.3). Consideration must be given to the overall strength of the examiner, joint position, and the location of applied resistance (McMahon, Burdett, and Whitney 1992; Wadsworth, Krishnan, Sear, Harrold, and Nielsen 1987; Wikholw and Bohannon 1991). Simple subjective manual muscle tests, functional testing, and other standard methods may also be used to assist in determining strength.

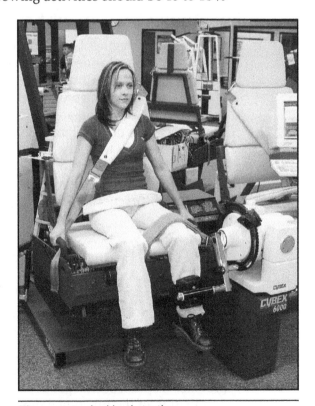

Figure 1.2 Isokinetic testing.

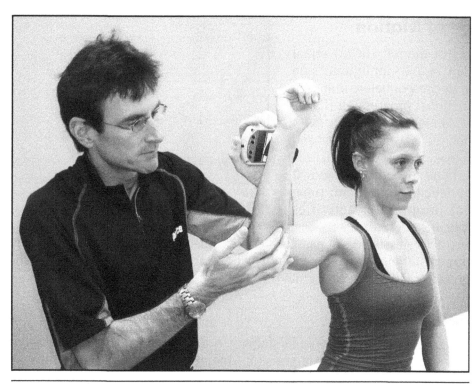

Figure 1.3   Upper extremity strength test with a handheld dynamometer.

Functional Movement Screening

Cook and colleagues have created the Functional Movement Screen (FMS). Designed to assess functional movement deficits, the FMS is based on proprioceptive and kinesthetic awareness principles (Cook, Burton, and Hoogenboom 2006). The evaluator assesses and grades seven fundamental dynamic movements, and the deficits are addressed through repeated movements and cues. Movements are done bilaterally and include deep squats, hurdle steps, in-line lunges, shoulder mobility exercises, active straight-leg raises, trunk stability push-ups, and rotary stability exercises. The FMS can be used as an adjunct to complete the rehabilitative process by addressing movement deficits before beginning a functional progression. The FMS is discussed in greater detail in chapter 4.

GUIDELINES FOR INITIATING FUNCTIONAL PROGRESSION

Perhaps the most important benefit of a functional progression is the ability to measure an athlete's tolerance to functional activity. More important, having the injured person proceed through an objective functional progression is an accurate assessment of her tolerance to a given activity. Tolerance to these activities provides a sport-specific gauge of progress.

Initiation of the functional progression begins with simple skills that are used as building blocks for the more-advanced skills. Throughout the program, the athlete is evaluated and reevaluated. If no problems are encountered, progression to the next step is allowed. However, if problems arise at a given stage, the athlete remains at that stage until the symptoms are resolved. The athlete can proceed to the next stage only after preceding skills are performed satisfactorily and are well tolerated. Guidelines for advancement during the functional progression include the following:

- Initiation of skills that require slow speed, with progression to faster speeds
- Initiation of simple skills, with progression to more-complex skills
- Initiation of skills at short distances, with progression to longer distances
- Initiation of unloaded skills, with progression to loaded skills

Slow Speeds Progressed to Fast Speeds

Initially, speed should be kept slow, with emphasis on proper form and skill execution. As the skill is mastered, it becomes more automatic, requiring less volitional and conscious effort. Once the skill can be performed properly, the speed may be increased. For example, jogging should be accomplished with symmetrical weight bearing and weight shift before beginning running and sprinting activities. The same principle applies to throwing, rowing, swimming, cycling, and other activities.

Simple Skills Progressed to Difficult Skills

The clinician needs to progress the athlete from simple rehabilitative exercises to more-difficult skills required for his sport activity. If a clinician does not know the specific requirements of the given sport, she should admit her limitations and try to become better informed. Other options are to send the athlete to a professional with better knowledge in the area or to work jointly with the athlete's coach. Examples that may require collaboration include simple countering moves in wrestling, the intricacies involved in diving or gymnastics (figure 1.4), or the footwork required in the football offensive backfield.

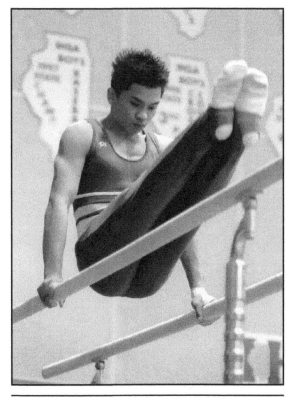

Short Distances Progressed to Longer Distances

Sport-specific anaerobic and aerobic endurance must be considered. Function must be automatic and efficient, and the skill must be performed for the duration of time required by a given sport. Without an adequate anaerobic or aerobic base, function suffers; more important, the athlete is at greater risk of reinjury as the duration of activity increases.

Figure 1.4 Before creating a functional rehabilitation program, the clinician must understand how movements occur in a particular sport.

Unloaded Activities Progressed to Loaded Activities

Unloaded skills are those in which no outside resistance is applied to the athlete. Examples of unloaded activities are running, assuming the down position in wrestling, and an American football player practicing agility drills while running with the football. These are contrasted with loaded activities in which extra resistance is added. Loaded activities are the same runner running with a weighted vest, the wrestler in a down position with another wrestler on top of him, and the football player being tackled by defenders. When progressing to loaded activities, the rehabilitation professional, the coach, or a trained observer should take extra care to regulate and supervise the athlete.

SUMMARY

The successful transition from clinical rehabilitation to a functional progression and an athlete's return to sport requires clinicians to be cognizant of the benefits of its implementation, clinical signs for advancement to functional exercise, and the gradual building of exercise principles during a functional progression. With these guidelines in mind, a clinician can successfully return the athlete to her sport activity.

2

Developing Successful Functional Progression Programs

As discussed in chapter 1, functional progressions play an integral role in both the rehabilitation of the injured athlete and the enhancement of performance in any individual or athlete. The tenets of a functional progression are outlined in that important chapter, which sets the stage for further discussion of the components of a successful functional progression program. To aid in better understanding how these progressions can be used, this chapter gives a few examples to illustrate where and when functional progressions are most often utilized. Additionally, clinical determinants of exercise progression, such as monitoring signs and symptoms and the application of clinical tests to guide exercise selection and progression rates, are also detailed using patient-relevant examples. Finally, the last part of the chapter details the vital interaction of the upper extremity, lower extremity, and trunk by reviewing the kinetic chain concept.

Clinical rehabilitation professionals are often faced with the challenge of rehabilitating an athlete or active person after an anterior cruciate ligament (ACL) reconstruction, a meniscal repair, or a microfracture procedure of the knee. Many articles and published texts can guide clinicians in the early postoperative and postinjury management of these patients. At some point in the rehabilitation (e.g., 4 to 6 weeks post-op), when the patient has regained some control of the quadriceps muscles, regained most or all of her range of motion, and demonstrates a normal gait pattern, the thought process of both the treating clinician and patient moves to the return of full function, and this most often means athletic or recreational activity. The functional progression program becomes extremely important at this point.

Another example of the importance of functional progression can be highlighted during the rehabilitation of a patient after an arthroscopic labral repair in the shoulder. Although the initial phase of rehabilitation is immeasurably important to regain range of motion and improve rotator cuff strength and scapular stabilization, there comes a point where the integration and advancement of the rehabilitation program requires functional progression to allow that patient to return to throwing or overhead function. Failure to provide this progression in the program often leads to delayed recovery times, overtraining, and an overall unsuccessful outcome after surgery or injury. Furthermore, if the clinician working with this person fails to properly analyze the future demands that his patient will place on her upper extremity in the throwing motion, it will likely lead to inappropriate exercise progressions, ineffective loading patterns, and extended rehabilitation times. These two examples show how important the design and integration of a functional progression program are in order to restore full function and achieve optimal success.

KEY COMPONENTS OF FUNCTIONAL PROGRESSION PROGRAMS

Many key components are inherent in a successful functional progression program. Since the program above all else has to be designed for a specific person, following one preset guideline or functional progression cannot be recommended. Therefore, it is important in this chapter to briefly review some of the key components in the rehabilitation process and the process of using and applying functional exercise progressions, and then introduce in the following chapters a detailed series of functional progressions, with supportive evidence and background information in anatomy and biomechanics, to empower the reader to develop his or her own progression for successful applications.

Monitoring Signs and Symptoms

The continued monitoring of the signs and symptoms of the patient during the functional progression is of critical importance for the success of any progression. This forms the basis for the rate and frequency of the progression of the program. Some of the key signs and symptoms are introduced in chapter 1 but are so important that they warrant repeating. For example, the presence of intra-articular swelling is one factor of critical importance in virtually all rehabilitation and functional progressions. Although it may be somewhat joint specific, intra-articular swelling can be palpated and measured or clinically observed in several key joints throughout the body. Swelling about the knee and ankle, for example, is easily monitored and in lower extremity progressions can be an extremely valuable marker for clinical progression. In other joints such as the glenohumeral and coxofemoral joints, swelling is much less noticeable and does not play a major role in the screening process. Progressing exercise and activities in the presence of joint swelling is contraindicated and clearly not recommended.

Other signs and symptoms that often occur with or without swelling are joint pain, significant muscular fatigue or loss of control, and decreased joint motion. The presence of any of these in isolation or combination slows down the functional progression. Using visual analog scales (VAS) or simply asking the person to rate his level of pain, fatigue, or improvement using a scale of 0 to 10 can help put an objective slant on otherwise subjective perceptions of the person's function and feelings during the progression.

Establishing Continuous Progression

The concept of continuous progression is apparent to most, but it is often not adhered to in many suboptimal programs. It is difficult and often encumbering to initially design the functional progression program. Continuing to adjust and progress the program, however, is required to successfully progress the person to optimize gains in strength, motion, and function. Frequent and periodic reevaluations of function as well as consistent monitoring of performance are required to allow continuous progression of the program once initiated. Each of the subsequent chapters on the upper and lower extremities and the trunk will outline specific progressions, complete with information about the methods commonly used and recommended for progressing the program. These form the basic elemental aspects of a functional progression program and can include increases in volume, frequency, duration, and of course exercise intensity.

Using Sport- and Activity-Specific Progression in Addition to Basic Progressions

This key concept highlights the need to balance specific training with the required basic progressions to ensure that optimal baseline strength, coordination, and other important factors remain present throughout the progression. To best illustrate this concept, here is a specific example. When a throwing athlete returns to pitching after rotator cuff tendinitis, baseball-specific progressions are used, including throwing drills that progressively increase the intensity and distance of the throwing motion as well as progress from throwing on flat ground to off the mound. Although this sounds like a very sound progression for a baseball pitcher (and from a throwing perspective, it is), failure to address rotator cuff and scapular strengthening—which for all intents and purposes may appear to be too basic— will likely result in inadequate emphasis on those important muscle groups and lead to muscular imbalance and suboptimal recovery. Additionally, ignoring core stability training and hip strengthening progressions during this return program would also be remiss because these programs (rotator cuff and scapular program, core stability, and hip strengthening) form the basis on which the functionally specific program can progress.

This example highlights the importance of combining sport- or activity-specific programs with more-basic programs to ensure strength development and muscular balance. Other examples include the continued emphasis on quadriceps strength development in the patient while cutting and running drills are concomitantly being progressed to ensure that this important muscle group is continuing to develop during the sport-specific progression. The basic progressions supplied in this book for key muscle groups, and concepts such as core stability, scapular stabilization, and rotator cuff strength, cannot be forgotten or deemphasized once the other sport-specific functional progressions are initiated.

Using Objective and Functional Tests to Guide Progression

Another key factor to consider with respect to functional progression is the integration and use of objective tests and functional tests to guide the progression of the program. The final three chapters of this book list key tests and measures that can help guide the clinician during the progression of a functional program. An example of the application of this type of testing helps support this concept. Frequently, a one-leg stability test or one-leg squat test is used during rehabilitation or preseason physical evaluation of an athlete. For this test, the athlete performs a one-leg squat while the clinician observes the quality of the motion. Often during this movement, the contralateral hip drops downward (termed a positive Trendelenburg sign) as the knee of the stance limb bends (figure 2.1). The presence of this

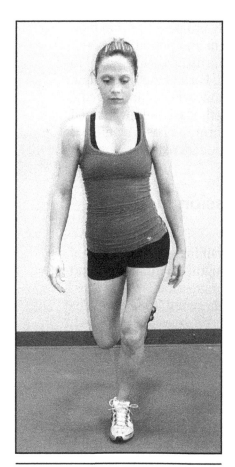

Figure 2.1   Trendelenburg sign.

finding indicates weakness of the stance limb's gluteus medius, as it is unable to properly stabilize the pelvis in a level orientation during the descent of the one-leg squat maneuver (Hardcastle and Nade 1985; Kibler, Press, and Sciascia 2006, Chimielewski et al. 2007).

More-detailed interpretation of functional testing has been reported by Piva et al. (2006) for a lower extremity step-down test. Compensatory movements of the arm, dropping of the pelvis, and inward (valgus) angulation of the knee while performing the step-down test can be objectively evaluated and provide key insight into the readiness of a person to return to lower extremity functional activities. The presence of a positive hip drop or Trendelenburg finding in a patient after knee injury indicates the need for more-specific and basic exercise progressions to increase core and gluteus medius strength before introducing more-advanced progressions. This test, then, can become a key part of the reevaluation process to ensure that adequate hip and core stability and pelvic control have been restored before moving on to more-functional and sport-specific programs.

A similar example in the upper extremity is the use and application of clinical tests such as impingement tests (Ellenbecker 2004) and the subluxation relocation test (Hamner, Pink, and Jobe 2000) coupled with isokinetic strength testing to determine readiness of a patient with rotator cuff tendinitis to return to more-advanced throwing progressions. In this example, progressing a patient who has pain in the position of 90° of abduction and 90° of external rotation to a throwing program would be inadvisable based on the findings of that objective test. Similarly, extensive weakness or an imbalance in the rotator cuff musculature identified with an isokinetic shoulder internal and external rotation test is another contraindication for progression. Frequent testing and retesting to gauge improvement not only ensures proper rates of progression in the functional programs but also empowers the person or athlete by demonstrating the effectiveness of the programs being applied to improve baseline function. Functional tests and objective measures of strength, range of motion, and anthropometric girth can form the basis for the thoughtful and educated progression of the programs contained in this book.

Evaluating Technique

The final section of this chapter deals with the importance of evaluating the person's technique as he progresses in the functional program. One of the key concepts in the evaluation of technique involves the kinetic link principle. Clinicians often focus so closely on the injured joint or segment during evaluation that other links and compensations in the kinetic chain are missed and not properly addressed in either the rehabilitation or functional progression program. Many methods can be used to evaluate technique, including simple clinical observation, expert consultation, and video analysis. All three of these methods can prove useful; it is difficult to always rely solely on clinical observation because of the high inherent speeds of human performance. Additionally, the varied sport performance background of the people being worked with often requires expertise beyond the specialty of the primary clinician. Outside exerts with established competence in the sport or activity in question can often offer critically important information relative to the development and implementation of the functional progression program.

Finally, the readily accessible use of digital video recorders and computer software, which allows for manipulation of those images to improve analysis as well as provide feedback to the athlete or person, is exceptionally important in this process. A discussion of the role the kinetic link plays in human performance closes this chapter and prepares the reader for the specific information contained in the second part of this book.

KINETIC LINK PRINCIPLE

The kinetic link (also referred to as the kinetic chain) principle provides both the framework for understanding and analyzing human movement patterns and the rationale for the utilization of exercise conditioning and rehabilitation programs that emphasize the entire body. The kinetic link principle highlights many of the concepts discussed in this book, and understanding this principle will assist the reader with application of the testing and training progressions presented later. The ability to break down and analyze human movement and critically evaluate movement and exercise patterns is an important part of functional progression. The purpose of this section of the chapter is to cover the concept of the kinetic chain or kinetic link principle and highlight the way the body segments work together to produce functional movement patterns, and how in the presence of pathology, this kinetic link system can be disrupted and abnormal.

The kinetic link principle describes how the human body can be considered in terms of a series of interrelated links or segments (figure 2.2). Movement of one segment affects segments both proximal and distal to the first segment. Kibler

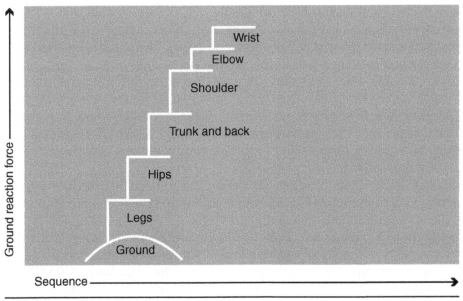

Figure 2.2 Kinetic link system.

Reprinted from J.L. Groppel, 1992, *High tech tennis,* 2nd ed. (Champaign, IL: Human Kinetics), 79. By permission of J.L. Groppel.

(1998) refers to the kinetic link system as a series of sequentially activated body segments. The kinetic link principle is predicated on a concept developed and described initially by Hanavan (1964), who constructed a computerized form of the adult human body. This computerized form comprises conical links that include the lower extremities, torso, and upper extremities. In reference to upper extremity skill performance, work in these upper extremity segments is transmitted to the trunk and spine via a large musculoskeletal surface. There is an exchange of forces across this musculoskeletal surface, which results in the generation of massive amounts of energy (Hanavan 1964).

Davies (1992) describes how the upper extremity can be viewed as a series of links. The links proposed by Davies include the trunk, scapulothoracic articulation, scapulohumeral or glenohumeral joints, and distal arm regions. Each of these links can be considered independent anatomically and biomechanically, but with reference to human function, they must be considered a unit.

Similar to the descriptions of the kinetic link by Hanavan (1964) and Davies (1992), Putnam (1993) has described the concept of proximal to distal sequencing. While ultimately utilized in the biomechanical analysis of human movement, the proximal to distal sequencing model has relevance in exercise both for rehabilitation and performance enhancement. The terms *kinetic link*, *proximal to distal sequencing*, and *summation of speed principle* (Bunn 1972), along with Plagenhoef's (1971) concept of acceleration–deceleration, all attempt to describe the complex interaction of the body's independent segments working together to form a sequence or unit of functional segments.

The goal of nearly all sport-related activities such as throwing, serving, and kicking a ball is to achieve maximal acceleration and hence the largest possible speed at the end of the linked segments (Bunn 1972). The concept ideally states that motion should be initiated with the more-proximal segments and proceed to the more-distal segments, with the more-distal segment initiating its motion at the time of the maximum speed of the proximal segment. Each succeeding segment would generate larger end-point speeds than the proximal segment. This proximal to distal sequencing has been demonstrated in research by examining the linear speeds of segment end points, joint angular velocities, and resultant joint moments (Marshall and Elliott 2000).

Several investigators have demonstrated the proper proximal to distal sequencing in kicking (Putnam 1993; Marshall and Wood 1986). The linear speeds in the lower extremity when kicking a ball in the sagittal plane follow the proximal to distal sequence. The hip, knee, and ankle joints all reach their peak speeds in sequence, with each peak greater than that of the proximal joint. Putnam (1993) believes that deceleration of the proximal segment occurs secondary to the acceleration of the distal segment. Other researchers (Marshall and Wood 1986) show a reversal of the proximal joint torques late in the motion, which apparently increases the speed of the distal segment.

Proximal to distal sequencing has been clearly identified in the tennis serve (Groppel 1992; Plagenhoef 1971; VanGheluwe and Hebbelinck 1985; Elliott, Marsh, and Blansby 1986; Elliott, Marshall, and Noffal 1995; Elliott et al. 2003) and the throwing motion (Feltner and Dapena 1986). Closely analyzing the literature in upper extremity throwing or striking sports shows a modification of the proximal to distal pattern. This modification occurs when the human body exploits the benefits of long-axis rotation of the humerus (internal rotation) and forearm (forearm pronation) to maximize end-point speed (Marshall and Elliott 2000).

Research consistently demonstrates that peak internal rotation of the shoulder (glenohumeral joint) follows the movement of the wrist and hand (VanGheluwe and Hebbelinck 1985; Elliot, Marshall, and Noffal 1995; Marshall and Elliot 2000). Additionally, the peak speed of pronation has been found to occur immediately before ball contact on the tennis serve and forehand groundstroke, suggesting that this long-axis rotation does not conform to traditional explanations of proximal to distal sequencing (Marshall and Elliott 2000).

Kibler (1998) provides an objective analysis of force generation during a tennis serve. Table 2.1 shows that 54% of the force development during a tennis serve comes from the legs and trunk, with only 25% coming from the elbow and wrist. Nonoptimal performance and increased risk of injury occur in tennis and other sport activities when the player attempts to utilize the smaller muscles and distal arm segments as a primary source of power generation (Kibler 1994; Groppel 1992).

The kinetic link principle is of paramount importance when analyzing sport performance or exercise movement patterns. Movement patterns that do not sequentially activate all portions of the kinetic link system or leave out a portion or link, such as trunk rotation, can lead to injury and nonoptimal performance (Kibler 1994; Groppel 1992). Examples of nonoptimal use of the kinetic link principle are depicted in figure 2.3. Figure 2.3a represents a segment missing from the normal sequential activation pattern, and figure 2.3b demonstrates improper timing of the sequential activation. These two examples are commonly encountered by clinicians when analyzing complex human movement patterns such as the tennis serve and throwing motion. It is very common for a person to perform an activity without hip rotation because of either improper foot positioning or inflexibility in the hip region. Additionally, inappropriate timing of trunk rotation can lead to disastrous consequences in segments proximal and distal to the trunk (Marshall, Noffal, and Legnani 1993).

Applying figure 2.3 to a functional movement pattern such as the tennis serve involves hitting the serve with little or no trunk rotation because the hips are precluded from rotating by an improper stance. This would produce greater loads and stresses to the shoulder and elbow and possibly result in injury. Additionally, if improper sequencing or timing of the rotation from the legs to the hip and trunk occurs, greater loads to the upper arm are again encountered. Marshall, Noffal, and Legnani (1993) used three-dimensional cinematography to analyze the mechanics of a highly skilled tennis player in order to analyze the torques

Table 2.1   Contribution of Specific Segments to Kinetic Energy and Force Production in the Tennis Serve

Segment	Velocity (m/s)	Kinetic energy [units, (%)]	Force [units, (%)]
Leg/trunk	2.7	197.1 (51%)	729 (54%)
Shoulder	2.2	49.1 (13%)	297 (21%)
Elbow	6.4	82 (21%)	212 (15%
Wrist	7.8	61 (15%)	130 (10%)

Adapted from W.B. Kibler, 1994, "Clinical biomechanics of the elbow in tennis: Implications for evaluation and diagnosis," *Medicine and Science in Sports and Exercise* 26(10): 1203-1206.

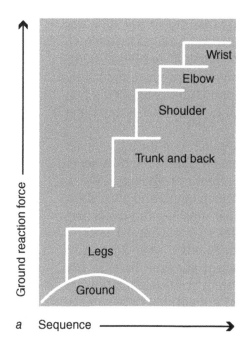
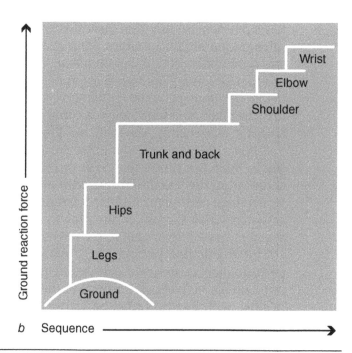

Figure 2.3   *(a)* Nonoptimal use of the kinetic link system because of a missing link. *(b)* Nonoptimal use of the kinetic link system because of improper timing.

Reprinted from J.L. Groppel, 1992, *High tech tennis,* 2nd ed. (Champaign, IL: Human Kinetics), 79. By permission of J.L. Groppel.

produced during the tennis serve. The effects of delaying internal shoulder rotation (until late in the total movement) were studied analytically on the medial aspect of the elbow, highlighting the underlying concept behind the kinetic link principle. The amount of valgus stress to the medial elbow was increased 53% immediately before ball impact when nonoptimal timing was utilized during the serving motion. This graphically displays the effects of manipulation of the normal kinetic link interaction on the human body during stressful upper body sport movement and exertion.

These studies help demonstrate the important role the kinetic link system plays in human movement and also demonstrate the importance of training the entire limb or entire kinetic link of the body when attempting to affect a specific segment or link in the kinetic link system.

Total Arm Strength Concept

Application of the kinetic link system in a clinical or rehabilitative way has led to the development of the total arm strength (TAS) concept (Davies and Ellenbecker 1993). This concept is predicated on the kinetic link system as well as demonstrated by the close clinical relationship between shoulder and elbow injuries in sport. Priest and Nagel (1976) studied 84 world-class tennis players and reported that 74% of men and 60% of women had a history of shoulder or elbow injury in the dominant arm that affected tennis play. Injuries to both the shoulder and elbow of the dominant arm were reported by 21% and 23% of the men and women, respectively. Another study by Priest, Braden, and Gerberich (1980) surveyed 2,633 recreational tennis players and found an incidence of tennis elbow of 31%. Additionally, there is a 63% greater incidence of shoulder injury in this population, as compared with those players who did not have a history of tennis elbow.

One further study of the total arm strength concept is that by Strizak et al. (1983). These researchers incorporated the isometric strength of the forearm (pronation and supination), wrist (radial and ulnar deviation; flexion and extension), and metacarpophalangeal (MCP) joints (flexion and extension) to create a total arm strength index. This index was compared among three groups: (1) a normal, noninjured, non-tennis-playing control population, (2) healthy recreational tennis players, and (3) recreational tennis players with tennis elbow. Results of this study show significantly greater dominant-arm total arm strength relative to body weight in the control group and tennis-playing group but no significant difference in the group with tennis elbow. The finding of greater total arm strength in both the control population and healthy tennis players and lack of this finding in the injured group supports the use of whole extremity (or, in this application, total arm strength) rehabilitation and conditioning programs. This concept is prevalent today in upper extremity rehabilitation and is reflected in the emphasis on both shoulder and elbow rehabilitation in trunk and scapular stabilization exercise programs. This is reflected in this book on functional progression and forms the basis for the whole extremity or total arm strength focus presented here.

Total Leg Strength Concept

The total arm strength concept is paralleled in the lower extremity by the total leg strength (TLS) concept. Nicholas, Strizak, and Veras (1976) created a TLS parameter by isokinetically testing the hip flexors, hip abductors, hip adductors, quadriceps, and hamstrings and adding all those individual strength measures together to create the TLS parameter. The researchers found proximal muscular weakness of the lower extremities with plantar flexion and inversion ankle sprains. Gleim, Nicholas, and Webb (1978) expanded on the original work of Nicholas, Strizak, and Veras by correlating individual muscle deficits and TLS deficits with 219 patients. Their research established that a 10% isolated muscular deficit was significant with regard to lower extremity injury. Of particular interest was the finding that a 5% deficit in the TLS parameter was significant with respect to lower extremity injury.

Additionally, Bullock-Saxton (1994) found local sensation changes and an alteration of proximal (gluteus maximus) hip muscle function after severe ankle sprains. Bolz and Davies (1984) tested isokinetic hip extension and flexion, hip abduction and adduction, knee extension and flexion, and ankle plantar flexion and dorsiflexion in 24 subjects. They found significant unilateral muscular weakness in the total leg strength factor (summing all measures from the eight motions tested) in 8 out of 24 subjects who had a leg length discrepancy of 0.5 cm or more. The total leg strength factor revealed a consistent weakness in the short leg in these subjects.

Continued emphasis on the total leg strength concept is reflected in the orthopedic and sports medicine literature today. Tyler et al. (2006) showed a significant relationship between increased hip flexibility and hip flexion strength and successful nonoperative treatment for patellofemoral pain syndrome. Improved hip flexion strength was a characteristic found in 93% of the patients successfully treated for patellofemoral pain during a total leg strength rehabilitation program. Hewett et al. (2005) studied the landing patterns of female athletes in high-risk lower extremity sports during a jump-landing task using three-dimensional analysis. Female athletes with ACL injury had significantly greater dynamic knee valgus and knee abduction torques as compared with the female athletes with no history of ACL injury. Hewett and colleagues found increases in hip and knee adduction in the injured group and showed the interrelationship of the kinetic chain segments of the hip and knee and their respective influence on ACL injury. Through their research and identification of biomechanical risk factors for ACL injury, total lower extremity evidence-based prevention programs have been developed that utilize total leg strength training and functional progressions contained in this book.

SUMMARY

Chapter 2 presents details of a successful functional exercise program and provides the framework for application of the specific regional progressions contained in part II of this book. These key components guide the clinician in selecting appropriate exercise progressions emphasizing function. Additionally, this chapter summarizes some of the relevant anatomical and biomechanical relationships of the kinetic link system of the human body, pointing out the potential benefits of exercises that work multiple joints and muscle groups and that stress and challenge the body's kinetic link system. Integration of the kinetic link system and total arm and total leg strength concepts provides the clinician with the functionally specific framework that can lead to optimal program design for both performance enhancement and injury rehabilitation. The following chapters focus on functional progressions for the upper and lower extremities and trunk that are based on the anatomy and biomechanics of the specific joint structures and demands placed on the musculoskeletal system during functional activities.

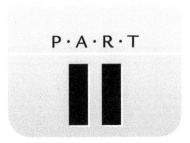

P·A·R·T II

Regional Functional Progressions

In this important part of the book, a regional presentation of exercise progressions is developed. Rather than just list the progressions of exercise, however, each author carefully reviews the clinically relevant anatomy and biomechanics of each area and applies that information to the exercise progressions that form the cornerstone of this text.

Each chapter in part II contains specific exercise progressions using a consistent descriptive approach. This will guide the reader in the use of these progressions by providing not only pertinent exercise descriptions but also pearls of performance when applicable. These pearls help the clinician apply these progressions to patients and athletes through the provision of additional insight into the exercise or often the person's response to the exercise, either during or after performing it. Although each progression focuses on one primary region of the body, it has significant kinetic chain carryover. Because of the critical role of core stability, the chapter on the trunk provides progressions that are particularly warranted for individuals who are undergoing extremity rehabilitation.

3

Upper Extremity

As mentioned in chapter 2, the focus in shoulder and elbow rehabilitation in the past decade has shifted from a predominantly joint-specific emphasis to a total extremity approach. This includes a significant emphasis on evaluation and treatment of the scapula and significant focus on scapular stabilization. The idea that proximal stability promotes distal mobility is clearly evident in current rehabilitation programs and as such forms the basis for functional progressions for the upper extremity. This chapter overviews the pertinent anatomy and biomechanics of the upper extremity as they relate specifically to function and to injury mechanics in particular, followed by specific upper extremity functional progressions. It is beyond the scope of this text to provide an exhaustive anatomical and biomechanical overview; however, the level of detail attempts to direct the reader into a greater understanding of the basis for the specific functional exercises recommended.

Compared with the loading used in the lower extremity and trunk chapters of this book, upper extremity loads are generally much lower, particularly when targeting the rotator cuff and scapular muscles that provide stabilization to the shoulder. Recent research (Bitter, Clisby, and Jones 2007) has identified the value of low loading and its relative effect on rotator cuff muscle activation.

Additionally, this chapter contains progressions utilizing both open and closed kinetic chain exercises. Ellenbecker and Davies (2001) have reviewed the strengths and weaknesses of both types of kinetic chain exercise, and based on their recommendations, both types of exercise are prevalent in the progressions for the upper extremity contained in this chapter.

ANATOMY OF THE UPPER EXTREMITY

To best understand the functional exercise progressions in this chapter, specific anatomical concepts of the shoulder and elbow are briefly outlined. Knowledge of these concepts will enhance the application of these exercises by providing in many cases the rationale for their inclusion and specific limitations described herein.

Bones

To begin with pertinent osteology, the important bones of the proximal aspect of the upper extremity are the scapula, clavicle, and humerus (figure 3.1). The clavicle forms a rigid strut from an engineering perspective and provides a firm stabilization

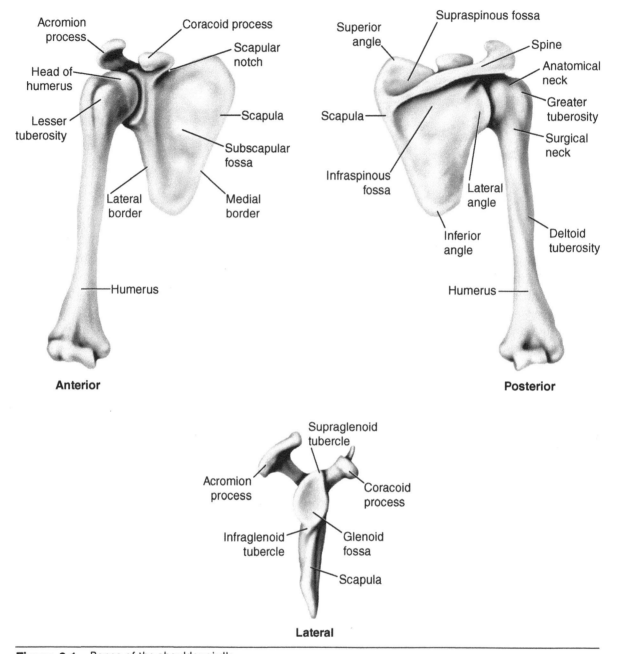

Figure 3.1 Bones of the shoulder girdle.

Reprinted from R. Behnke, 2006, *Kinetic anatomy,* 2nd ed. (Champaign, IL: Human Kinetics), 37.

against excessive protraction of the scapula at rest. The scapula forms the basis for many muscular attachments about the shoulder girdle. The glenoid, which is part of the scapula, is angled 30° anteriorly relative to the coronal, or frontal, plane of the body (Saha 1983). This anterior orientation of the glenoid coupled with the posterior, or retroverted, proximal humeral head leads to the formation of the scapular plane. The scapular plane is an ideal location for exercise and human movement because it is the place where maximal congruity between the humeral head and glenoid occurs, rendering it more stable than human movement in other planes (Saha 1983). This osseous relationship formed by the retrotorsion of the humeral head relative to the shaft of the humerus and anteversion of the glenoid fossa is a critically important anatomical concept that is applied throughout the progressions contained in this chapter.

Both open and particularly closed kinetic chain exercise movement patterns frequently position the shoulder in the scapular plane (30° anterior to the coronal, or frontal, plane) to optimize bony congruity; minimize focal stress on the anterior capsular structures; and mimic or specifically re-create functional positions used during serving, throwing, and other activity- and sport-specific movements. Utilization of the sagittal plane position during closed kinetic chain exercises for the upper extremity can subject the glenohumeral joint to undue posterior shear stresses and are often contraindicated in many people after injury.

Distally, the humerus contains two major articulating structures, the capitellum laterally and the trochlea medially (figure 3.2). The trochlea, or medial aspect of the distal humerus, projects further distally, thereby creating the normal anatomical "carrying angle," which is characterized by a valgus angulation of the ulnohumeral joint. The radius and ulna terminate against the carpal bones and have distal projections called styloid processes.

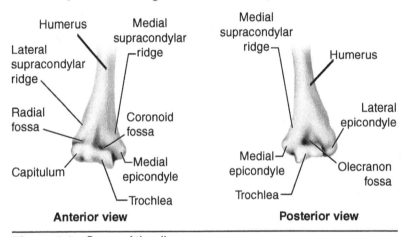

Figure 3.2 Bones of the elbow.

Reprinted from R. Behnke, 2006, *Kinetic anatomy*, 2nd ed. (Champaign, IL: Human Kinetics), 62.

Ligaments

From a ligamentous perspective, several very important ligaments provide support to the very mobile glenohumeral (shoulder) joint (figure 3.3). These are called the glenohumeral capsular ligaments and are located in superior, middle, and inferior portions of the anterior capsule of the shoulder. These important ligaments help prevent excessive anterior translation of the humerus on the glenoid and can become injured in both overuse and traumatic sport activity.

The coracoacromial ligament is a key part of the coracoacromial arch and forms the top, or superior, part of the shoulder joint. This ligament is the site of primary impingement, in addition to the anterior aspect of the acromion, and can create mechanical rotator cuff compression or impingement if unbalanced muscle function or lack of glenohumeral dynamic stabilization is coupled with excessive overuse. Functionally, this ligament can create impingement of the rotator cuff tendons during arm elevations greater than 90°. Upper extremity exercise progressions recommended in this chapter for overhead athletes are typically characterized by movement patterns that position the shoulder below 90° of elevation to minimize the compressive forces of this ligament and the overlying acromion on the rotator cuff tendons.

The acromioclavicular (AC) ligaments (conoid and trapezoid) stabilize the AC joint and can become attenuated during a fall on the lateral aspect of the shoulder or a lateral collision, creating an unstable AC joint and a characteristic

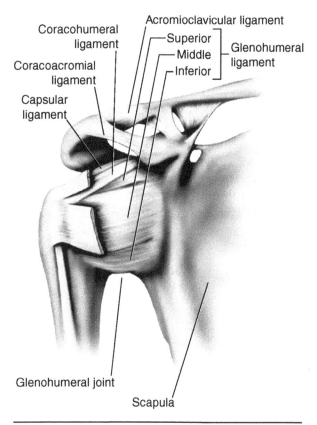

Figure 3.3 Ligaments of the shoulder.

step-down or piano key sign when attenuated. When performing functional exercise progressions after AC joint injury, patients must take care in the movement patterns of cross-arm adduction, as this increases joint loading and creates impingement.

Ligamentous support of the elbow comes primarily from the medial and lateral ulnar collateral ligaments (figure 3.4). The medial ulnar collateral ligament has three distinct bands. The anterior and posterior bands are the primary support against valgus loads encountered during throwing and also support the joint in near extension (anterior band) and in flexion (posterior band) (Morrey 1993). The radial collateral ligament does not provide the primary lateral stabilization as would be expected; instead, this function is provided by the lateral ulnar collateral ligament. The annular ligament stabilizes the proximal radial head against the ulna and allows for pronation and supination while stabilizing the radial head against distal migration and excessive translation.

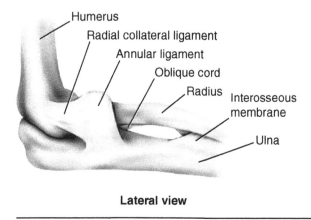

Lateral view

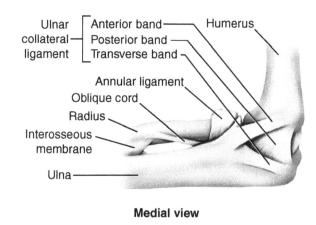

Medial view

Figure 3.4 Ligaments of the elbow.

Reprinted from R. Behnke, 2006, *Kinetic anatomy*, 2nd ed., (Champaign, IL: Human Kinetics), 65.

MUSCULAR STABILIZATION OF THE UPPER EXTREMITY

Muscular stabilization of the proximal aspect of the upper extremity has significant overlap with the discussion of the trunk (chapter 5) and arises from many muscles that originate on the torso and insert onto the scapula. These muscles, known as scapular stabilizers, play an extremely important role in functional exercise programming, as they form the base required for any distal shoulder, elbow, wrist, or hand movement. The primary scapular stabilizers are the trapezius, rhomboids, and serratus anterior (figure 3.5). The trapezius and rhomboids are the primary muscles to retract the human scapula, while the serratus anterior is the primary protractor, assisted to a lesser degree by the pectoralis minor. The upper trapezius, with the assistance of the levator scapulae, elevates the scapula superiorly, while the lower trapezius depresses the scapula inferiorly. These muscles also work together to provide scapular rotation, which is discussed at length in the biomechanics section of this chapter.

The rotator cuff consists of four muscles originating on the scapula and inserting into the greater and lesser tuberosities of the humerus. Considered part of the scapulohumeral muscle group, these four muscles are primary stabilizers of the glenohumeral joint. The supraspinatus, which is primarily an abductor, is the most centrally located of the rotator cuff tendons and is most susceptible to mechanical compression, or impingement, of its tendon against the overlying coracoacromial arch. The subscapularis originates on the anterior aspect of the scapula and inserts into the lesser tuberosity; it is a powerful internal rotator and stabilizer of the glenohumeral joint. The infraspinatus and teres minor are the most posteriorly located rotator cuff muscles and are external rotators inserting with the supraspinatus onto the greater tuberosity. In addition to internal and external rotation, the subscapularis, infraspinatus, and teres minor provide a downward, or caudally directed, pull to fight the effects of deltoid contraction during arm elevation and can help minimize the force of impingement (Wuelker, Plitz, and Roetman 1994). Additionally, these muscles can also assist with elevation of the humerus (Otis et al.1994).

The other scapulohumeral muscles include the three heads of the deltoid (anterior, middle, and posterior), teres major, and coracobrachialis; they provide important muscular contributions to the prime movements of the glenohumeral joint.

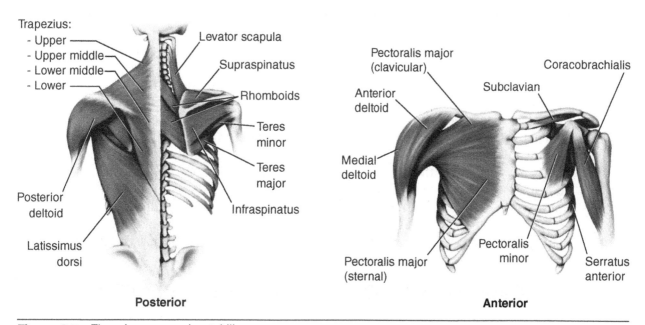

Figure 3.5 The primary scapular stabilizers.

The axiohumeral muscles (i.e., latissimus dorsi, pectoralis major, and pectoralis minor) are prime movers of the shoulder complex and are active in flexion, extension, and horizontal abduction and adduction movements of the shoulder joint. These muscles are not considered stabilizers, and often with overtraining, they can overpower the stabilizing muscles (rotator cuff and scapular stabilizers), resulting in muscular imbalances and nonoptimal function of the shoulder. This chapter gives specific examples highlighting the importance of muscle balance and describes upper extremity strength progressions designed to improve muscular balance by emphasizing the rotator cuff and scapular musculature.

In the upper arm, or brachium, the elbow flexors (biceps, brachialis, and brachioradialis) cover the anterior aspect and primarily provide strong elbow flexion force (see figure 3.6). Posteriorly, the triceps is the primary elbow extensor, joined by the anconeus on the lateral aspect of the elbow. Although the biceps and triceps cross both the shoulder joint and elbow joint, they do not significantly affect shoulder flexion and extension from the standpoint of muscular force contribution.

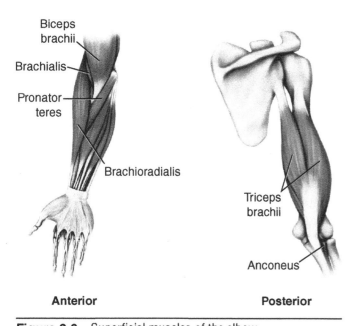

Biceps brachii

Brachialis

Pronator teres

Brachioradialis

Triceps brachii

Anconeus

Anterior   **Posterior**

Figure 3.6   Superficial muscles of the elbow.

Reprinted from R. Behnke, 2006, *Kinetic anatomy,* 2nd ed. (Champaign, IL: Human Kinetics), 66.

Yamaguchi et al. (1997) and others have shown that the biceps long head contributes minimally (1 to 3% maximal voluntary contraction, or MVC) to shoulder flexion. In addition to elbow flexion, the biceps provides essential forearm supination along with the supinator muscle. Distally, two muscles provide pronation, the pronator teres and pronator quadratus, with the pronator teres originating at the medial epicondyle of the distal humerus. Additionally, on the medial epicondyle the wrist and finger flexors originate from a conjoined tendon and are very prone to overuse from activities of daily living as well as sport. Specific progressions for the distal muscles are included in this chapter.

Laterally, the wrist and finger extensors take origin from the lateral epicondyle; like the medially oriented muscle–tendon units, they can become prime targets for overuse injury (humeral epicondylitis). An and colleagues (1981) provide a detailed biomechanical analysis of muscular function about the elbow joint. They found that the anconeus, brachioradialis, extensor carpi radialis, and extensor carpi ulnaris muscles create the primary valgus moment (which resists elbow varus stress). In contrast, the pronator teres, flexor carpi radialis, and flexor carpi ulnaris all create a varus moment and are the primary dynamic stabilizers against valgus stress of the elbow. Valgus stress of the elbow is discussed later in this chapter relative to the overhead throwing motion.

BIOMECHANICS OF THE UPPER EXTREMITY

This brief overview of upper extremity biomechanics attempts to lay out the key concepts relevant in the design and execution of functional exercise progressions for individuals and athletes. Concepts such as scapulohumeral rhythm, the scapular plane, obligate translation, and valgus extension overload are of critical importance relative to the design and implementation of these exercise programs. Knowledge of the force-couple concepts for the shoulder and scapulothoracic joints is also of key importance in program development.

Scapulothoracic Motion

Scapulothoracic movement was initially described in clinical terms as "scapulohumeral rhythm" by both Codman (1934) and Inman, Saunders, and Abbot (1944). Inman states that "the total range of scapular motion is not more than 60 degrees" and that the total contribution from the glenohumeral joint is not greater than 120°. The scapulohumeral rhythm was described for the total arc of elevation of the shoulder joint to contain 2° of glenohumeral motion for every degree of scapulothoracic motion (Inman, Saunders, and Abbot 1944).

In addition to this ratio of movement, Inman identified what he termed a "setting phase," occurring during the first 30 to 60° of shoulder elevation and characterized by minimal scapular movement. Once 30° of abduction and 60° of flexion are reached, the relationship of scapulothoracic to glenohumeral joint motion remains remarkably constant (Inman, Saunders, and Abbot 1944).

Later research using three-dimensional analysis and other laboratory-based methods has confirmed Inman's early descriptions of scapulohumeral rhythm (Doody, Freedman, and Waterland 1970; Bagg and Forrest 1988). These studies also provide more-detailed descriptions of the exact contribution of the scapulothoracic and glenohumeral joint during arm elevation in the scapular plane. Doody, Freedman, and Waterland (1970) found the ratio of glenohumeral to scapulothoracic motion to change from 7.29:1 in the first 30° of elevation to 0.78:1 between 90 and 150°. Bagg and Forrest (1988) found similar differences based on the range of motion examined. In the early phase of elevation, 4.29° of glenohumeral joint motion occurred for every 1° of scapular motion, with 1.71° of glenohumeral motion occurring for every 1° of scapular motion between the functional arc of 80 and 140°.

Bagg and Forrest (1988) also clearly identified the instantaneous center of rotation (ICR) of the scapulothoracic joint at various points in the range of motion. The ICR moves from the medial border of the spine of the scapula, with the shoulder at approximately 20° of elevation very near the side of the body, and migrates superolaterally to the region near the acromioclavicular (AC) joint at approximately 140°. Bagg and Forrest's research also identified an increased muscular stabilization role of the lower trapezius and serratus anterior force couple at higher, more-functional positions of elevation.

The cooperative muscular role between the trapezius and serratus anterior can be termed a *force couple* and refers to two or more muscles working synchronously, either as synergists or in agonist–antagonist pairing, to enable a particular motion to occur. In this case, the serratus anterior and upper trapezius provide the essential muscular component in the early phases of arm elevation to optimize the upward scapular rotation needed for the movement. Nearing 90° of glenohumeral joint abduction, the lower trapezius and serratus anterior force couple provide the key scapular stabilization and continued upward rotation for overhead movement. This is just one example of a muscular force couple and explains the emphasis placed on these muscles in the exercise progressions later in this chapter.

Scapular Motion

Typical movement of the scapula occurs in the coronal, sagittal, and transverse planes. Brief descriptions here will provide an understanding of how the scapula moves.

The movements of upward and downward rotation occur in the coronal or frontal plane. The angle typically used to describe the position of scapular rotation is formed between the spine and medial border of the scapula. Poppen and Walker (1978) have reported normal elevation of the acromion to be approximately 36° from the neutral position to maximum abduction. Sagittal plane motion of the scapula is referred to as anterior and posterior tilting. Transverse plane movement of the scapula is referred to as internal and external rotation. Abnormal increases in the internal rotation angle of the scapula lead to changes in the orientation of the glenoid. This altered position of the glenoid, called antetilting, allows for an opening up of the anterior half of the glenohumeral articulation (Kibler 1991). The antetilting of the scapula has been shown by Saha (1983) to be a component of the subluxation or dislocation complex in patients with microtrauma-induced glenohumeral instability.

Finally, the composite movements of protraction and retraction occur literally around the curvature of the thoracic wall (Kibler 1998). Retraction typically occurs in a curvilinear fashion around the wall, while protraction may proceed in a slightly upward or downward motion, depending on the position of the humerus relative to the scapula (Kibler 1998). Depending on the size of the person and the vigorousness of the activity, the translation of the human scapula during protraction and retraction can occur over distances of 15 to 18 cm (6 to 7 inches) (Kibler 1993). The scapula can move in the coronal plane along the thoracic wall superiorly and inferiorly in movements typically called elevation and depression, respectively. Evaluation of a person with rotator cuff weakness often identifies excessive early scapular elevation as a compensatory movement to optimize humeral movement (Kibler 1998).

In summary, scapular motion is closely governed by the muscular force couple formed by the serratus anterior and trapezius muscles. Recent research best clarifies and summarizes the scapular movement during arm elevation, concluding that 44° of posterior tilting, 49° of upward rotation, and 27° of external rotation occur to allow for normal glenohumeral movement (Bourne et al. 2007). Specific exercises ensure that optimal strength and muscular endurance are present in the important muscles that control these movements.

Deltoid–Rotator Cuff Force Couple

In addition to the muscular force-couple relationship governing scapular motion, another extremely important force couple involves the deltoid and rotator cuff. Inman, Saunders, and Abbot (1944) first outlined the integral relationship between the human deltoid muscle and the four muscle–tendon units of the rotator cuff (figure 3.7). The deltoid muscle provides force primarily in a superior direction when contracting unopposed during arm elevation (Rathburn and McNab 1970). This resultant superior force

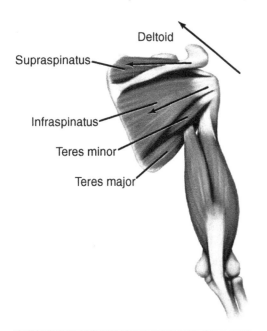

Supraspinatus

Deltoid

Infraspinatus

Teres minor

Teres major

Figure 3.7 Arrows depicting the direction of force from the deltoid and rotator cuff muscles, demonstrating the force-couple relationship in the human shoulder.

creates proximal, or superior, migration of the humeral head. To offset this superior pull, the muscle–tendon units of the rotator cuff must provide both a compressive force and an inferior, or caudally directed, force to minimize superior migration and minimize contact or impingement of the rotator cuff tendons against the overlying acromion (Inman, Saunders, and Abbot 1944). Failure of the rotator cuff to maintain humeral congruency leads to glenohumeral joint instability and rotator cuff impingement, resulting in rotator cuff tendon pathology and labral injury (Burkart, Morgan, and Kibler 2003).

Imbalances in the deltoid–rotator cuff force couple, which primarily occur during inappropriate and unbalanced strength training as well as through repetitive overhead sport activities, can lead to development of the deltoid without concomitant increases in rotator cuff strength and can increase the superior migration of the humeral head provided by the deltoid, leading to rotator cuff impingement. Specific emphasis in shoulder rehabilitation programs (Ellenbecker 2006; Wilk, Arrigo, and Andrews 2003) on restoring muscular balance between the rotator cuff and deltoid—typically by increasing the relative strength of the very frequently underdeveloped rotator cuff muscles—forms the basis of exercise prescription and current treatment strategies utilized by therapists and trainers for people with shoulder pathology.

Additionally, most well-intentioned patients and athletes faced with either shoulder discomfort or a desire to increase shoulder strength using traditional gym-based exercise training utilize exercise patterns that emphasize deltoid, upper trapezius, and pectoral strengthening and often lead to improper muscle balance between the larger deltoid and prime mover and the rotator cuff. Exercise progressions in this chapter focus strongly on rotator cuff and scapular muscular strength development and provide balanced alternatives to programs biased toward deltoid, upper trapezius, and pectoral strength contained in popular magazines or prevalent among many gym-based exercise programs.

Scapular Plane Concept

Another key in upper extremity strength development and rehabilitation is the scapular plane concept. The scapular plane has ramifications in treatment, evaluation, and even functional activity in sports. According to Saha (1983), the scapular plane is 30° anterior to the coronal, or frontal, plane of the body. Placement of the glenohumeral joint in the scapular plane optimizes the osseous congruity between the humeral head and the glenoid and is widely recommended as an optimal position for both performing various evaluation techniques and during many rehabilitation exercises (Saha 1983; Ellenbecker 1995). With the glenohumeral joint placed in the scapular plane, bony impingement of the greater tuberosity against the acromion does not occur because of the alignment of the tuberosity and acromion in this orientation (Saha 1983). Additionally, during glenohumeral joint abduction, humeral external rotation must occur to clear the greater tuberosity during overhead movement. During shoulder flexion in the sagittal plane, internal rotation of the humerus must accompany arm elevation for this clearance to occur. According to Saha (1983), specific humeral rotation does not need to occur to clear the greater tuberosity and hence minimizes true bony impingement when this position of arm elevation (scapular plane) is used. Therefore, the scapular plane position is recommended for use with shoulder elevation exercises for strength training in performance enhancement and during rehabilitation.

Glenohumeral Joint Arthrokinematics and Obligate Translation

Another important biomechanical principle that is relevant to shoulder function is joint arthrokinematics. During normal glenohumeral joint motion, rotation, sliding, and rolling all occur (Kessler and Hertling 1983). Rotation is defined as movement occurring about a longitudinal axis of the bone. Rolling can simply be thought of as occurring when certain points at certain intervals along one joint surface contact points of another bone at the same intervals on the opposing surface. This is analogous to a car tire rolling along the street. Sliding also occurs, which is analogous to a car tire sliding on ice where one point on one joint surface contacts various points on another joint surface. For normal shoulder motion to occur, all three of these component parts—rotation, rolling, and sliding—need to take place.

The glenohumeral joint can be thought of as a convex humeral head moving on a concave glenoid. That being said, it falls into the convex on concave arthrokinematic pattern, which states that rolling and sliding have to occur in opposite directions. For example, during arm elevation, the humerus is rolling upward as the humerus elevates but must have a component of caudal, or inferior, slide or glide to minimize the intensity of abutment or impingement against the overlying acromion. In people with range of motion loss after injury or surgery, this caudal slide or glide is often deficient and hence requires specific mobilization to restore. Loss of normal joint arthrokinematics among many people who have had shoulder surgery or injury supports the recommendation of many functional exercise patterns emphasized in this chapter to utilize patterns with less than 90° of arm elevation to protect the rotator cuff from judicious impingement against the superior surfaces (coracoacromial arch).

Obligate translation is another important concept that can be applied to the shoulder during specific arm movements. In the shoulder, movement of the humeral head can be thought of as moving "away" from the side of capsular tightness. For example, when the shoulder is brought into external rotation, the anterior capsule tightens and causes posterior translation of the humeral head away from the tightness in the anterior capsule (Harryman, Sidles, and Clark 1990; Karduna, Williams, and Williams 1996). Conversely, when the shoulder is brought into internal rotation, the posterior capsule tightens and causes obligate translation anteriorly away from the tightness in the posterior capsule.

Elbow: Valgus Extension Overload

Although it is beyond the scope of this chapter to completely review biomechanics of the elbow, one specific biomechanical aspect—valgus extension overload—deserves discussion. Repeated overhead throwing or serving activity can lead to characteristic patterns of osseous and osteochondral injury in the athletic elbow. These injuries are commonly referred to as valgus extension overload injuries (Wilson et al. 1983) (figure 3.8). As a result of the valgus stress incurred during throwing or the serving motion, traction placed via the medial aspect of the elbow can create bony spurs, or osteophytes, at the medial epicondyle or coronoid process of the elbow (Bennet 1959; Indelicato et al. 1979; Slocum 1978). Additionally, the valgus stress during elbow extension creates impingement, which leads to osteophyte formation at the posterior and posteromedial aspects of the olecranon tip, causing chondromalacia and loose body formation (Wilson et al. 1983). The combined motion of valgus pressure with the powerful extension of the elbow leads to posterior osteophyte formation because of impingement of the posteromedial aspect of the ulna against the trochlea and olecranon fossa.

Figure 3.9 shows the valgus loading of the athletic elbow and the site of medial tension injury or valgus tensile overload response. Injury to the ulnar collateral ligament and medial muscle–tendon units of the flexor–pronator group can also occur with this type of repetitive loading (Indelicato et al. 1979; Wolf and Altchek 2003). Additionally, in the pediatric throwing athlete, separation of the medial epicondylar growth plate (Little League elbow) occurs during the forceful valgus stress and tensile loading produced by the repetitive forceful muscular contractions of the wrist flexors and forearm pronators during throwing or serving activities.

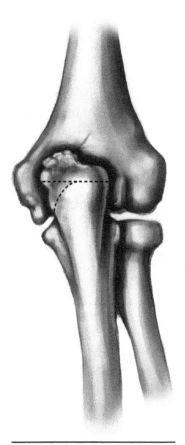

Figure 3.8 Posterior view of the elbow showing olecranon osteophyte from valgus extension overload. The dotted lines indicate the portion of the osteophyte often removed during arthroscopic surgery to gain extension range of motion and minimize bony compression and pain with throwing.

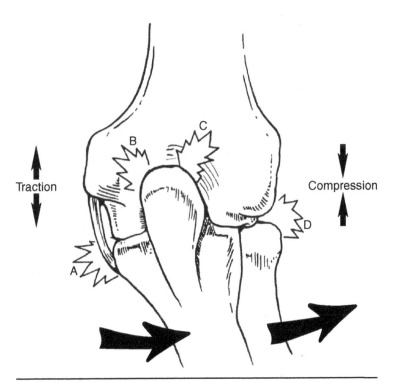

Figure 3.9 Valgus extension overload. Arrows represent the valgus stress and rotations that occur during the acceleration phase of throwing or the tennis serve: *(a)* medial aspect (traction); *(b)* contact of the posteromedial aspect of the olecranon, leading to osteochondral injury; *(c)* loose body formation; and *(d)* lateral aspect (compression).

During the valgus stress that occurs to the human elbow during the acceleration phase of both the throwing and serving motions, lateral compressive forces occur in the lateral aspect of the elbow, specifically at the radiocapitellar joint. Of great concern in the immature pediatric throwing athlete is osteochondritis dissecans (Joyce, Jelsma, and Andrews 1995; Ellenbecker and Mattalino 1997b). However in the older adult elbow, the radiocapitellar joint can be the site of joint degeneration and osteochondral injury from the compressive loading (Indelicato et al. 1979). This lateral compressive loading is increased in the elbow with medial ulnar collateral ligament laxity or ligament injury (Ellenbecker and Mattalino 1997b).

Overhead Throwing Motion

For the purposes of this chapter, throwing mechanics are discussed broken into the traditional stages (Glousman et al. 1992) for ease of analysis and discussion, with both typical and abnormal or injury-producing pathomechanics discussed for each stage. The throwing motion has been divided into four primary phases: windup, cocking, acceleration, and follow-through (figure 3.10). The windup phase begins with the initial motion of the pitcher and ends when the ball leaves the glove (Glousman et al. 1992; Fleisig, Dillman, and Andrews 1989). Very little muscular activation is required in the throwing shoulder during this phase, and therefore few injuries or episodes of pain provocation typically occur.

One essential aspect to analyze and evaluate during the windup phase, however, is the presence of proper balance (Fleisig, Dillman, and Andrews 1989). The lead leg (left leg in a right-handed throwing athlete) is lifted and rotated around the plant leg (right leg in a right-handed throwing athlete). This rotation must be achieved in a balanced fashion and should be evaluated in reference to the shoulder. An unstable base during this phase of throwing may have drastic consequences as the player moves into external rotation and begins the sequential segmental rotation during acceleration later in the throwing motion. This has significant ramifications for the throwing athlete and ties in the functional balance and proprioceptive exercise progressions discussed in the lower extremity chapter of this book.

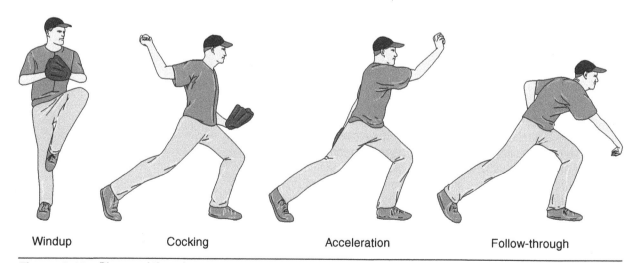

| Windup | Cocking | Acceleration | Follow-through |

Figure 3.10 Phases of throwing.

The cocking phase is often divided into two phases (Glousman et al. 1992; Fleisig, Dillman, and Andrews 1989). The early cocking phase begins as the ball leaves the glove and continues until the lead foot contacts the ground. During the early cocking phase, the arm is brought backward away from the body coupled with a forward drive of the lead leg. As the lead leg is extended forward, it strikes the mound. This is termed *foot contact*. At front foot, or lead foot, contact, another critical marker or evaluation point takes place. At the time the foot strikes the mound, the throwing elbow should be flexed 90° and the throwing shoulder should be externally rotated to at least the neutral position (Fleisig, Dillman, and Andrews 1989). Failure of the athlete to achieve this arm position at foot contact can lead to a "lagging" behind of the arm as the hips rotate forward in preparation for ball release. This places the arm in a "catch-up" situation because the rest of the body is too far ahead of the arm at this point in the movement pattern.

Additional information critically important to the glenohumeral joint is the stride characteristics of the lower extremity during the foot contact portion of the throwing motion. Fleisig et al. (2000) outline the stride characteristics during baseball pitching. They describe stride length (distance from ankle to ankle) as ranging between 70 and 80% of an athlete's height. Fleisig et al. (2000) also report that at foot contact the angle of the lead foot should be closed (angled inward) between 5 and 25° rather than pointing straight ahead toward home plate. An open stance, or stride angle, would increase opening or early rotation of the pelvis and may lead to hyperangulation and arm lag, increasing stress on the medial elbow and shoulder. Excessively closed stride angles would block rotation of the pelvis and decrease the contribution from the lower extremity segments.

Additionally, the lead foot should land directly in front of the rear foot or in a position with a closed stance of a few centimeters (lead foot a few centimeters to the right of the rear foot in a right-handed thrower). Again, if the lead foot lands in a position too closed, pelvic rotation will be impeded, forcing the pitcher to throw across his body, which minimizes the contribution from the lower extremity (Fleisig et al. 2000). Consequently, landing in a too-open position leads to early pelvic rotation and dissipation of the ground reaction forces and lower extremity contribution, resulting in arm fatigue and throwing with "too much arm" (Fleisig et al. 2000). Careful evaluation of foot position can again give valuable insight into possible mechanisms of arm injury stemming from lower extremity pathomechanics.

Late cocking occurs after foot contact and continues until maximal external rotation of the throwing shoulder occurs (Glousman et al. 1992). By the end of the cocking phase, the shoulder can obtain a nearly horizontal position of 180° of external rotation. This amount of external rotation, however, is combined with scapulothoracic and trunk articulation and gives the appearance of an artificially high external rotation value at the shoulder joint (Fleisig, Dillman, and Andrews 1989).

At the time of maximal external rotation in the throwing arm, it is important to note that the scapulothoracic joint must be in a retracted position (Kibler 1998; Burkhart, Morgan, and Kibler 2003). The scapula actually translates 15 to 18 cm (6 to 7 inches) during the throwing motion (Kibler 1998). Failure to retract the scapula leads to an increase in the antetilting of the glenoid because of the protracted scapular position and can exacerbate the instability continuum and create anterior instability and suboptimal performance, leading to injury (Kibler 1998; Burkhart, Morgan, and Kibler 2003).

Recent research demonstrates that in late cocking, the abduction and external rotation position places the posterior band of the inferior glenohumeral ligament in a "bowstrung" position under the humeral head. Tightness in this structure can lead to a posterosuperior shift in the humeral head, which can lead to rotator cuff and labral pathology (Burkhart, Morgan, and Kibler 2003). Improper scapular positioning coupled with increases in horizontal abduction during late cocking and the transition into the acceleration phase has been termed *hyperangulation* and leads to aggravation of undersurface rotator cuff impingement and labral injury derangement.

The acceleration phase begins after maximal external rotation and ends with ball release. During the delivery phase, the arm initially starts in –30° of horizontal abduction (30° behind the coronal plane) (Dillman 1991). As acceleration of the arm continues, the glenohumeral joint is moved forward to a position of + 10° of horizontal adduction (10° of horizontal adduction anterior to the coronal plane) and nears the scapular plane position (Dillman 1991). During acceleration, the arm moves from a position of 175 to 180° of composite external rotation to a position of nearly vertical (105°) of external rotation at release. When viewed from the side, the forearm will be in a nearly vertical position; however, the arm will appear to be 10 to 15° behind the trunk because the trunk is flexed forward at ball release. This internal rotation occurs at more than 7,000° per second (Dillman 1991; Fleisig, Dillman, and Andrews 1989).

Research has consistently shown that the abduction angle for the throwing motion ranges between 90 and 110° (Dillman 1991; Atwater 1979). This angle is relative to the trunk, with varying amounts of trunk lateral flexion changing the actual release position while keeping the abduction angle remarkably consistent across individuals and major pitching styles (Dillman 1991; Fleisig, Dillman, and Andrews 1989; Atwater 1979). Elevation of the glenohumeral abduction angle to greater than 110° can subject the rotator cuff to impingement stresses from the overlying acromion.

Follow-through is the stage after ball release and contains very high levels of eccentric muscular activity in the posterior rotator cuff and scapular region (Fleisig et al. 2000). Additional movements of the entire body to help dissipate the energy of the arm are necessary. Critical monitoring during this stage of the throwing motion is also recommended to ensure that the pitcher does not assume an abrupt upright posture and that he gradually dissipates the forward momentum by wrapping the arm across the body with trunk rotation. Additionally, the rear leg should come forward to assist in this process, leaving the pitcher again in a balanced finish position.

Failure at any one of these stages in the throwing motion can have profound implications on the throwing shoulder.

INJURIES

Although it is beyond the scope of this text to discuss in detail all the upper extremity injuries typically encountered during rehabilitation and functional progression of an athlete or active person, this section overviews several of the most common injuries in the shoulder and elbow to give some background for the reader when applying functional progressions. The multiple mechanisms of injury described in this chapter can help the clinician understand the potential forces and stresses the human shoulder receives during functional movement patterns. This section is heavily referenced to direct the reader to more-extensive resources.

Rotator Cuff

Injuries to the rotator cuff are common in overhead sports and nearly always occur from repetitive overuse. For years, the primary mechanism by which the rotator cuff became injured was thought to be impingement. With advances and increased basic science research, there is a greater understanding of how the rotator cuff becomes injured. These mechanisms include impingement, tensile overload, and instability. Restoration of optimal strength and muscular endurance is an integral part of the treatment of rotator cuff injury from each of these mechanisms and forms the basis for many of the functional progressions in this book. Each mechanism is briefly overviewed here to give important background on injuries to this important structure.

Impingement, also known as compressive disease or outlet impingement, is a direct result of compression of the rotator cuff tendons between the humeral head and the overlying anterior third of the acromion, coracoacromial ligament, coracoid, or acromioclavicular joint (Neer 1973, 1983). The physiological space between the inferior acromion and superior surface of the rotator cuff tendons is called the subacromial space, and it has been reported to be only 7 to 13 mm (Golding 1962). During arm elevation, peak forces against the acromion were measured in a range of motion between 85 and 136° of elevation (Wuelker, Plitz, and Roetman 1994). This position is functionally important for activities of daily living and is inherent in sport-specific movement patterns (Fleisig et al. 1995; Elliott, Marsh, and Blanksby 1986) as well as commonly incurred in ergonomic activities. The position of the shoulder in forward flexion, horizontal adduction, and internal rotation during the acceleration and follow-through phases of the throwing motion is likely to produce subacromial impingement, due to abrasion of the supraspinatus, infraspinatus, or biceps tendon against the overlying structures (Fleisig et al. 1995).

Neer's Stages of Impingement

Neer (1973, 1983) has outlined three stages of primary impingement as it relates to rotator cuff pathology. Stage I, "edema and hemorrhage," results from mechanical irritation of the tendon from the impingement incurred with overhead activity. This is characteristically observed in younger patients who are more athletic and is described as a reversible condition with conservative physical therapy. The primary symptoms and physical signs of this stage of impingement are similar to the other two stages and consist of a positive impingement sign, painful arc of movement, and varying degrees of muscular weakness (Neer 1983).

The second stage of compressive disease outlined by Neer is "fibrosis and tendonitis." This occurs from repeated episodes of mechanical inflammation and can include thickening, or fibrosis, of the subacromial bursae. The typical age range for this stage of injury is 25 to 40 years. Neer's stage III impingement lesion, called "bone spurs and tendon rupture," is the result of continued mechanical compression of the rotator cuff tendons. Full-thickness tears of the rotator cuff, partial-thickness tears of the rotator cuff, biceps tendon lesions, and bony alteration of the acromion and acromioclavicular joint may be associated with this stage (Neer 1973, 1983).

Secondary Impingement

Impingement, or compressive, symptoms may be secondary to underlying instability of the glenohumeral joint (Jobe and Kvitne 1989; Andrews and Alexander 1995). Although relatively common knowledge today, this concept was not well understood or recognized in the medical community even through the late 1980s. The idea that impingement could occur secondary to impingement, rather than as a primary cause, has had significant ramifications, altering evaluation methods, treatment, and rehabilitation (Wilk and Arrigo 1993; Ellenbecker 1995).

Attenuation of the static stabilizers of the glenohumeral joint, such as the capsular ligaments and labrum, from the excessive demands incurred in throwing or overhead activities can lead to anterior instability of the glenohumeral joint. Because of the increased humeral head translation, the biceps tendon and rotator cuff can become impinged secondary to the ensuing instability (Jobe and Kvitne 1989; Andrews and Alexander 1995). A progressive loss of glenohumeral joint stability is created when the dynamic stabilizing functions of the rotator cuff are diminished from fatigue and tendon injury (Andrews and Alexander 1995; Nirschl 1988). The effects of secondary impingement can lead to rotator cuff tears as the instability and impingement continue (Jobe and Kvitne 1989; Andrews and Alexander 1995).

Posterior, Internal, or Undersurface Impingement

An additional type of impingement more recently discussed as an etiology for rotator cuff pathology is posterior, internal (or inside), or undersurface impingement; it can often progress to an undersurface tear of the rotator cuff in the young athletic shoulder (Jobe and Pink 1994; Walch et al. 1992). Placement of the shoulder in a position of 90° of abduction and 90° of external rotation causes the supraspinatus and infraspinatus tendons to rotate posteriorly. This more-posterior orientation of the tendons aligns them such that the undersurface of the tendons rub on the posterosuperior glenoid lip and become pinched between the humeral head and the posterosuperior glenoid rim (Walch et al. 1992). In contrast to patients with traditional outlet impingement (either primary or secondary), the area of the rotator cuff tendon that is involved in posterior or undersurface impingement is the articular side of the rotator cuff tendon. Traditional impingement involves the superior or bursal surface of the rotator cuff tendon or tendons. Patients presenting with posterior shoulder pain brought on by positioning of the arm in 90° of abduction and 90° or more of external rotation, typically from overhead positions in sport or industrial situations, may be considered potential candidates for undersurface impingement.

Tensile Overload

One additional mechanism of rotator cuff injury that should be discussed here is tensile overload. During the throwing motion, repetitive eccentric muscular contractions of the posterior rotator cuff are required to keep the humeral head centered in the glenoid and prevent excessive anterior humeral head translation (Andrews and Alexander 1995). Repetitive stress to the rotator cuff tendons from eccentric overload can lead to rotator cuff tendinosis and progress to tearing on the undersurface of the rotator cuff (Nakajima et al. 1994).

Glenoid Labrum

The glenoid labrum has several important functions, including deepening the glenoid fossa to enhance concavity and serving as the attachment for the glenohumeral capsular ligaments. Injury to the labrum can compromise the concavity compression phenomenon by as much as 50% (Matsen, Harryman, and Sidles

1991). People with increased capsular laxity and generalized joint hypermobility have increased humeral head translation, which can subject the labrum to increased shear forces (Kvitne et al. 1995). In the throwing athlete, large anterior translational forces are present at levels up to 50% of body weight during arm acceleration of the throwing motion with the arm in 90° of abduction and external rotation (Fleisig et al. 1995). This repeated translation of the humeral head against and over the glenoid labrum can lead to labral injury. Labral injury can occur as either tearing or actual detachment from the glenoid.

Tears of the glenoid labrum can occur at virtually any point in the circumference of the labrum. These occur from acute injury, such as falls on an outstretched arm, as well as from overuse—the humeral head is scoured over the labrum over many, many repetitions.

In addition to the tearing that can occur in the labrum, actual detachment of the labrum from the glenoid rim can occur. The two most common labral detachments encountered clinically are the Bankart lesion and the SLAP lesion. Perthes (1906) was the first to describe the presence of a detachment of the anterior labrum in patients with recurrent anterior instability. Bankart (1923, 1938) described a method for surgically repairing this lesion that now bears his name.

A Bankart lesion is found in as many as 85% of dislocations (Gill et al. 1997) and is described as a labral detachment occurring between 3 o'clock and 6 o'clock on a right shoulder and between the 6 and 9 o'clock positions on a left shoulder. This anteroinferior detachment decreases glenohumeral joint stability by interrupting the continuity of the glenoid labrum and compromising the glenohumeral capsular ligaments (Speer et al. 1994). Detachment of the anteroinferior glenoid labrum increases anterior and inferior humeral head translation, a pattern commonly found in patients with glenohumeral joint instability (Speer et al. 1994).

In addition to labral detachment in the anteroinferior aspect of the glenohumeral joint, similar labral detachment can occur in the superior aspect of the labrum. SLAP lesions are defined as superior labrum anterior posterior. Snyder et al. (1990) classified superior labral injuries into four main types. The most common of these four types is the type II lesion (Morgan et al. 1998). Type II SLAP lesions have been described as complete labral detachment from the anterosuperior to posterosuperior glenoid rim, with instability of the biceps long head tendon noted.

One of the consequences of a superior labral injury is the involvement of the biceps long head tendon and the biceps anchor in the superior aspect of the glenoid. The compromised integrity of both the superior labrum and the biceps anchor leads to significant losses in the static stability of the human shoulder. Cheng and Karzel (1997) demonstrated the important role the superior labrum and biceps anchor play in glenohumeral joint stability by experimentally creating a SLAP lesion between the 10 and 2 o'clock positions. They found 11 to 19% decreases in the glenohumeral joint's ability to withstand rotational force, as well as 100 to 120% increases in strain on the anterior band of the inferior glenohumeral ligament. This demonstrates a significant increase in the load on the capsular ligaments in the presence of superior labral injury.

One final area of discussion is the proposed mechanism of superior labral injury. This is particularly relevant as it will help the clinician understand the positions used during functional progressions as well as the mechanisms that could cause stress or reinjury. Andrews and Gillogly (1985) first described labral injuries in throwers and postulated tensile failure at the biceps insertion as the primary mechanism of failure. Their theory was based on the important role the biceps plays in decelerating the extending elbow during the follow-through phase of pitching, coupled with the large distractional forces present during this violent phase of the throwing motion. Recent hypotheses have developed based on the finding by Morgan et al. (1998) of a more commonly located posterior type II SLAP lesion in the throwing or overhead athlete. This posterior-based lesion can best be explained by the "peel-back mechanism" described by Burkhart and Morgan (1998). The torsional force created when the abducted arm is brought into external rotation is thought to "peel back" the biceps and posterior labrum. Several of the tests for identifying patients with a superior labral injury utilize the position of abduction and external rotation similar to the position Burkhart and Morgan (1998) describe for the peel-back mechanism.

Humeral Epicondylitis

Overuse injuries constitute most of the elbow injuries in the athletic elbow, with humeral epicondylitis, or tennis elbow as it is more popularly known, being one of the most common (Ellenbecker and Mattalino 1997b; Nirschl and Sobel 1981). The repetitive overuse reported as one of the primary etiological factors is particularly evident in the history of most athletes with elbow dysfunction. Epidemiological research on tennis-playing adults reports incidences of humeral epicondylitis ranging from 35 to 50% (Carroll 1981; Kamien 1990; Kitai et al. 1986; Hang and Peng 1984; Priest et al. 1977). This incidence is actually far greater than that reported in elite junior players (11 to 12%) (Winge, Jorgensen, and Nielsen 1989; USTA unpublished data).

Reported in the literature as early as 1873 by Runge, humeral epicondylitis has been extensively studied by many researchers. In 1936, Cyriax listed 26 causes of tennis elbow (Cyriax and Cyriax 1983), while an extensive study of this overuse disorder by Goldie in 1964 reported hypervascularization of the extensor aponeurosis and an increased quantity of free nerve endings in the subtendinous space (Goldie 1964). More recently, Leadbetter (1992) described humeral epicondylitis as a degenerative condition consisting of a time-dependent process, including vascular, chemical, and cellular events that lead to a failure of the cell-matrix healing response in human tendons. This description of tendon injury differs from earlier theories where an inflammatory response was considered a primary factor, hence the term *tendinitis*.

Nirschl (1992, 1993) defines humeral epicondylitis as an extra-articular tendinous injury characterized by excessive vascular granulation and an impaired healing response in the tendon, which he has termed *angiofibroblastic hyperplasia*. In the most recent and thorough histopathological analysis, Nirschl and colleagues (Kraushaar and Nirschl 1999) studied specimens of injured tendon obtained from areas of chronic overuse and reported that they do not contain large numbers of lymphocytes, macrophages, and neutrophils. Instead, tendinosis appears to be a degenerative process characterized by large populations of fibroblasts, disorganized collagen, and vascular hyperplasia (Kraushaar and Nirschl 1999). It is not clear why tendinosis is painful, given the lack of inflammatory cells, and it is also unknown why the collagen does not mature.

Nirschl (1992) describes the primary structure involved in lateral humeral epicondylitis as the tendon of the extensor carpi radialis brevis. Approximately one third of cases involve the tendon of the extensor communis (Kraushaar and Nirschl 1999). Additionally, the extensor carpi radialis longus and extensor carpi ulnaris can be involved as well. The primary site of medial humeral epicondylitis is the flexor carpi radialis, pronator teres, and flexor carpi ulnaris tendons (Nirschl 1992, 1993).

Valgus Extension Overload and Ulnar Collateral Ligament Injury

Repeated overhead throwing or serving activity can lead to characteristic patterns of osseous and osteochondral injury. These injuries are commonly referred to as valgus extension overload injuries (Wilson et al. 1983). As a result of the valgus stress incurred during the throwing or serving motion, traction placed via the medial aspect of the elbow can create bony spurs, or osteophytes, at the medial epicondyle or coronoid process of the elbow (Bennet 1959; Indelicato et al. 1979; Slocum 1978). Additionally, the valgus stress during elbow extension creates impingement, which leads to the development of osteophyte formation at the posterior and posteromedial aspects of the olecranon tip, causing chondromalacia and loose body formation (Wilson et al. 1983). The combination of valgus pressure and powerful extension of the elbow leads to posterior osteophyte formation, due to impingement of the posteromedial aspect of the ulna against the trochlea and olecranon fossa. Joyce (Joyce, Jelsma, and Andrews 1995) has reported the presence of chondromalacia in the medial groove of the trochlea, which often precedes osteophyte formation. Erosion to subchondral bone is often witnessed when olecranon osteophytes are initially developing.

The anterior band of the ulnar collateral ligament is the primary ligamentous restraint against valgus stress during the acceleration phase of the throwing motion. Injury to this ligament can occur from overuse, especially when accompanied by improper mechanics or inadequate rest. Additionally, traumatic valgus stress can create injury to this important stabilizing ligament.

FUNCTIONAL TESTING OF THE UPPER EXTREMITY

After rehabilitation from any upper extremity injury, the application of clinical and functional tests helps determine the person's readiness for functional exercise progressions. A complete evaluation program cannot possibly be covered in any of the last three chapters of this text (upper extremity, lower extremity, and trunk); however, key functional measures that can be used to monitor progression and appropriateness of the individual athlete for exercise progressions are covered. For complete functional evaluation information, refer to Magee 1997; Ellenbecker 2004; and Loudon, Jenkins, and Loudon 1996.

Scapular Evaluation

The specific sequence recommended for scapular evaluation includes both static and dynamic aspects. Statically, the evaluator should note the outline of the scapulae and compare the prominence and positioning of the scapulae bilaterally. Although many variations exist in standing posture, the clinician should be particularly discriminating when there are bilateral differences in scapular posture and, most notably, when greater prominence of the scapula is present on the dominant side in a throwing athlete. After examining the athlete with the arms at the side of the body, the clinician then examines the athlete in the hands-on-hips position (hands on the hips with the thumbs pointing backward). Again, symmetrical positioning and prominence of the scapulae are evaluated.

After the static inspection, the clinician asks the athlete to bilaterally elevate the shoulders using a self-selected plane of elevation. The evaluator should be positioned directly behind the athlete to best observe the movement of the scapulae during concentric elevation and especially during eccentric lowering. Excessive superior movement of the scapula during concentric arm elevation, as well as inferior angle and medial border prominence during the eccentric phase, is commonly encountered in people with scapular dysfunction. Repeated bouts of arm elevation to confirm initial observations, as well as to determine the presence of any symptoms (location in or on the shoulder as well as the range of motion where symptoms occur), are recommended. Additionally, the effect of repeated movements is also of critical importance to assess the effects of fatigue on scapular stabilization.

Finally, scapular provocation tests are recommended to monitor the person's ability to keep the scapulae firmly affixed to the thoracic wall during shoulder loading. Two such positions include leaning into a wall with the shoulders flexed to 90° and pressing against a wall with the hands at waist level. During both positions, the evaluator should examine the response of the scapulae during shoulder loading and look for the winging, or protrusion, of the scapulae from the thoracic wall (see figure 3.11). Other functional positions for these provocations include weight bearing on all fours (quadruped position).

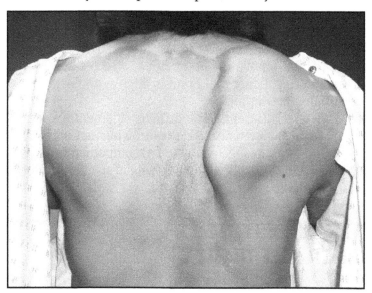

Figure 3.11   Winging of the right scapula during shoulder loading.

Muscular Strength Testing

Objective assessment of muscular strength in the upper extremity is indicated to determine the presence of muscular strength deficiencies as well as to monitor progress during exercise progression. Although not always feasible, the use of a handheld dynamometer or isokinetic dynamometer is recommended to provide the highest degree of accuracy and represent muscular strength relationships (e.g., bilateral comparisons and unilateral strength ratios). Specific test positions have been described by Daniels and Worthingham (1980) and Kelly, Kadrmas, and Speer (1996) for testing the rotator cuff and scapular musculature. Of key importance is the close monitoring of external and internal rotation strength in the neutral position as well as in 90° of glenohumeral joint abduction. These can be tested bilaterally and compared. Close monitoring of the medial scapular border is also necessary, specifically during external rotation testing. If the evaluator notes significant movement of the medial border of the scapula away from the thorax during testing of external rotation with the arm in neutral abduction or adduction at the side, this constitutes a "flip sign." This indicates a lack of scapular stabilization and points the evaluator to include scapular stabilization exercise progressions in the person's exercise programming.

Additionally, the empty can test has been used to test for supraspinatus strength and can also be used as a provocation test to evaluate rotator cuff pathology (Itoi et al. 1999). Although all muscles of the upper extremity can be tested manually, the rotator cuff and scapular muscles are perhaps of greatest importance during functional screening. Distal strength testing using a hand-grip dynamometer should reveal significantly greater dominant-arm strength in baseball pitchers and tennis players (Ellenbecker and Mattalino 1997b).

Isokinetic testing performed at 90° of glenohumeral joint abduction is recommended for screening overhead athletes. This joint position more-specifically addresses muscular function required for overhead activities (Bassett, Browne, and Morrey 1994). Descriptive data profiles for throwing athletes (Wilk et al. 1993; Ellenbecker and Mattalino 1997b) as well as for elite junior tennis players (Ellenbecker and Roetert 2003) are listed in tables 3.1 through 3.5. These data provide objective information regarding the normal torque-to-body-weight ratios as well as external rotation and internal rotation (ER/IR) ratios used in the interpretation of instrumented upper extremity strength testing.

Table 3.1 Isokinetic Peak Torque-to-Body-Weight and Work-to-Body-Weight Ratios for 147 Professional Baseball Pitchers

Speed	INTERNAL ROTATION		EXTERNAL ROTATION	
	Dominant arm	Nondominant arm	Dominant arm	Nondominant arm
210°/sec				
Torque	21%	19%	13%	14%
Work	41%	38%	25%	25%
300°/sec				
Torque	20%	18%	13%	13%
Work	37%	33%	23%	23%

Data were obtained on a Cybex 350 concentric isokinetic dynamometer.

Data from T.S. Ellenbecker and A.J. Mattalino, 1997, "Concentric isokinetic shoulder internal and external rotation strength in professional baseball pitchers," *Journal of Orthopaedic Sports Physical Therapy* 25: 323-328.

Table 3.2 Isokinetic Peak Torque-to-Body-Weight Ratios for 150 Professional Baseball Pitchers

Speed	INTERNAL ROTATION		EXTERNAL ROTATION	
	Dominant arm	Nondominant arm	Dominant arm	Nondominant arm
180°/sec	27%	17%	18%	19%
300°/sec	25%	24%	15%	15%

Data were obtained on a Biodex isokinetic dynamometer.

Data from K.E. Wilk et al., 1993, "The strength characteristics of internal and external rotator muscles in professional baseball pitchers," *American Journal of Sports Medicine* 21: 61-66.

Table 3.3 Isokinetic Peak Torque-to-Body-Weight Ratios and Single Repetition Work-to-Body-Weight Ratios in Elite Junior Tennis Players

	DOMINANT ARM		NONDOMINANT ARM	
	Peak torque (%)	Work (%)	Peak torque (%)	Work (%)
External rotation (ER)				
Male, 210°/sec	12	20	11	19
Male, 300°/sec	10	18	10	17
Female, 210°/sec	8	14	8	15
Female, 300°/sec	8	11	7	12
Internal rotation (IR)				
Male, 210°/sec	17	32	14	27
Male, 300°/sec	15	28	13	23
Female, 210°/sec	12	23	11	19
Female, 300°/sec	11	15	10	13

A Cybex 6000 series isokinetic dynamometer and 90° of glenohumeral joint abduction were used. Data are expressed in foot-pounds per unit of body weight for ER and IR.

Data from T.S. Ellenbecker and E.P Roetert, 2003, "Age specific isokinetic glenohumeral internal and external rotation strength in elite junior tennis players," *Journal of Science and Medicine in Sport* 6(1): 63-70.

Table 3.4 Unilateral External Rotation and Internal Rotation Ratios in Professional Baseball Pitchers

	Dominant arm	Nondominant arm
210°/sec[a]		
Torque	64	74
Work	61	66
300°/sec[a]		
Torque	65	72
Work	62	70
180°/sec[b]		
Torque	65	64
300°/sec[b]		
Torque	61	70

[a]Data from, T.S. Ellenbecker and A.J. Mattalino, 1997, "Concentric isokinetic shoulder internal and external rotation strength in professional baseball pitchers," *Journal of Orthopaedic Sports Physical Therapy* 25: 323-328. [b]Data from W.E. Wilk et al., 1993, "The strength characteristics of internal and external rotator muscles in professional baseball pitchers," *American Journal of Sports Medicine* 21: 61-66.

Table 3.5   Isokinetic External Rotation/Internal Rotation Ratios in Elite Junior Tennis Players

ER/IR ratio	DOMINANT ARM		NONDOMINANT ARM	
	Peak torque (%)	Work (%)	Peak torque (%)	Work (%)
Male, 210°/sec	69	64	81	81
Male, 300°/sec	69	65	82	83
Female, 210°/sec	69	63	81	82
Female, 300°/sec	67	61	81	77

A Cybex 6000 series isokinetic dynamometer and 90° of glenohumeral joint abduction were used. Data are expressed as ER/IR ratios representing the relative muscular balance between the external and internal rotators.

Data from T.S. Ellenbecker and E.P. Roetert, 2003, "Age specific isokinetic glenohumeral internal and external rotation strength in elite junior tennis players," *Journal of Science and Medicine in Sport* 6(1): 63-70.

Muscular imbalances caused by repetitive and forceful internal rotation during the acceleration of the throwing motion, tennis serve, and forehand can lead to unilateral muscular imbalances on the dominant arm between the external and internal rotators and jeopardize optimal muscular stabilization. Careful monitoring of the external and internal rotation unilateral strength ratio is an integral measure of musculoskeletal testing programs for return to sport as well as injury prevention and assists in the determination of optimal application of exercise programs for the overhead athlete.

Range of Motion Testing

A thorough objective documentation of the cardinal movements of the glenohumeral, elbow, and distal joints using a goniometer is recommended. Refer to Berryman-Reese and Bandy (2002) and Norkin and White (1995) for a more-complete discussion.

One of the most important measures for the overhead athlete is humeral rotation. Several important principles should be discussed to optimize its measurement. One of these is the contribution of the scapulothoracic joint to glenohumeral motion, which has been widely documented (Inman, Saunders, and Abbott 1944; Mallon et al. 1996). This is one of the variables that can lead to extensive variation of rotational measurement in the human shoulder. Ellenbecker, Roetert, and Piorkowski (1993) assessed active rotational range of motion measures bilaterally in 399 elite junior tennis players using two differing measurement techniques and a universal goniometer. In this study, 252 subjects were measured in the supine position for internal and external rotation with 90° of glenohumeral joint abduction, using no attempt to stabilize the scapula, and 147 elite junior tennis players were measured for internal and external rotation active range of motion in 90° of glenohumeral joint abduction using scapular stabilization. This stabilization was provided by a posteriorly directed force applied by the examiner's hand placed over the anterior aspect of the shoulder (over the anterior acromion and coracoid process) (figure 3.12). Results of the two groups showed significantly less internal rotation range of motion when using the measurement technique with scapular stabilization (18 to 28% reduction in range of motion). Changes in external rotation range of motion were smaller between groups, with 2 to 6% reductions in active range of motion measured.

Confirmed in this research is the finding of significantly less (approximately 10 to 15°) dominant-arm glenohumeral joint internal rotation in elite junior tennis players (Ellenbecker 1992; Ellenbecker et al. 1996). The significance of this research, however, lies in the fact that this difference between extremities in internal rotation range of motion was identified only when the scapula was stabilized. Failure to stabilize the scapula did not produce glenohumeral joint internal rotation range of motion measurements that identified a deficit. Only measuring this population with scapular stabilization identified the characteristic range of motion limitation in internal rotation. This study clearly demonstrates the importance of using consistent measurement techniques when documenting range of motion of glenohumeral joint rotation.

For interpretation and application to the overhead athlete, the total rotation range of motion should be discussed. Simply combine the glenohumeral joint internal and external rotation range of motion measures by adding the two numbers to get a numerical representation of the total rotation range of motion available at the glenohumeral joint. Research by Kibler et al. (1996) and Roetert, Ellenbecker, and Brown (2000) has identified decreases in the total rotation range of motion arc in the dominant extremity of elite tennis players correlated with increasing age and number of competitive years of play.

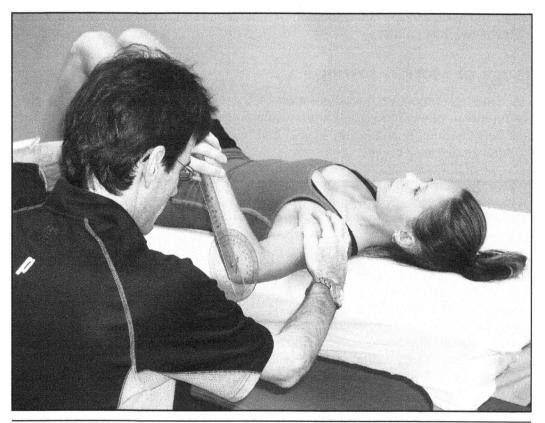

Figure 3.12 Measurement of glenohumeral joint internal rotation with 90° of abduction in the coronal plane with scapular stabilization.

Ellenbecker et al. (2002) measured bilateral total rotation range of motion in professional baseball pitchers and elite junior tennis players. The findings of this study show the professional baseball pitchers to have greater dominant-arm external rotation and significantly less dominant-arm internal rotation when compared with the contralateral nondominant side. The total rotation range of motion, however, was not significantly different between extremities in the professional baseball pitchers (145° dominant arm, 146° nondominant arm). This research shows that, despite bilateral differences in the actual internal or external rotation range of motion in the glenohumeral joints of baseball pitchers, the total arc of rotational motion should remain the same. In the 117 elite male junior tennis players, significantly less internal rotation range of motion was found in the dominant arm (45° versus 56°) as well as significantly less total rotation range of motion in the dominant arm (149° versus 158°). The total rotation range of motion did differ between extremities. Approximately 10° less total rotation range of motion can be expected in the dominant arm of the noninjured elite junior tennis player, as compared with the nondominant extremity.

Use of normative data from population-specific research such as this study can assist clinicians in interpreting normal range of motion patterns and identify when sport-specific adaptations or clinically significant maladaptations are present. Table 3.6 contains the descriptive data from the professional baseball pitchers and elite junior tennis players (Ellenbecker et al. 2002). Further research on additional subject populations is needed to further outline the total rotation range of motion concept.

Upper Extremity Functional Testing

Unlike the lower extremity, where many functional tests exist in the scientific and medical literature, the upper extremity has very few true functional screening tests. One of the gold standards in physical education for gross assessment of upper extremity strength is the push-up. This test has been used to generate sport-specific normative data in noninjured populations (Ellenbecker and Davies 2001; Roetert and Ellenbecker 2007) but is not typically considered appropriate

Table 3.6 Bilateral Comparison of Isolated and Total Rotation ROM of Professional Baseball Pitchers and Elite Junior Tennis Players

Subjects	Dominant arm	Nondominant Arm
Baseball pitchers		
ER	103.2 +/– 9.1 (1.34)	94.5 +/– 8.1 (1.19)
IR	42.4 +/– 15.8 (2.33)	52.4 +/– 16.4 (2.42)
Total rotation	145.7 +/– 18.0 (2.66)	146.9 +/– 17.5 (2.59)
Elite jr. tennis players		
ER	10 +/– 10.9 (1.02)	101.8 +/– 10.8 (1.01)
IR	45.4 +/– 13.6 (1.28)	56.3 +/– 11.5 (1.08)
Total rotation	149.1 +/– 18.4 (1.73)	158.2 +/– 15.9 (1.50)

All measurements are expressed in degrees. Standard error of the mean is in parentheses.

Adapted, by permission, from T.S. Ellenbecker et al, 2002, "Glenohumeral joint total rotation range of motion in elite tennis players and baseball pitchers," *Medicine and Science in Sports and Exercise* 34(12): 2052-2056.

for use in patient populations with shoulder dysfunction. Positional demands placed on the anterior capsule and increased joint loading limit the effectiveness of this test in musculoskeletal rehabilitation. Modification of the push-up has been reported and used clinically as an acceptable alternative for assessing closed-chain function in the upper extremities.

Davies developed the closed kinetic chain (CKC) upper extremity stability test in an attempt to more-accurately assess the functional ability of the upper extremity (Ellenbecker and Davies 2001; Goldbeck and Davies 2000). The test is initiated in the starting position of a standard push-up for males and modified (off knees) push-up for females. Two strips of tape are placed parallel to each other, 3 feet (0.9 m) apart on the floor (figure 3.13). The subject then moves both hands back and forth, touching each line alternately as many times as possible in 15 seconds. Each touch of the line is counted and tallied to generate the CKC upper extremity stability test score. Normative data have been established, with men averaging 18.5 touches in 15 seconds and females averaging 20.5 touches. The CKC upper extremity stability test has been assessed for test–retest reliability, generating an intraclass correlation coefficient (ICC) of .927, indicating high clinical reliability between sessions with this examination method (Goldbeck and Davies 2000).

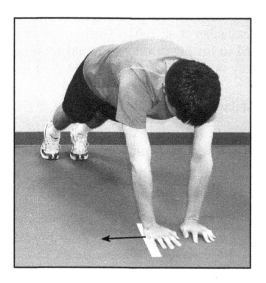
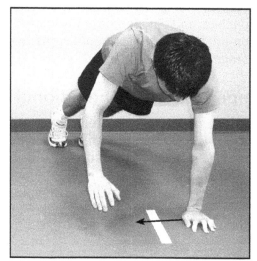
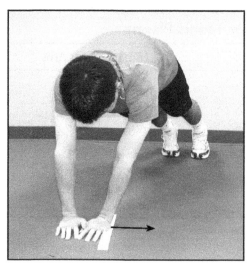

Figure 3.13 Closed kinetic chain functional test.

The brief overview of functional testing for the upper extremity provided here is meant to provide examples of evidence-based test procedures that can be used before and after application of the functional exercise progressions in this book. This section cannot be used in isolation because even in the functional evaluation of an overhead throwing athlete, the ability to perform a functional squat, measured using the one-leg stability test (Wilson et al. 2006), is of critical relevance and should be obtained and applied to the overall testing and training sequence. The remainder of this chapter is devoted to the exercise progressions for the upper extremity.

FUNCTIONAL EXERCISE PROGRESSIONS

The functional progressions in this section of the text provide detailed instructions for the person performing the exercise. Primary muscle groups, indications, contraindications, and pearls of performance are presented to guide the clinician. Some of the exercise progressions contain stages that provide further progression between groupings of exercises. In each instance, stage 1 exercises typically precede stage 2 exercises, and so on. In some instances there are only stage 1 exercises because these exercises are not directly associated with a further obvious progression. This section also includes progressions containing modifications of traditional upper body exercises most applicable for overhead athletes and for people who have had shoulder pathology for which protected or modified exercise is recommended.

ROTATOR CUFF PROGRESSION 1

This progression forms the basis for rotator cuff strengthening. It primarily utilizes a neutral adducted shoulder position to minimize compression of the cuff under the coracoacromial arch. In general, multiple sets of 15 to 20 repetitions should be performed unless otherwise noted.

Side-Lying External Rotation

PROGRESSION NAME: Rotator Cuff Progression 1

STAGE: 1

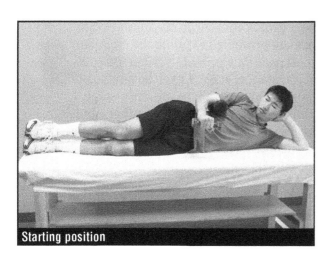
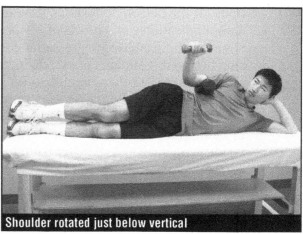

Starting position   Shoulder rotated just below vertical

Starting position: Lie on your side, with a towel roll or pillow under your armpit and your arm resting against your abdomen.

Exercise action: Slowly externally rotate your shoulder by raising the hand and forearm upward until they are just below vertical. Slowly return to the starting position and repeat.

Primary muscle groups: Posterior rotator cuff

Indications: Strengthens the rotator cuff—important base exercise

Contraindications: Shoulder joint pain during exercise

Pearls of performance: Ensure that the patient uses a low-weight, high-repetition format and does not cheat or compensate by using larger muscle groups.

Prone Extension

PROGRESSION NAME: Rotator Cuff Progression 1

STAGE: 1

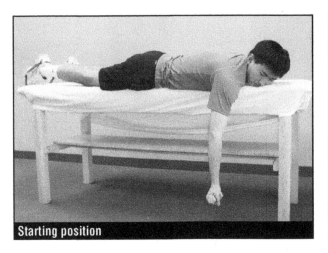

Starting position

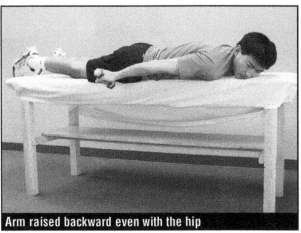

Arm raised backward even with the hip

Starting position: Lie facedown on a plinth or exercise table. Begin with your arm pointing straight down toward the ground (90° of shoulder flexion). The arm should be externally rotated such that the thumb is pointing outward.

Exercise action: Raise your arm backward into extension, keeping the elbow straight until it comes to a level parallel to the floor or even with the hip as pictured. Slowly return to the starting position.

Primary muscle groups: Posterior rotator cuff, scapular stabilizers

Indications: Strengthens the rotator cuff and scapular stabilizers—important base exercise

Contraindications: Extending the shoulder beyond neutral position (above the hip), as this stresses the anterior capsule

Prone Horizontal Abduction

PROGRESSION NAME: Rotator Cuff Progression 1

STAGE: 2

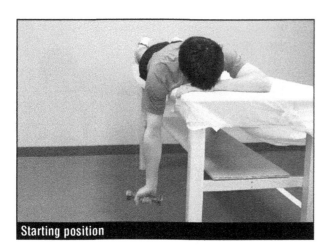

Starting position

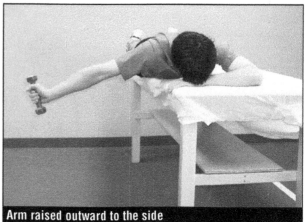

Arm raised outward to the side

Starting position: Lie facedown on a plinth or exercise table. Begin with your arm pointing straight down toward the ground (90° of shoulder flexion). The arm should be externally rotated such that the thumb is pointing outward.

Exercise action: Keeping your elbow straight and thumb pointing outward, raise your arm outward directly to the side until it is just below parallel to the ground. Slowly return to the starting position.

Primary muscle groups: Rotator cuff, scapular stabilizers

Indications: Strengthens the rotator cuff and scapular stabilizers—important base exercise

Contraindications: Raising the arm outward beyond parallel, as this increases stress on the anterior capsule

Pearls of performance: Advanced patients can do this exercise while lying on an exercise ball to increase core stabilization.

Standing External Rotation

PROGRESSION NAME: Rotator Cuff Progression 1

STAGE: 1

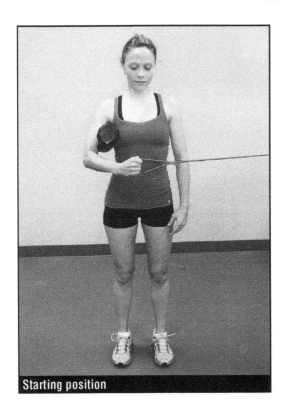

Starting position

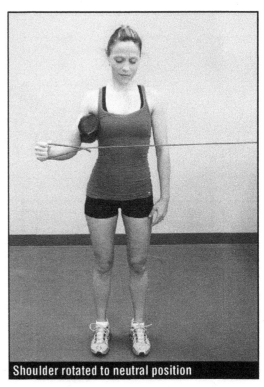

Shoulder rotated to neutral position

Starting position: Stand with your arm at your side, with a towel roll placed under the axilla as pictured. Your hand should be nearly touching your abdomen. Secure a piece of elastic tubing in a door at waist height, with the opposite end in your hand. Your elbow should be bent at a 90° angle and remain in that position during the entire exercise.

Exercise action: Rotate your hand and forearm outward externally, rotating the shoulder to neutral position (straight out in front). Slowly return to the starting position.

Primary muscle groups: Posterior rotator cuff

Indications: Strengthens the rotator cuff—important base exercise

Contraindications: Shoulder joint pain

Pearls of performance: Ensure that the patient does not use tubing that is too heavy in resistance, as this leads to over-recruitment of the deltoid muscle and unwanted compensatory movement patterns.

Standing Internal Rotation

PROGRESSION NAME: Rotator Cuff Progression 1

STAGE: 1

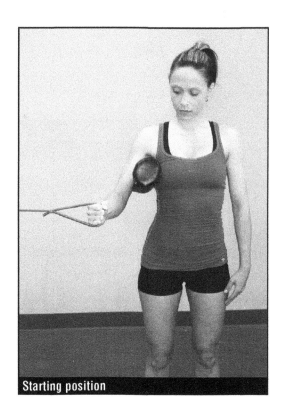
Starting position

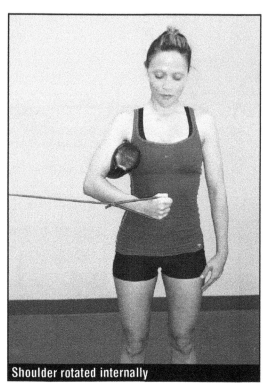
Shoulder rotated internally

Starting position: Stand with your arm at your side, with a towel roll placed under the axilla as pictured. Secure a piece of elastic tubing at waist level in a door or stable object. Begin with your arm straight out in front of you (neutral shoulder rotation). Your elbow should be bent at a 90° angle and remain in that position during the entire exercise.

Exercise action: Move your hand toward the abdomen, internally rotating the shoulder. Slowly return to the starting position.

Primary muscle groups: Subscapularis, pectoralis major, teres major

Indications: Strengthens the anterior portion of the rotator cuff

Contraindications: Overuse in many athletes who have increased development of this muscle group

Pearls of performance: Ensure that no body rotation or shrugging of the shoulder occurs during this exercise.

External Rotation Oscillation

PROGRESSION NAME: Rotator Cuff Progression 1

STAGE: 2

Starting position: Stand with your arm at your side, with a towel roll placed under the axilla as pictured. Secure a piece of elastic tubing in a door at waist height, with the opposite end in your hand. Your elbow should be bent at a 90° angle and remain in that position during the entire exercise. Grasp an oscillating device such as a Bodyblade or Thera-Band FlexBar in your exercising hand.

Exercise action: Keeping the shoulder in a neutral rotation position (hand and forearm directly in front of you), oscillate the bar or blade quickly for a preset time period. Multiple sets of 30 seconds are recommended.

Primary muscle groups: posterior rotator cuff, scapular stabilizers

Indications: increases local muscular endurance by increasing the number of activations of the muscle over the exercise period; requires proximal stabilization from the scapular muscles to allow distal oscillation to occur

Starting position using a FlexBar

Contraindications: shoulder joint pain

Pearls of performance: When performed properly, minimal movement of the hand and forearm occurs; device oscillation is the primary movement, with a stabilized upper extremity.

Side-Lying Bodyblade

PROGRESSION NAME: Rotator Cuff Progression 1

STAGE: 2

Starting position: Lie on your side with a pillow or towel roll under the axilla. Grasp a Bodyblade or oscillating device in one hand. Keep your elbow bent at a 90° angle during the entire exercise.

Exercise action: Perform small rotational movements, oscillating the Bodyblade in 6- to 10-inch (15 to 25 cm) oscillations. Perform multiple sets of 30 seconds.

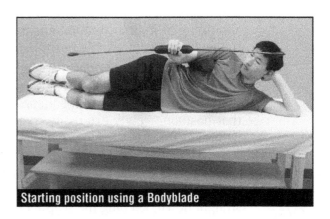
Starting position using a Bodyblade

(continued)

Side-Lying Bodyblade   *(continued)*

Primary muscle groups: Rotator cuff, scapular stabilizers

Indications: Increases local muscular endurance of the rotator cuff and scapular stabilizers

Contraindications: Shoulder joint pain

Pearls of performance: In addition to holding one position of rotation during the 30-second sets, the patient can oscillate while performing a range of internal and external rotation.

ROTATOR CUFF PROGRESSION 2

This set of progressions contains exercises that focus on rotator cuff strengthening with the shoulder in a 90° abducted position. This is an integral exercise progression for any overhead athlete.

Prone External Rotation

PROGRESSION NAME: Rotator Cuff Progression 2

STAGE: 1

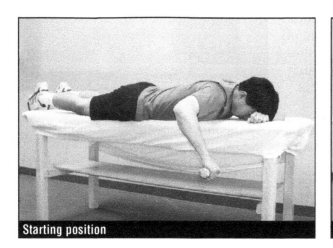 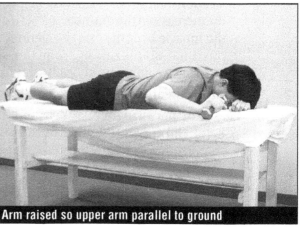

Starting position | Arm raised so upper arm parallel to ground

Starting position: Lie facedown on a plinth or exercise table. Begin with your arm pointing straight down toward the ground (90° of shoulder flexion). The arm should be in neutral rotation such that the thumb is pointing inward toward the body in a comfortable position.

Exercise action: Raise your arm upward, bending the elbow to 90° until the upper arm is parallel to the ground. As this motion occurs, the shoulder blade or scapula will be retracted, or squeezed toward the midline of the body. Holding that position, slowly externally rotate the shoulder by raising the back of the hand upward until the forearm is also parallel to the floor if possible. (Clinician: If the patient does not have full range of external rotation, instruct him or her to use whatever amount of external rotation is available.) Return the shoulder to neutral rotation by lowering the hand and forearm downward until it is pointing straight down, keeping the scapula in a retracted position. Then lower the arm downward slowly, releasing the scapular muscles to the starting position.

Primary muscle groups: Rotator cuff, scapular musculature—important base exercise for overhead athletes

Indications: Strengthens the rotator cuff and scapular stabilizers

Contraindications: Shoulder joint pain or impingement due to 90° position used during exercise

Standing 90/90 External Rotation

PROGRESSION NAME: Rotator Cuff Progression 2

STAGE: 1

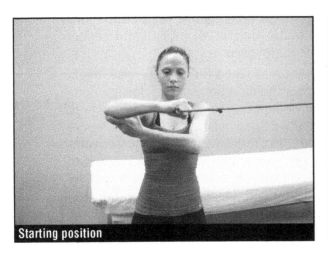
Starting position

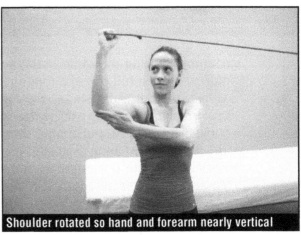
Shoulder rotated so hand and forearm nearly vertical

Starting position: Secure a piece of elastic tubing in a door or secure object at approximately waist level. Grasp one end of the elastic tubing in your hand. Stand facing the door or attachment site for the elastic tubing, with your arm elevated 90° in the scapular plane (30° forward from the frontal, or coronal, plane). Your elbow should be bent 90° and remain in that position during the entire exercise. Use the opposite hand to support the elbow of the exercising arm in 90° of elevation. The starting position for this exercise is with the shoulder in full internal rotation (forearm horizontal or parallel to the ground).

Exercise action: Rotate the forearm and hand back externally, rotating the shoulder until the hand and forearm are nearly vertical. Slowly return to the starting position.

Primary muscle groups: Posterior rotator cuff, scapular musculature

Indications: Strengthens the rotator cuff and scapular muscles in 90° of elevation

Contraindications: Shoulder pain

Pearls of performance: This exercise can be performed using the opposite hand to stabilize under the elbow during the external rotation movement. This helps decrease unwanted compensatory movements and isolates the desired external rotation muscle activation. As competency increases or for variation, the patient can perform the exercise without the other arm's assistance to increase the amount of scapular stabilization required during execution.

(continued)

Standing 90/90 External Rotation   *(continued)*

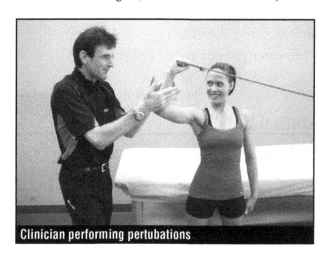

Clinician performing pertubations

Variation 1: After performing five repetitions, hold the forearm in a vertical position against the resistance of the tubing. The clinician then performs pertubations, or challenges, in all directions by pushing the forearm into multiple directions. (Clinician: Cue the patient by saying, "Hold that position—don't let me move you." Challenge the patient for 5 to 10 seconds or until he or she fatigues and cannot hold against the pertubations being delivered.) Rest, and repeat multiple sets.

Variation 2: Using the same initial positioning as listed for this exercise, begin the exercise in full external rotation against the resistance of the elastic tubing (forearm in vertical position). Rapidly move the extremity into internal rotation, and immediately move back to the externally rotated position using an explosive movement pattern and timing sequence. This movement sequence activates the stretch-shortening cycle and uses a plyometric-type training facilitation to initially activate the external rotators eccentrically, followed immediately by an abrupt concentric external rotation movement. Hold the end position (full external rotation) for 1 or 2 seconds, then repeat the exercise.

Standing 90/90 Internal Rotation

PROGRESSION NAME: Rotator Cuff Progression 2

STAGE: 1

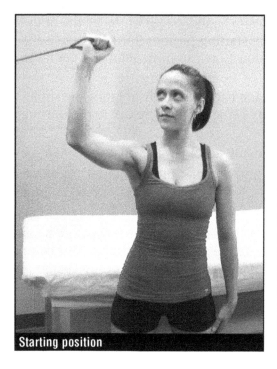

Starting position

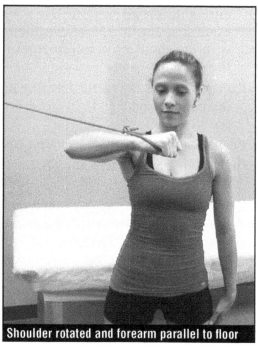

Shoulder rotated and forearm parallel to floor

Starting position: Secure a piece of elastic tubing in a door or secure object at approximately shoulder level. Grasp one end of the elastic tubing in your hand. Stand with your back toward the door or attachment site of the elastic tubing, with your arm elevated 90° in the scapular plane (30° forward from the frontal, or coronal, plane). Your elbow should be bent 90° and remain in that position during the entire exercise. The starting position for this exercise is in the 90/90 position, with your forearm in a vertical position.

Exercise action: Rotate your shoulder internally by moving the hand and forearm forward toward the floor until the forearm is nearly parallel to the ground. Slowly return to the starting position and repeat.

Primary muscle groups: Subscapularis, pectoralis major, teres major, latissimus dorsi

Indications: Strengthens the anterior rotator cuff and internal rotators (accelerators of the throwing and serving motion)

Contraindications: People who are very internal rotation dominant and have very weak external rotation strength

Statue of Liberty

PROGRESSION NAME: Rotator Cuff Progression 2

STAGE: 2

Starting position: Secure a piece of elastic tubing in a door or secure object at approximately waist level. Stand facing the door or attachment site of the elastic tubing with your arm elevated 90° in the scapular plane (30° forward from the frontal, or coronal, plane). Your elbow should be bent 90° and remain in that position during the entire exercise. Grasp a FlexBar or Bodyblade (oscillatory device) in your hand, with the tubing looped around your wrist. Your forearm should be in a vertical position, with the hand pointing toward the ceiling. When first learning this exercise, it may be advantageous to support the elbow with the nonexercising arm as pictured to ensure greater isolation of the rotational movements inherent in this exercise. However, as skill is acquired and proper form is verified, performing the exercise without the assistance of the opposite extremity supported is allowed.

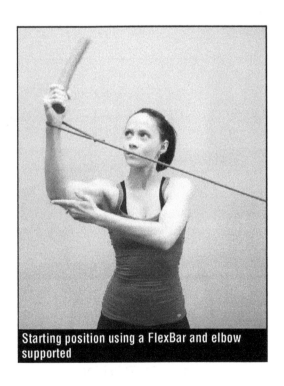
Starting position using a FlexBar and elbow supported

Exercise action: Keeping the arm in the 90/90 position (90° of external rotation, 90° of abduction), oscillate the bar or blade for 30 seconds or until fatigue prevents you from continuing with proper form. Repeat.

Primary muscle groups: Posterior rotator cuff, scapular musculature

Indications: Increases local muscle endurance of the rotator cuff in the position used in overhead sports

(continued)

Statue of Liberty   *(continued)*

Contraindications: Shoulder pain; inability to stabilize shoulder and scapula in 90/90 position

Pearls of performance: This exercise can be performed with the opposite hand placed under the exercising arm's elbow. This results in increased isolation of the external rotation movement pattern and minimizes the use of compensatory movement patterns. Use of the 90/90 position without stabilization from the opposite arm requires greater stabilization and increases scapular muscle firing. Progression from the stabilized position initially to no stabilization from the other arm is recommended with guidance from the clinician.

PLYOMETRIC ROTATOR CUFF PROGRESSION

This progression follows the first two rotator cuff progressions, which form the basis for more-explosive upper extremity function. Failure to perform RCP 1 and 2 would not warrant advancing to the plyometric progression outlined here. These exercises position the arm in an abducted position and simulate overhead functional activities.

90/90 Prone Plyos

PROGRESSION NAME: Plyometric Rotator Cuff Progression

STAGE: 2

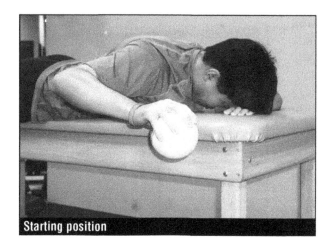

Starting position

Starting position: Lie facedown on a plinth or supportive surface. The shoulder is abducted 90° and the elbow bent 90°. Hold a small medicine ball (0.5 or 1 kg) in your hand. The shoulder should be in 90° of external rotation such that the forearm is nearly parallel to the ground.

Exercise action: Rapidly drop and catch the ball by opening and closing the hand around it, allowing the ball to move very little (several inches (or cm) up and down) during the timed set of exercise. Repeat several sets of 20 to 30 seconds in duration.

Primary muscle groups: Posterior rotator cuff, scapular musculature

Indications: Strengthens the rotator cuff and scapular stabilizers in the 90/90 functional position

Contraindications: Shoulder pain; inability to hold the 90/90 position at start of exercise

90/90 Plyo Reverse Catches

PROGRESSION NAME: Plyometric Rotator Cuff Progression

STAGE: 2

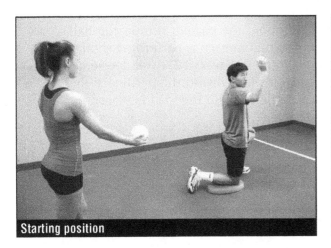
Starting position

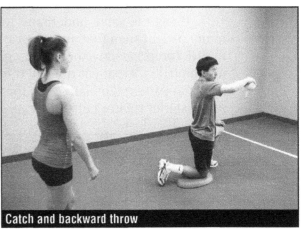
Catch and backward throw

Starting position: Kneel on one knee (right knee for right shoulder exercise, left knee for left shoulder exercise) with the arm in 90° of abduction and 90° of elbow flexion. The shoulder is positioned in 90° of external rotation such that the forearm is in a vertical position. The palm should be facing forward, with the wrist extended slightly. A partner is needed to stand 4-5 feet (1.5 m) behind the patient with a small medicine ball (0.5 to 1 kg). The patient looks backward toward the partner, waiting to accept the tossed ball.

Exercise action: The partner tosses the ball underhand to the patient, who catches the ball and continues into a motion of internal rotation until the forearm is nearly horizontal (parallel to the floor). As the ball is decelerated, the patient immediately and explosively throws the ball backward using a forceful concentric external rotation movement. The partner catches the ball and returns the ball back to the patient using another underhand toss.

Primary muscle groups: Posterior rotator cuff, scapular muscles

Indications: Strengthens the rotator cuff and scapular muscles in the position of throwing and overhead function

Contraindications: Shoulder joint pain; inability to control the movement with the ball to gain the benefit from a plyometric series of muscle activation

Pearls of performance: Ensure that the patient's elbow remains high during the exercise (indicating the upper arm is parallel to the floor and the shoulder is hence abducted 90°).

(continued)

90/90 Plyo Reverse Catches *(continued)*

Variation: The patient assumes the same single-knee starting position. The partner stands slightly to the outside of the patient (farther to the right of a right-handed person, left of a left-handed person). The patient waits for the ball with the elbow straight and the shoulder elevated approximately 100 to 110°. Using the same underhand tossing motion, the partner throws the ball to the patient such that after the catch a diagonal motion is performed similar to PNF (proprioceptive neuromuscular facilitation) diagonal 2. After decelerating the ball, the patient quickly throws it backward toward the partner in the diagonal pattern simulating the throwing motion. Again the load is placed on the posterior rotator cuff and scapular muscles.

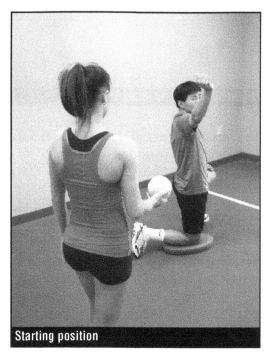

Starting position

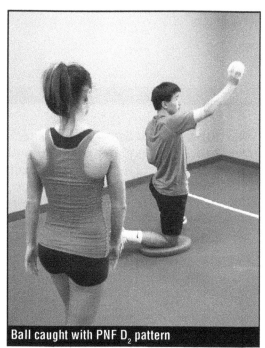

Ball caught with PNF D$_2$ pattern

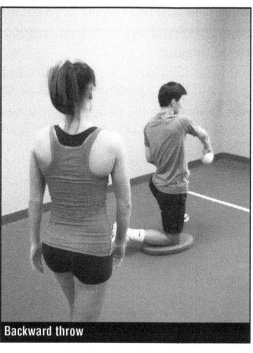

Backward throw

Internal Rotation Plyos at 90° Abduction

PROGRESSION NAME: Plyometric Rotator Cuff Progression

STAGE: 2

Starting position: Stand facing a wall about 1 foot (0.3 m) away. Raise (abduct) the shoulder to 90° and bend the elbow to 90°. Place a small medicine ball (2 to 4 pounds; 1 to 2 kg) in your hand. (For optimal results, the medicine ball should be a gel-based or bounceable variety.) The exercise starts in 90° of external rotation (forearm vertical position).

Exercise action: Throw the ball forcefully against the wall, and catch the ball upon rebound. Repeat the exercise for several timed sets to increase strength and local muscle endurance.

Primary muscle groups: Subscapularis, pectoralis major, latissimus dorsi, teres major

Indications: Increases explosive internal rotation strength as well as wrist flexion strength

Contraindications: Shoulder pain; overly developed internal rotation strength and external rotation weakness

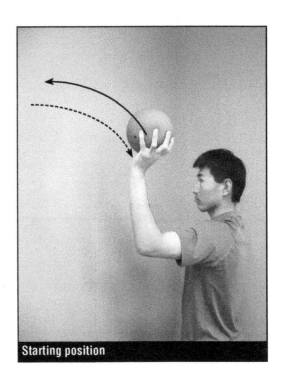

Starting position

Windshield Wiper

PROGRESSION NAME: Plyometric Rotator Cuff Progression

STAGE: 2

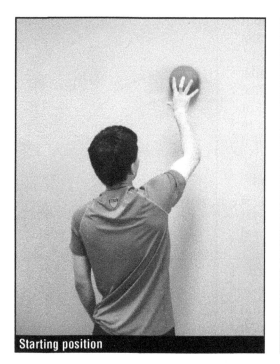

Starting position

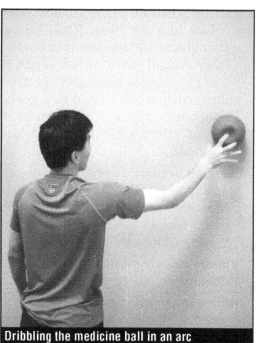

Dribbling the medicine ball in an arc

Starting position: Stand facing a wall about 1 foot (0.3 m) away. Raise (abduct) the shoulder to 90° and bend the elbow to 90°. Place a small medicine ball (2 to 4 pounds; 1 to 2 kg) in your hand. (For optimal results, the medicine ball should be a gel-based or bounceable variety.) The exercise starts in 90° of external rotation (forearm vertical position).

Exercise action: Throw the ball against the wall forcefully as in the internal rotation drill just described. However, in this exercise, progress the dribbling along an arc from approximately the 2 to 3 o'clock position up to the 10 to 12 o'clock position (right-handed exercise). The ball and hand move back and forth like a windshield wiper on a car for multiple sets.

Primary muscle groups: Subscapularis, pectoralis major, latissimus dorsi, teres major

Indications: Improves strength of the muscles that internally rotate and horizontally adduct the shoulder; also provides a training stimulus for the wrist flexors

Contraindications: Shoulder pain; difficulty in overhead positions (this exercise includes overhead reaching while performing the dribbling)

Pearls of performance: In addition to performing the exercise with the elbow flexed 90°, the patient can perform this exercise with an extended elbow.

SCAPULAR STABILIZATION PROGRESSION I

These exercises provide a training stimulus for the important trapezius–serratus anterior force couple components and provide dynamic stabilization of the scapula. These exercises help provide the proximal platform of strength for the upper extremity and are the first stage in the scapular progression series.

External Rotation With Retraction

PROGRESSION NAME: Scapular Stabilization Progression I

STAGE: 1

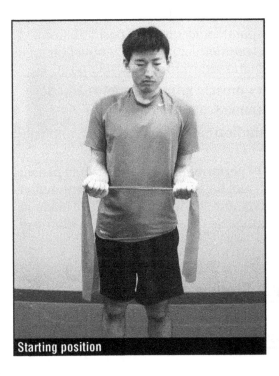
Starting position

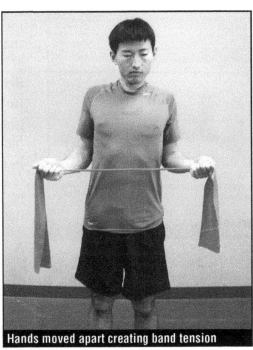
Hands moved apart creating band tension

Starting position: Stand with your arms in front of your body, elbows flexed 90° and a piece of elastic band or tubing placed across the hands in the palm-up position. Shoulders are in neutral rotation such that the hands are directly in front of you.

Exercise action: With light tension in the band, externally rotate both shoulders by moving the hands apart about 3 to 6 inches (8 to 15 cm) against the resistance of the band. While holding this position, maximally retract and depress (squeeze shoulder blades together and downward), holding this end position for 1 to 2 seconds. Return to the starting position by relaxing the shoulder blades and moving the hands back toward each other.

Primary muscle groups: Scapular stabilizers, rotator cuff

Indications: Excellent exercise to recruit the lower trapezius with little activation of the upper trapezius

Contraindications: Shoulder pain

Pearls of performance: Ensuring that the patient maximally retracts the scapulae is an important guide in this exercise. Giving feedback by palpating the scapular medial border is recommended during skill acquisition of this exercise.

Serratus Punch (Serratus Press)

PROGRESSION NAME: Scapular Stabilization Progression I

STAGE: 1

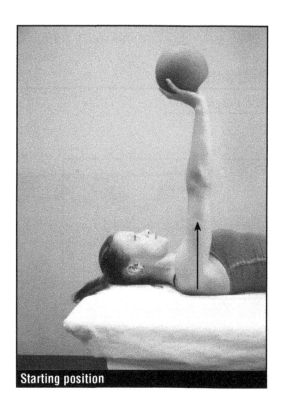

Starting position

Starting position: Lie in the supine position on a supportive surface. Shoulder is flexed to 90°. Place a 4-6 lb (2-3 kg) medicine ball or weight in the hand. The elbow remains in extension and does not move during this exercise.

Exercise action: Using a relatively small motion of 4 to 6 inches (10 to 15 cm) typically, punch the ball upward by protracting the scapula. Hold the end position (termed the *plus position*) of maximal protraction for a second, and return to the starting position.

Primary muscle groups: Serratus anterior

Indications: Scapular stabilization

Contraindications: Shoulder pain; impingement

Pearls of performance: Ensure that the patient is only moving the scapula into protraction by feeling and guiding the shoulder blade at first during this exercise. Compensation can devalue this exercise.

Supine Rhythmic Stabilization

PROGRESSION NAME: Scapular Stabilization Progression I

STAGE: 1

Starting position: Lie supine with your shoulder in 90° of flexion. The shoulder should be in slight external rotation (thumb pointing up toward you, palm facing inward).

Exercise action: The clinician provides challenges in multiple directions by slapping or pressing your arm, first in a nonrandom then a random direction. (Clinician: Cue the patient by saying, "Hold that position—don't let me move you." Increase the intensity as the patient gains strength and stabilization.)

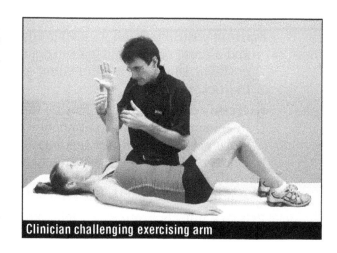

Clinician challenging exercising arm

Primary muscle groups: Scapular stabilizers, biceps, triceps

Indications: General scapular stabilization; general upper extremity strengthening

Contraindications: Shoulder pain

Pearls of performance: Increase the speed of the challenges or pertubations as the level of competency increases during training. Placing the shoulder in a more-protracted position increases the difficulty of the exercise.

Lawn Mower

PROGRESSION NAME: Scapular Stabilization Progression I

STAGE: 1

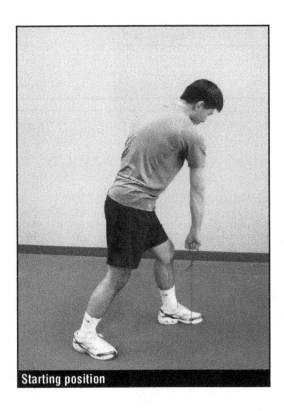
Starting position

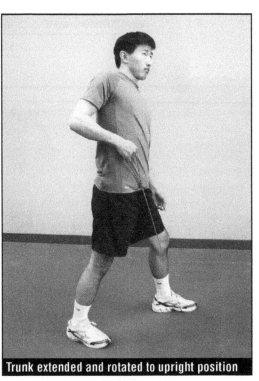
Trunk extended and rotated to upright position

Starting position: Stand with your left foot approximately 12 to 18 inches (30 to 46 cm) in front of your right (right-handed exercise). Place a piece of elastic tubing or band under the left foot, and grasp the other end of the tubing with the right hand at a level near the outside (lateral side) of the left knee. The trunk is bent 45 to 60° and in slight left rotation.

Exercise action: Extend and rotate the trunk toward an upright position while rocking back onto the right foot. As this whole-body motion occurs, bring the right hand toward the base of the right side of the rib cage as you move the shoulder blade into retraction and depression. Emphasis is again on squeezing the shoulder blades together as this exercise motion occurs. Return to the starting position and repeat.

Primary muscle groups: Scapular stabilizers, back extensors, core

Indications: Scapular stabilization; core stability

Contraindications: Shoulder pain; history of low back and sacroiliac dysfunction

(continued)

Lawn Mower   *(continued)*

Pearls of performance: This open kinetic chain exercise has a primary emphasis on scapular stabilization but offers a training stimulus for the core as well. Ensure that the patient does not drive the elbow farther back than the side of the body (shoulder extension) or abduct the shoulder away from the side of the body. These compensations decrease the scapular stabilization emphasis during the exercise.

Robbery

PROGRESSION NAME: Scapular Stabilization Progression I

STAGE: 1

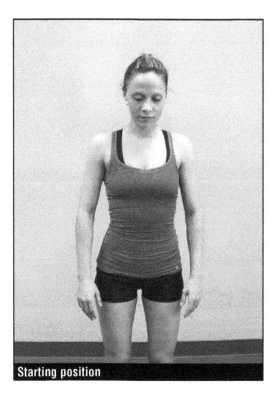
Starting position

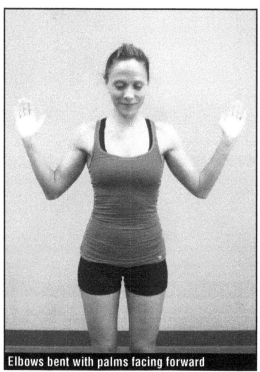
Elbows bent with palms facing forward

Starting position: Stand with your arms at your sides, initially with no weight; as strength progresses, hold small dumbbells in hands with the forearms pronated (palms back).

Exercise action: Bend the elbows and bring the hands upward while retracting and depressing the scapulae (squeezing together and downward). The hands stop in a "don't shoot" type of position seen in a robbery situation in movies. The elbows remain fairly close to the sides during this exercise.

Primary muscle groups: Scapular stabilizers

Indications: Scapular stabilization

Contraindications: Shoulder pain

Bilateral Shoulder Extension

PROGRESSION NAME: Scapular Stabilization Progression I

STAGE: 1

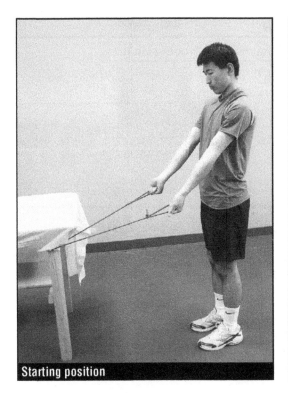

Starting position

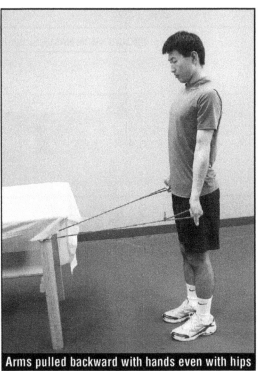

Arms pulled backward with hands even with hips

Starting position: Stand facing a door or stable object. Secure tubing at midlength safely in a doorway or around a pole or nonmovable object. Stand with ends of tubing in each hand, with light tension in the band such that the shoulders are in approximately 45° of flexion. The shoulders are externally rotated such that the thumbs are pointing outward away from the body in the starting position. The elbows are fully extended and remain so during the duration of this exercise.

Exercise action: Keeping the elbows straight, bring the shoulders bilaterally into extension until the hands are even with the sides of the body. As you bring the arms back into extension, pinch the scapulae together and downward (retracted and depressed). Slowly return to the starting position.

Primary muscle groups: Scapular stabilizers, triceps

Indications: Scapular stabilization

Contraindications: Shoulder pain

SCAPULAR STABILIZATION PROGRESSION II

This progression contains additional scapular stabilization exercises that use both open and closed kinetic chain environments.

Row

PROGRESSION NAME: Scapular Stabilization Progression II

STAGE: 1

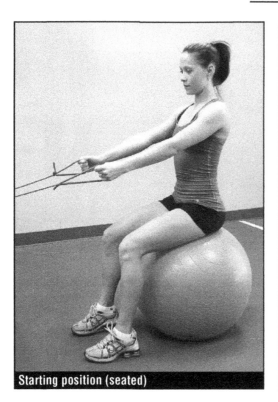

Starting position (seated)

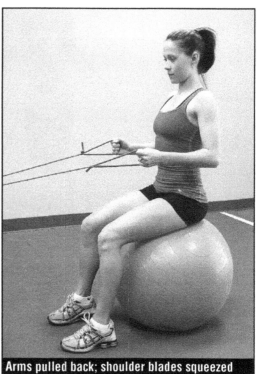

Arms pulled back; shoulder blades squeezed

Starting position: Stand or sit facing a door, post, or stable object with tubing secured in the door or around the post or stable object. Grasp ends of tubing loops or handles in each hand. Start with hands out in front of you, reaching forward such that there is light tension in the tubing.

Exercise action: Pull your arms backward toward your sides. As you bring the arms backward, squeeze the shoulder blades together forcefully while pushing your upper chest outward. Hold the position, with shoulder blades squeezed together and elbows near your sides. Don't pull the arms back such that the elbows protrude past the sides of your body. Slowly return to the starting position and repeat.

Primary muscle groups: Scapular stabilizers, middle trapezius, serratus anterior, rhomboids

Indications: Strengthens scapular stabilizers

Contraindications: Shoulder pain

Pearls of performance: This exercise can also be performed while sitting or on an exercise ball to increase activation of the core muscles of the trunk.

Step-Ups

PROGRESSION NAME: Scapular Stabilization II

STAGE: 1

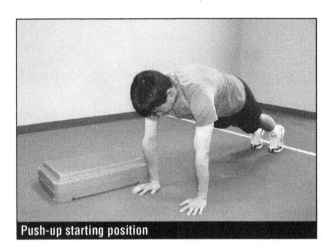
Push-up starting position

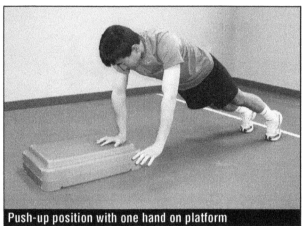
Push-up position with one hand on platform

Starting position: Start on your hands and knees with your hips and pelvis positioned slightly in front of the knees such that greater body weight is placed on the upper body. Position yourself just beside an 8- to 12-inch (20 to 30 cm) platform or step.

Exercise action: Reach up and place one hand on the platform, then put the other hand on top of the first hand so they are on top of each other. Once your hands are positioned on the platform, push yourself upward such that your back rounds like a cat. (This protracts, or slides, the scapulae forward on the upper back). One at a time return each hand back to the floor and repeat.

Progression: Begin this exercise as described. Then progress to doing it from a standard push-up starting position (pictured). This increases the load on the upper body and scapular region.

Primary muscle groups: Serratus anterior, triceps

Indications: Scapular stabilization

Contraindications: Shoulder pain

Pearls of performance: The key to this exercise is placing the shoulder blades into protraction by rounding the back upward like a cat. This is termed the *plus position* and has been proven to increase muscle activation of the serratus anterior.

Step-Up Monster Walk

PROGRESSION NAME: Scapular Stabilization II

STAGE: 2

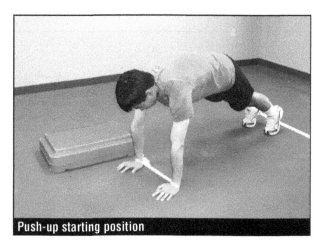

Push-up starting position

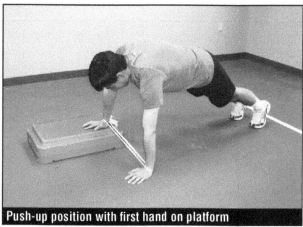

Push-up position with first hand on platform

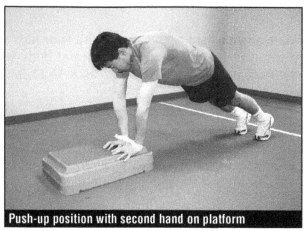

Push-up position with second hand on platform

Starting position: Start on your hands and knees with your hips and pelvis positioned slightly in front of the knees such that greater body weight is placed on the upper body. Position yourself just beside an 8- to 12-inch (20 to 30 cm) platform or step. Loop a piece of Thera-Band around your hands in about an 8- to 12-inch (20 to 30 cm) diameter loop.

Exercise action: Reach up and place one hand on the platform, positioning that hand in the center of the platform. This will place tension in the band between the hand that moves initially and the hand that remains on the floor. Slowly and with control move the hand from the floor onto the near edge of the platform, keeping slight tension in the band as you position the second hand on the platform. Once your hands are positioned on the platform, push yourself upward such that your back rounds like a cat. (This protracts, or slides, the scapulae forward on the upper back). One at a time return each hand back to the floor, keeping tension in the band, and repeat.

Primary muscle groups: Serratus anterior, triceps

Indications: Scapular stabilization

Contraindications: Shoulder pain

Pearls of performance: The patient can progress to performing this exercise from a standard push-up position to increase loading.

Scapular Plane Oscillation

PROGRESSION NAME: Scapular Stabilization II

STAGE: 1

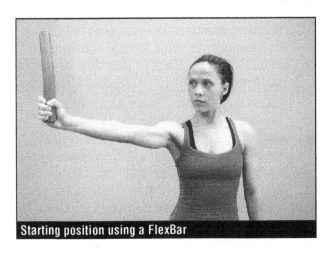

Starting position using a FlexBar

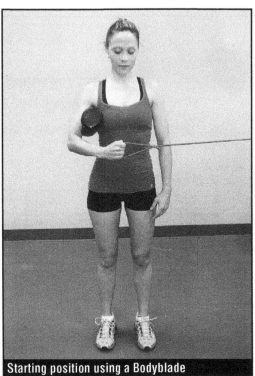

Starting position using a Bodyblade

Starting position: Stand holding an oscillation device (such as a FlexBar or Bodyblade). Elevate your arm to shoulder level (90°) in the scapular plane (30° forward from the coronal, or frontal, plane).

Exercise action: Oscillate the device, maintaining this position. Repeat several sets of 30 seconds of the exercise.

Primary muscle groups: Scapular stabilizers, biceps, triceps

Indications: Base scapular stabilization

Contraindications: Shoulder pain

Pearls of performance: This exercise can be progressed by challenging the patient's balance system. First ask the patient to perform the exercise off one leg, then off one leg on a balance platform or BOSU ball.

Medicine Ball Balance

PROGRESSION NAME: Scapular Stabilization II

STAGE: 2

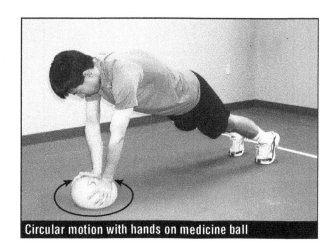

Circular motion with hands on medicine ball

Starting position: Position yourself on the ground on your hands and toes, similar to the starting position of a push-up.

Exercise action: Place your hands on each side of a large medicine ball, and balance on top of the ball while keeping the shoulder blades rounded forward (scapular protraction). When you are able to hold this position successfully, begin making small circles with the ball in clockwise and counterclockwise directions.

Primary muscle groups: Scapular stabilizers, pectoralis major, triceps

Indications: Scapular stabilization with emphasis on balance

Contraindications: Shoulder pain; history of posterior instability

Pearls of performance: Careful monitoring of the patient is important during this exercise to ensure that the scapulae remain fixed against the thorax through muscular contraction. Any evidence as the exercise continues of the scapulae protruding, or winging, should result in discontinuation of that set of the exercise. After the patient rests, the proper scapular position can be reset in the next set. Increase the length of each set as the patient increases strength and competence.

SCAPULAR PLYOMETRICS

This progression contains explosive upper extremity exercises that target many muscle groups but are particularly effective in improving scapular stabilization.

Chest Pass

PROGRESSION NAME: Scapular Plyometrics

STAGE: 1

Starting position: Stand 3 feet (1 m) in front of a rebound device or 6-8 feet (1.8-2.4 m) away from a partner if a rebound device is not available. Holding a 4- to 6-pound (2 to 3 kg) medicine ball in both hands, prepare to throw the ball forward using a chest-pass motion as seen in basketball.

Exercise action: Explosively pass the ball into the rebound device or to a partner, and prepare for the rapid return of the ball. Immediately upon catching the ball, throw it back explosively. Repeat for either a preset number of repetitions or a timed set.

Primary muscle groups: Scapular stabilizers, pectorals, triceps, wrist flexors

Indications: General upper body strengthening to improve explosive strength

Contraindications: Shoulder pain

Pearls of performance: This exercise can be made more challenging by having the patient stand on a BOSU ball or balance platform.

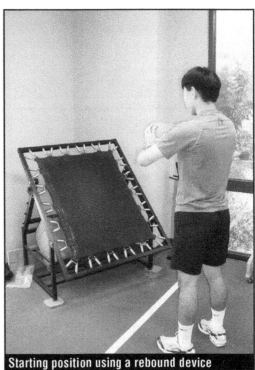

Starting position using a rebound device

Wood Chops

PROGRESSION NAME: Scapular Plyometrics

STAGE: 1

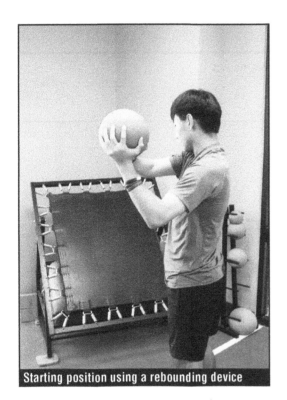

Starting position using a rebounding device

Starting position: Stand 3 feet (1 m) in front of a rebound device or 6-8 feet (1.8-2.4 m) away from a partner. Grasp a 4- to 6-pound (2 to 3 kg) medicine ball in both hands. Position the ball directly over the left shoulder such that the elbows are bent 90 to 120° and the shoulders are flexed 45 to 60°. Rotate your trunk slightly to the left to preload this exercise.

Exercise action: Throw the ball using a chopping motion with both arms in a diagonal pattern such that the ball is thrown downward and to the right. The partner or rebound device quickly returns the ball. Upon catching and absorbing the impact of the ball, immediately direct it forward again toward the device or partner. Several timed sets or sets of multiple repetitions are recommended to improve both strength and muscular endurance. After completing one set of this exercise, reverse the direction such that the movement consists of a downward movement toward the right.

Primary muscle groups: Scapular and core stabilizers, triceps

Indications: General upper body strengthening to improve explosive strength

Contraindications: Shoulder pain

Wall Plyos

PROGRESSION NAME: Scapular Plyometrics

STAGE: 1

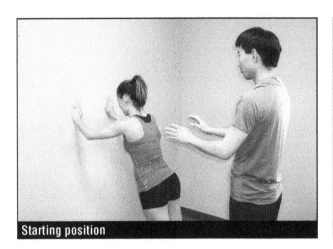

Starting position

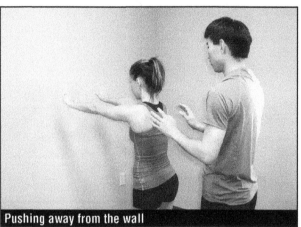

Pushing away from the wall

Starting position: Stand about 2 to 3 feet (.6 to 1 m) away from a wall, facing toward the wall. Put your palms on the wall about shoulder level. A trusted partner should stand behind you in a position of readiness.

Exercise action: Push yourself away from the wall toward the partner behind you. The partner quickly pushes you back toward the wall rather forcefully, and upon contacting the wall, you rapidly explode back off the wall toward the partner.

Primary muscle groups: Scapular stabilizers, pectorals, triceps, wrist flexors

Indications: General upper body strengthening to improve explosive strength

Contraindications: Shoulder pain

Unilateral Quadruped Ball Catches

PROGRESSION NAME: Scapular Plyometrics

STAGE: 2

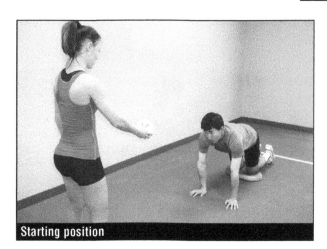

Starting position

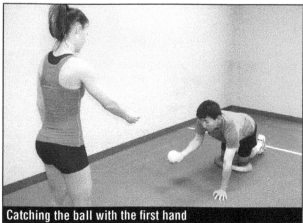

Catching the ball with the first hand

Starting position: Begin in the quadruped position (on hands and knees, with hands directly under shoulders and knees under hips). A partner stands approximately 3 feet (1 m) in front of you with a 2- to 4-pound (1 to 2 kg) medicine ball, the size of which you can easily handle in one hand.

Exercise action: The partner tosses the ball toward one of your hands using an underhand toss. You catch the ball and immediately toss it underhand back to the partner. The partner tosses the ball toward your other hand, and the sequence is repeated.

Primary muscle groups: Scapular and core stabilizers, biceps

Indications: General scapular and core stabilization

Contraindications: Shoulder pain; posterior shoulder instability

Pearls of performance: This exercise can be made much more difficult by progressing the patient to the hands and toes push-up position as tolerated. The main goal of the exercise is to load the weight-bearing upper extremity in a rapid fashion to increase muscular activation in the scapular muscles.

Quadruped Ball Slaps

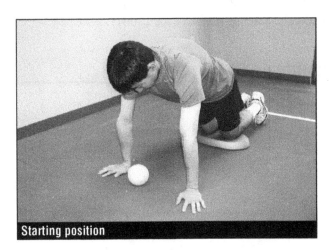
Starting position

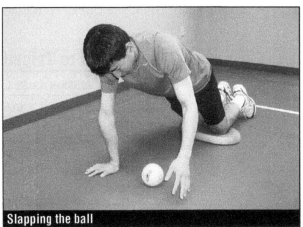
Slapping the ball

Starting position: Begin in the quadruped position (on hands and knees, with hands directly under shoulders and knees under hips). A 4- to 6-pound (2 to 3 kg) medicine ball is between the hands.

Exercise action: In a rapid and alternating fashion, slap the ball from side to side by shifting weight from one extremity to the other as quickly as possible. The medicine ball typically traverses approximately 6 inches (15 cm) between the hands as it is moved quickly from side to side.

Primary muscle groups: Scapular and core stabilizers, triceps

Indications: General scapular and core stabilization

Contraindications: Shoulder pain; posterior shoulder instability

Pearls of performance: This exercise can be made much more difficult by progressing the patient to the hands and toes push-up position as tolerated. The main goal of the exercise is to load the weight-bearing upper extremity in a rapid fashion to increase muscular activation in the scapular muscles.

CLOSED KINETIC CHAIN PROGRESSION

This progression uses closed kinetic chain environments and progresses the exercise by limiting the number of bases of support as well as using implements to decrease the stability afforded by the supportive surface. For data and evidence about the muscle activation, see Uhl et al. (2003) and Ellenbecker and Davies (2001).

Quadruped to Triped Rhythmic Stabilization

PROGRESSION NAME: Closed Chain Progression

STAGE: 1, 2

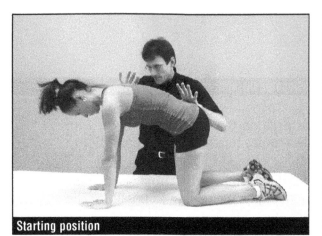

Starting position

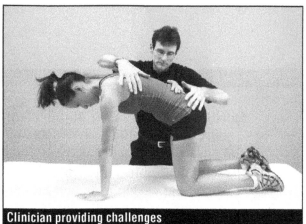

Clinician providing challenges

Starting position: Begin in the quadruped position (on hands and knees, with hands directly under shoulders and knees under hips).

Exercise action: The clinician provides challenges in all directions and diagonals to the trunk, shoulders, and hips, repeatedly challenging your balance. (Clinician: Cue the patient by saying, "Hold that position—don't let me move you." Increase the intensity based on the competency of the patient. Once the quadruped stabilization exercise is mastered, instruct the patient to place one upper extremity in the lumbar region [extension and internal shoulder rotation], and impart challenges against only three limbs of support.)

Progression: Placing a medicine ball or stability platform under the weight-bearing upper extremity increases the amount of difficulty for the patient during the application of the challenges by the clinician.

Primary muscle groups: Scapular and core stabilizers

Indications: Scapular and core stabilization

Contraindications: Shoulder pain; posterior shoulder instability

Pearls of performance: Placing the weight-bearing shoulders or shoulder in a protracted position will increase the activation levels of the serratus anterior during this exercise.

Triped to Pointer

PROGRESSION NAME: Closed Chain Progression

STAGE: 1, 2

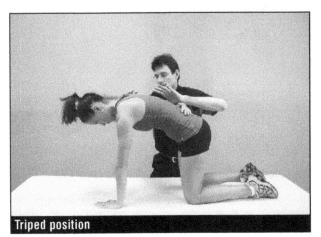

Triped position

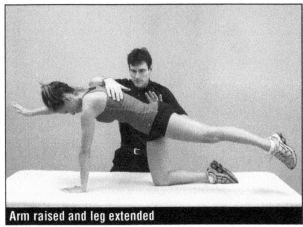

Arm raised and leg extended

Starting position: Begin in a triped position, with involved or targeted upper extremity as the weight-bearing limb.

Exercise action: The clinician provides challenges in all directions and diagonals to the trunk, shoulders, and hips, repeatedly challenging your balance. (Clinician: Cue the patient by saying, "Hold that position—don't let me move you." Increase the intensity based on the competency of the patient. Once the triped position is mastered, instruct the patient to raise one arm and extend the contralateral limb's hip and knee outward, maintaining balance. Impart challenges once the pointer position can be successfully maintained.)

Progression: In the pointer position, an unstable ball (medicine ball) can be inserted under the weight-bearing upper limb, while an oscillatory device such as a Bodyblade or FlexBar can be placed in the non-weight-bearing upper limb. Performing oscillations while on the unstable platform further challenges the musculature.

Primary muscle groups: Scapular and core stabilizers

Indications: Scapular and core stabilization

Contraindications: Shoulder pain; posterior shoulder instability

Pearls of performance: Placing the weight-bearing shoulder in a protracted position will increase the activation levels of the serratus anterior during this exercise.

Upper Extremity BOSU or Exercise Ball Stabilization

PROGRESSION NAME: Closed Chain Progression

STAGE: 1, 2

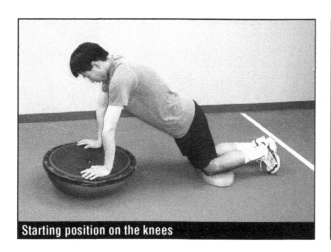

Starting position on the knees

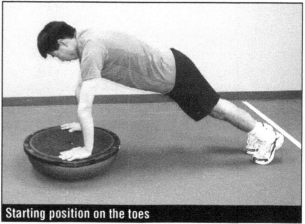

Starting position on the toes

Starting position: Start with your hands on the edges of a BOSU ball platform or on top of an exercise ball.

Exercise action: Try to stabilize while taking your body weight via the upper extremities. Attempts to perform circular movements while maintaining balance increase the difficulty of this exercise. Progress from knees (easiest) to toes (most difficult) depending on your competency and strength development.

Progression: Progressing not only from knees to toes but also from bilateral upper extremity weight bearing to unilateral weight bearing is recommended. Additionally, while on the BOSU platform, alternately raising the extended leg upward 6 inches (15 cm) off the ground while the upper extremity adjusts to the challenge is a further progression of this exercise. Finally, the highest level of difficulty involves placing an excise ball under the pelvis or midfemur while the upper extremities are on the BOSU platform. This significantly increases the whole-body muscular activation aspect of this exercise.

Primary muscle groups: Scapular and core stabilizers

Indications: Scapular and core stabilization

Contraindications: Shoulder pain; posterior shoulder instability

Pearls of performance: Placing the weight-bearing upper extremities in a protracted position will increase the activation levels of the serratus anterior muscle.

Upper Extremity on Ball Over Edge

PROGRESSION NAME: Closed Chain Progression

STAGE: 2

Starting position: Lie on your abdomen on a treatment table or elevated supportive surface. The top one third of your body should protrude over the lead edge of the table. Place one hand on top of an exercise ball next to the edge of the treatment table; place the opposite hand on the lower back.

Exercise action: Stabilize your upper body on top of the ball, bearing weight into the ball. Increase difficulty of the exercise by sliding your body further off the supportive surface such that a greater amount of weight is taken by the weight-bearing upper extremity.

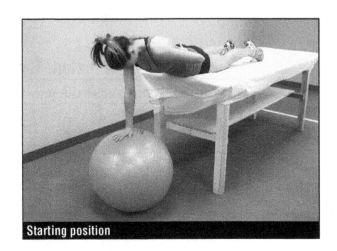

Starting position

Primary muscle groups: Scapular stabilizers, triceps

Indications: Scapular and core stabilization

Contraindications: Shoulder pain; posterior shoulder instability

BASE ELBOW AND WRIST PROGRESSION

This base progression can be applied to any athlete or person who uses extensive distal upper extremity muscular activation, such as tennis and baseball players. The base progression forms the platform for the more-challenging and dynamic exercises in the next progression.

Flexion–Extension Curls

PROGRESSION NAME: Base Elbow and Wrist Progression

STAGE: 1

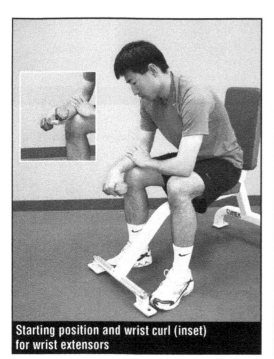

Starting position and wrist curl (inset) for wrist extensors

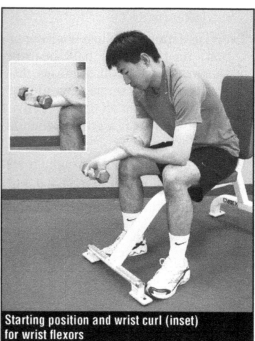

Starting position and wrist curl (inset) for wrist flexors

Starting position: In a seated position, stabilize your forearm over your thigh such that the wrist is protruding just over the knee to allow unrestricted wrist motion. The elbow is typically flexed 60 to 75° in this position. You may want to stabilize the forearm with the opposite hand to further isolate wrist motion during this exercise. To focus on the wrist extensors, the forearm should be pronated (palm down); for the flexors, use a supinated forearm (palm up).

Exercise action: In an isolated fashion, slowly curl your wrist upward against resistance. Hold for one count, and return to the starting position.

Primary muscle groups: Wrist and finger flexors and extensors

Indications: Distal upper extremity

Contraindications: Elbow or wrist pain

Pearls of performance: The patient begins by performing the wrist flexion–extension exercises with the elbow in a flexed position and progresses to using a nearly extended (straightened) position, which mimics the position of many sport-specific movement patterns.

Radial Ulnar Deviation

PROGRESSION NAME: Base Elbow and Wrist Progression

STAGE: 1

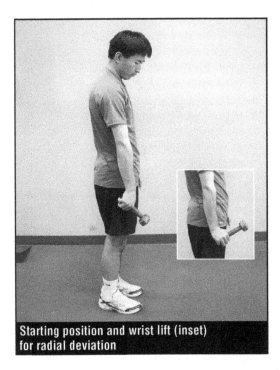

Starting position and wrist lift (inset) for radial deviation

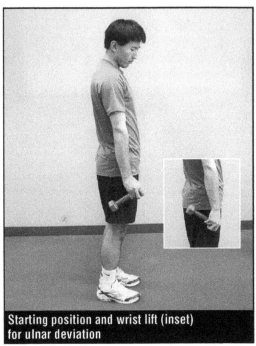

Starting position and wrist lift (inset) for ulnar deviation

Starting position: Stand with your arm at your side, holding a counterbalanced weight (2-3 lb or 0.9-1.4 kg weight at only one end) in your hand. For radial deviation, the weight should be in front of (anterior to) the hand; for ulnar deviation, the weight should be behind (posterior to) the hand.

Exercise action: Pointing the weight initially downward and keeping the elbow extended and forearm in neutral position (not supinated, not pronated), move the weight upward to the end range of available wrist motion. Hold for one count, and slowly return to the starting position.

Primary muscle groups: Wrist and finger flexors and extensors

Indications: Distal upper extremity strengthening

Contraindications: Elbow or wrist pain

Pearls of performance: Normal radial deviation at the wrist involves less range of motion than does ulnar deviation. Therefore, patients often compensate to try to use more motion during this exercise. It is far better to use a small, isolated range of motion without compensation.

Forearm Pronation and Supination

PROGRESSION NAME: Base Elbow and Wrist Progression

STAGE: 1

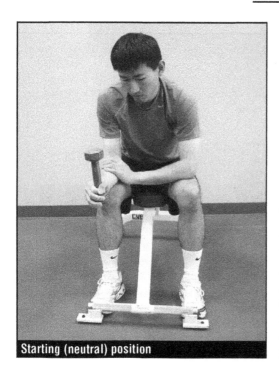

Starting (neutral) position

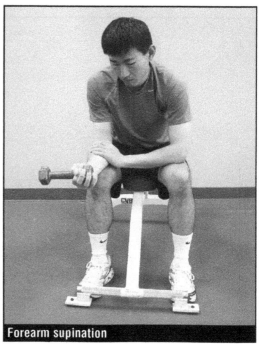

Forearm supination

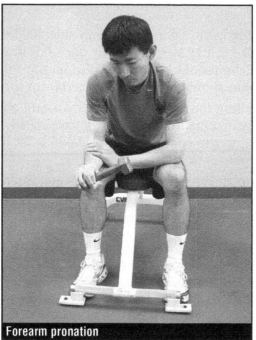

Forearm pronation

Starting position: In a seated position, stabilize your forearm over your thigh such that the wrist is protruding just over the knee to allow unrestricted wrist motion. The elbow is typically flexed approximately 60 to 75° in this position. Using a counterbalanced weight (2-3 lb or 0.9-1.4 kg weight on only one end) grasp the end opposite the weight. Exercise begins in neutral position (weight stick is vertical).

Exercise action: From the neutral position, move the weight by supinating the forearm (turning the palm upward) until the stick is in the horizontal position. Hold this position for 1 s and return to neutral. Repeat supination for desired number of sets and repetitions. For forearm pronation exercise, rotate the forearm (turning palm downward) until the stick is again in the horizontal direction. Hold that position for 1 s, and return to neutral starting position.

Primary muscle groups: Pronator teres, pronator quadratus, supinator, biceps

Indications: Distal upper extremity strengthening

Contraindications: Elbow or wrist pain

Pearls of performance: The patient should avoid simply moving or swinging the weight from pronation to supination. The exercise is most effective when only half the arc of motion (i.e., supination or pronation) is utilized. Initially this exercise typically uses a flexed position at the elbow of approximately 60 to 75°. As the patient progresses, increase the difficulty of this exercise to include a nearly extended (straight) elbow position.

ADVANCED ELBOW AND WRIST

Once the base progression of wrist and elbow exercises is integrated into the program, a progression to these more-dynamic and more-challenging exercises is indicated to better produce distal muscle power and local muscle endurance.

Ball Dribbles (Floor)

PROGRESSION NAME: Advanced Elbow and Wrist Progression

STAGE: 2

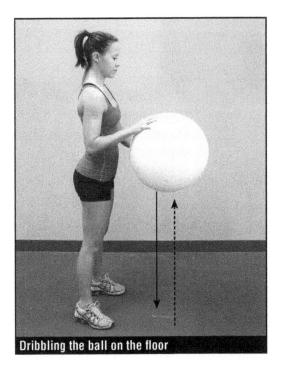
Dribbling the ball on the floor

Starting position: Stand with your trunk flexed, holding a small exercise ball (18 inches or 45 cm is the size most recommended).

Exercise action: Rapidly dribble the ball against the floor as quickly as possible, emphasizing the wrist snap to fatigue the wrist flexors. Several sets of 30 seconds of exercise are recommended to improve local muscle endurance.

Primary muscle groups: Wrist and finger flexors, triceps

Indications: Distal wrist and forearm strengthening

Contraindications: Elbow or wrist pain

Ball Dribbles (Wall)

PROGRESSION NAME: Advanced Elbow and Wrist Progression

STAGE: 2

Starting position: Stand holding a small exercise ball (18 inches or 45 cm is the size most recommended).

Exercise action: Rapidly dribble the ball against the wall, with your shoulder at approximately 90° of flexion and elbow bent 90°. Dribble the ball as quickly as possible, emphasizing the wrist snap to fatigue the wrist flexors. Several sets of 30 seconds of exercise are recommended.

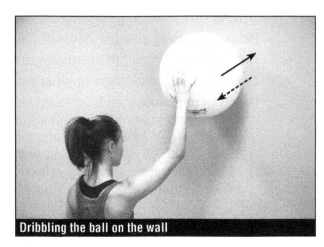

Dribbling the ball on the wall

Primary muscle groups: Wrist and finger flexors, triceps

Indications: Distal wrist and forearm strengthening

Contraindications: Elbow or wrist pain

Pearls of performance: Make sure the patient places the hand just under the front portion of the ball to keep the ball elevated in the optimal position against the wall. Significant fatigue ensues with the wall-dribble exercise. Movement of the ball in a pattern similar to a windshield wiper is a variation that can be applied.

Snaps

PROGRESSION NAME: Advanced Elbow and Wrist Progression

STAGE: 2

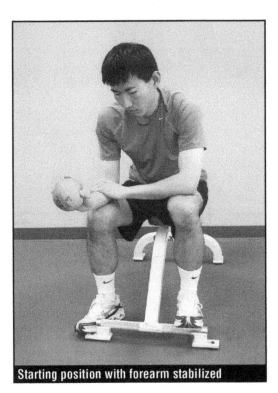

Starting position with forearm stabilized

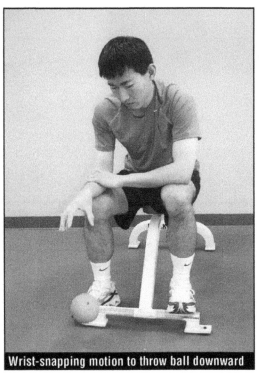

Wrist-snapping motion to throw ball downward

Starting position: In a seated position, stabilize your forearm over your thigh such that the wrist is protruding just over the knee to allow unrestricted wrist motion. The elbow is typically flexed 60 to 75° in this position. You may want to stabilize the forearm with the opposite hand to further isolate wrist motion during this exercise. Place the forearm in a palm-down (pronated) position. Hold a 0.5 to 1 kg exercise ball that can fit comfortably in the palm of the hand. A gel-based bounceable ball is recommended to optimize this exercise.

Exercise action: Extend the wrist backward (up toward the ceiling in a cocking motion), then forcibly thrust the ball down toward the ground using only a wrist-snapping motion. Catch the ball upon its return, and repeat the exercise. Be sure to localize the exercise to the wrist, as simply throwing the ball downward by extending the elbow is very easy. Several sets to fatigue are recommended.

Primary muscle groups: Wrist and finger flexors

Indications: Distal wrist and forearm strengthening

Contraindications: Elbow or wrist pain

Flips

PROGRESSION NAME: Advanced Elbow and Wrist Progression

STAGE: 2

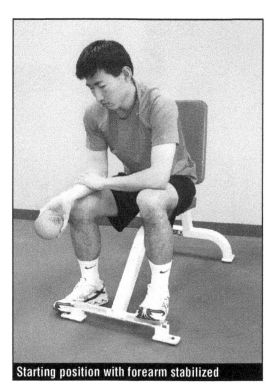

Starting position with forearm stabilized

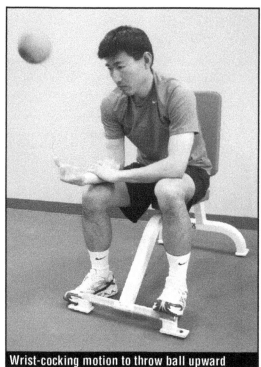

Wrist-cocking motion to throw ball upward

Starting position: In a seated position, stabilize your forearm over your thigh such that the wrist is protruding just over the knee to allow unrestricted wrist motion. The elbow is typically flexed 60 to 75° in this position. You may want to stabilize the forearm with the opposite hand to further isolate wrist motion during this exercise. The forearm is in a palm-up (supinated) position. Hold a 0.5 to 1 kg exercise ball that can fit comfortably in the palm of the hand.

Exercise action: Cock the wrist downward to preload the flexor muscles, and then forcibly flip the ball upward straight into the air as high as possible, trying then to catch the ball on the descent. Repeat for several sets. Be sure to try to isolate the motion at the wrist, as simply throwing the ball upward by bending the elbow is very easy.

Primary muscle groups: Wrist and finger flexors

Indications: Distal wrist and forearm strengthening

Contraindications: Elbow or wrist pain

Pearls of performance: It may take some practice to optimally time the release of the ball to get a vertical flip such that the ball can be caught perfectly on the descent. This exercise has an element of precision as well as power and explosiveness.

Blade Oscillation

PROGRESSION NAME: Advanced Elbow and Wrist Progression

STAGE: 2

Starting position: In a seated position, stabilize your forearm over your thigh such that the wrist is protruding just over the knee to allow unrestricted wrist motion. The elbow is typically flexed 60 to 75° in this position. You may want to stabilize the forearm with the opposite hand to further isolate wrist motion during this exercise. Grasp a Bodyblade or oscillation device in your hand. To work the extensors to a greater extent, use a pronated, or palm-down, position for the exercise. To increase work for the flexors, use a supinated, or palm-up, position.

Exercise action: Oscillate the Bodyblade using only the motion of wrist flexion and extension, keeping the rest of the upper extremity stable. Timed sets of 30 or more seconds are recommended to increase strength and muscle endurance.

Primary muscle groups: Wrist and finger flexors and extensors

Indications: Distal wrist and forearm strengthening

Contraindications: Elbow or wrist pain

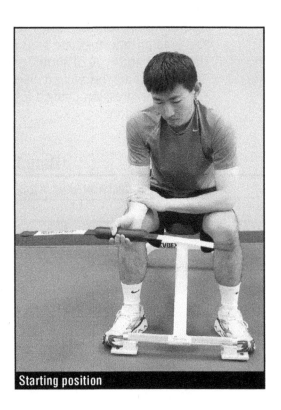

Starting position

MODIFIED ANTERIOR CHEST AND SHOULDER PROGRESSION

This progression is geared toward the person who has limitations after shoulder injury or surgery and must take precautions when returning to the weight room for traditional training. The exercises utilize protected ranges of motion and often serve as an intermediate step to returning to full lifting activities depending on the extent and type of shoulder injury. Be sure to start with a weight that is often 50% less than the weight used before the injury occurred for these exercises. Gradual progression using a low load, higher repetition base is recommended for this progression.

Bench Press Narrow Grip

PROGRESSION NAME: Modified Anterior Chest and Shoulder Progression

STAGE: 1

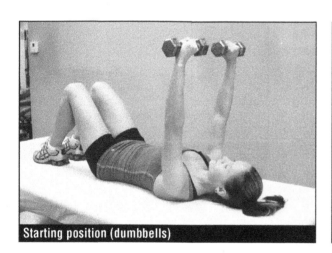
Starting position (dumbbells)

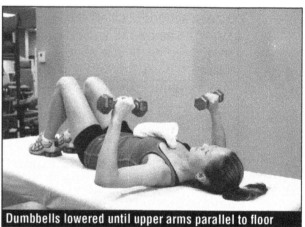
Dumbbells lowered until upper arms parallel to floor

Starting position: Lie on your back, assuming the traditional bench press position. You can use either a bar or dumbbells.

Exercise action: Hold the dumbbells shoulder-width apart and lower them toward the chest, stopping just before the upper arms become parallel to the floor. A positioning cue such as a rolled towel can be used to limit downward movement of the bar toward the chest.

Primary muscle groups: Pectoralis major, triceps

Indications: General chest and upper body strengthening

Contraindications: Shoulder pain; performance before return of rotator cuff strength

Pearls of performance: Use of a wider grip on the bar increases the likelihood of greater anterior shoulder load and is contraindicated for patients with anterior instability.

Chest Fly

PROGRESSION NAME: Modified Anterior Chest and Shoulder Progression

STAGE: 2

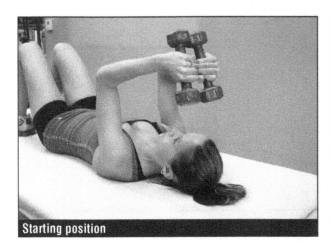
Starting position

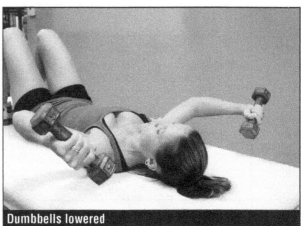
Dumbbells lowered

Starting position: Lie on your back, dumbbells in hands, with shoulders flexed to 90° and elbows slightly bent.

Exercise action: Slowly lower dumbbells toward the floor, stopping once the arms are 30° before parallel. Return to the starting position and repeat.

Primary muscle groups: Pectoralis major

Indications: General chest and upper body strengthening

Contraindications: Shoulder pain; performance before return of rotator cuff strength

Military Press Modification

PROGRESSION NAME: Modified Anterior Chest and Shoulder Progression

STAGE: 2

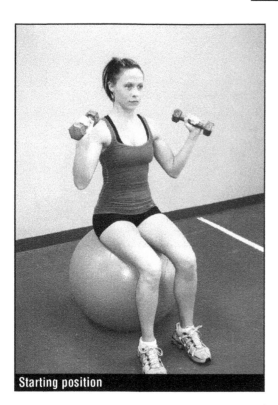

Starting position

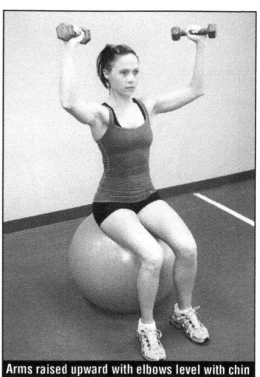

Arms raised upward with elbows level with chin

Starting position: Begin in a seated position with dumbbells in hands, elbows at sides. Position your elbows and shoulders such that elevation takes place in the scapular plane (30° anterior to the coronal plane).

Exercise action: Slowly raise your arms upward, flexing the shoulders until the elbows reach a level in line with your chin. Hold this position for 1-2 s and return to the starting position.

Primary muscle groups: Anterior deltoid

Indications: General upper body strengthening

Contraindications: Shoulder pain

Pearls of performance: Using a limited range of motion decreases the impingement and amount of rotator cuff compression under the acromion typically encountered with a full-ROM military press maneuver. Use of the scapular plane decreases the stress on the anterior capsule of the shoulder.

Scaption 0 to 90°

PROGRESSION NAME: Modified Anterior Chest and Shoulder Progression

STAGE: 2

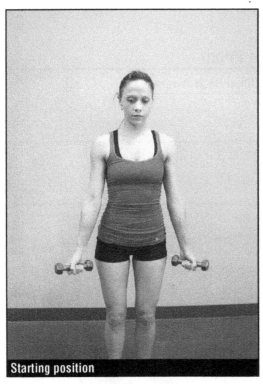

Starting position

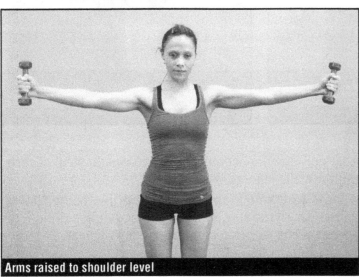

Arms raised to shoulder level

Starting position: Stand with dumbbells in each hand with shoulders in external rotation (thumb-up position).

Exercise action: Slowly raise your arms upward in thumb-up position as pictured until the arm is at shoulder level (90°). Slowly return to the starting position.

Primary muscle groups: Deltoid, rotator cuff

Indications: General shoulder strengthening

Contraindications: Shoulder pain

Pearls of performance: Use of the scapular plane increases joint congruity, decreases stress on the anterior capsule, and places the shoulder in an optimal position to exercise. Limiting the range of motion to only 90° decreases subacromial contact pressures but still allows for deltoid strengthening in a safe range of motion. Research shows that this externally rotated shoulder position improves the position of the scapula during exercise.

MODIFIED BACK PROGRAM

Modifications to these exercises are meant to protect the key stabilizing structures of the shoulder while allowing for recruitment of the muscles in the upper back. These modifications can allow the individual the ability to perform key exercises while minimizing loading the shoulder joint.

Lat Pull in Front

PROGRESSION NAME: Modified Back Program

STAGE: 2

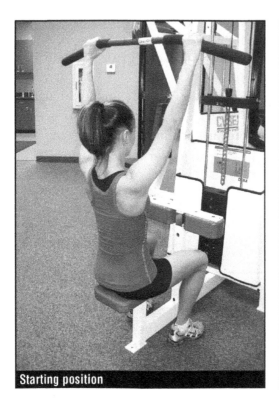
Starting position

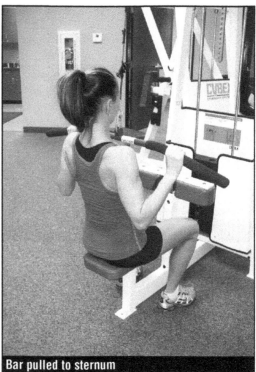
Bar pulled to sternum

Starting position: Sit at a lat pull-down machine, facing the weight stack. Grasp the bar in overhead position while leaning back slightly.

Exercise action: Pull the bar toward your sternum in front of the body. Slowly and with control, return the bar to the starting position, avoiding a rapid jerk of the arms upward that can occur if poor technique is used. Repeat.

Primary muscle groups: Latissimus dorsi, biceps

Indications: General upper body strengthening

Contraindications: Shoulder pain

Pearls of performance: The lat pull-down exercise in front decreases the stress on the anterior capsule of the shoulder and places the shoulder in a far better position compared with the traditional lat pull exercise where the bar is pulled down behind the neck.

Unilateral Bent-Over Row

PROGRESSION NAME: Modified Back Program

STAGE: 2

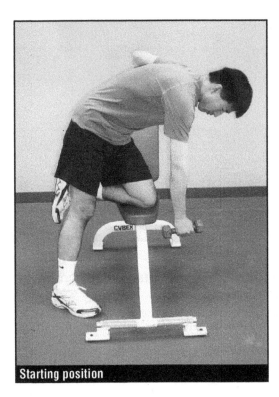
Starting position

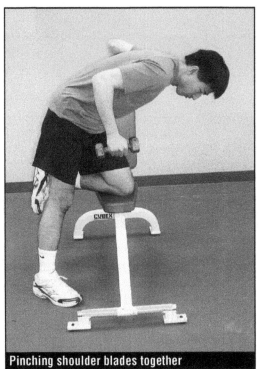
Pinching shoulder blades together

Starting position: Position yourself with one knee on a weight bench or the seat of a chair. Bend over at the waist, with your shoulder in an approximately vertical position and weight in hand.

Exercise action: Bring your hand toward the body while pinching the shoulder blades together. Do not bring the arm back to the extent where the elbow protrudes behind the plane of the body. This protrusion position can increase loading on the front of the shoulder. Slowly return the arm to the starting position and repeat.

Primary muscle groups: Scapular stabilizers, biceps

Indications: Scapular stabilization performed in traditional gym setting

Contraindications: Shoulder pain

Pearls of performance: Monitor the movement and control of the patient's scapula during exercise. Ensure that this exercise is not simply a biceps curl by making sure the scapula is retracted back toward the spine during the ascent phase of this exercise.

Prone Flys

PROGRESSION NAME: Modified Back Program

STAGE: 2

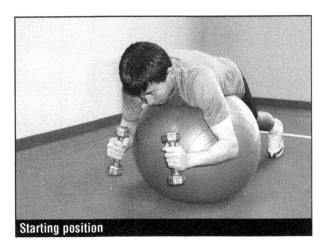
Starting position

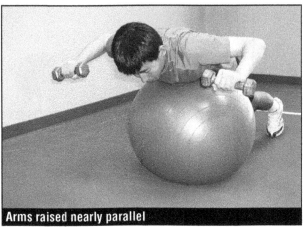
Arms raised nearly parallel

Starting position: Lie on an exercise bench in the prone (facedown) position. Grasp dumbbells in hands and keep elbows bent approximately 60°. The shoulders should be flexed to approximately 90°, with the tips of the elbows pointing toward the ground.

Exercise action: Raise your arms backward in a fly movement pattern until the upper arms are just shy of parallel to the floor. Hold this position for 1 s and return to the starting position.

Primary muscle groups: Posterior deltoid, middle trapezius, rhomboids

Indications: Scapular stabilization and deltoid strengthening in a traditional gym format

Contraindications: Shoulder pain

Pearls of performance: Limiting the range of motion to just below parallel minimizes the load on the anterior capsule of the shoulder, essential in patients with a shoulder injury history or history of anterior instability.

Seated Row Variation

PROGRESSION NAME: Modified Back Program

STAGE: 2

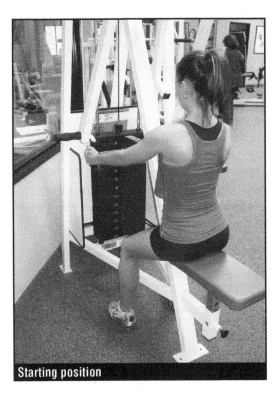

Starting position

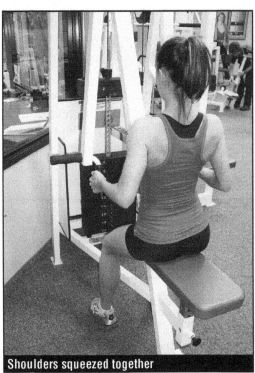

Shoulders squeezed together

Starting position: Sit in front of a rowing machine or cable system. Put hands on handles or grasp handle system.

Exercise action: Move your arms toward the sides of your body, ensuring as the motion is performed that the scapulae are being retracted (squeezed together). Ensure that the elbows do not protrude behind the body but stop in the body's midline. Hold that position with maximal squeezing together of the shoulder blades. Slowly return to the starting position. Use of handles in a horizontal direction will lead to rowing with greater amounts of internal shoulder rotation and slightly higher abduction angles (close to 90°); use of more-vertical handles will allow the rowing to be performed with the elbows closer to the sides of the body (less abduction).

Primary muscle groups: Middle trapezius, rhomboids, posterior deltoids

Indications: General scapular stabilization

Contraindications: Shoulder pain

RETURN TO SPORT: SPECIFIC PROGRAMS

The following interval return programs provide sport-specific functional progressions for returning to golf, tennis, and baseball. Each has specific instructions for returning based on the demands and activities required for successful performance in that sport. Reviewing the stages, and in many instances working with the person as he or she progress through the stages, is recommended to ensure an optimal result or return to participation. The programs listed here are designed to be given to the injured athlete and provide an overview of the progression of activity that is recommended for this functional return.

Of critical importance is the continued use of functional tests and objective measures to determine proper strength and range of motion before initiating the interval return program. Integration of continued functional exercise progression during the execution of the return programs is also recommended. Each of the programs in this section of the text provides step-by-step progressions of the key aspects of functional performance in these sports. Evaluation of proper sport biomechanics or technique is also of critical importance to decrease loading and ensure optimal progression in these functional return programs.

Tennis

Key Factors in an Interval Tennis Program

Frequency: Alternate-day performance

Supervision: Emphasis on proper stroke mechanics

Stroke progression: Groundstrokes → volleys → serves → overheads → match play

Impact progression: Low pre-impact ball velocity to higher pre-impact ball velocity

Ball progression: Low compression (foam) to regulation tennis ball

Sequencing: Proper warm-up, interval tennis program, cool-down and cryotherapy

Timing: Supplemental rotator cuff and scapular exercises performed either on rest day after interval tennis program or after execution of interval tennis program on the same day to minimize the effects of overtraining and overload

Interval Tennis Program Guidelines

- Begin at the stage indicated by your therapist or doctor.
- Do not progress or continue the program if joint pain is present.
- Always stretch your shoulder, elbow, and wrist before and after the interval program, and perform a whole-body dynamic warm-up before performing the interval tennis program.
- Play on alternate days, giving your body a recovery day between sessions.
- Do not use a wallboard or backboard as it leads to exaggerated muscle contraction without rest between strokes.
- Ice your injured arm after each stage of the interval tennis program.
- It is highly recommended to have your stroke mechanics formally evaluated by a USPTA teaching professional.

- Do not attempt to impart heavy topspin or underspin to your groundstrokes until the later stages of the interval program.
- Contact your therapist or doctor if you have questions about or problems with the interval program.
- Do not continue to play if you encounter localized joint pain.

Preliminary Stage

Start with foam-ball impacts, beginning with ball feeds from a partner. Perform 20 to 25 forehands and backhands, assessing initial tolerance to groundstrokes only. Presence of pain or abnormal movement patterns in this stage indicates you are not ready to progress to the actual interval tennis program. Continued rehabilitation would be emphasized.

Interval Tennis Program

Perform each stage _____ times before progressing to the next stage. Do not progress to the next stage if you had pain or excessive fatigue in your previous outing—remain at the previous level until you can perform that part of the program without fatigue or pain.

Stage 1

a. Have a partner feed 20 forehand groundstrokes to you from the net. (Partner must use a slow, looping feed that results in a waist-high ball bounce.)

b. Have a partner feed 20 backhand groundstrokes as in 1a.

c. Rest 5 minutes.

d. Repeat 20 forehand and backhand feeds.

Stage 2

a. Begin as in Stage 1, with a partner feeding 10 forehands and 10 backhands from the net.

b. Rally with a partner from the baseline, hitting controlled groundstrokes until you have hit 50 to 60 strokes. (Alternate between forehand and backhand, allowing 20 to 30 seconds rest after every two or three rallies.)

c. Rest 5 minutes.

d. Repeat 2b.

Stage 3

a. Rally groundstrokes from the baseline for 15 minutes.

b. Rest 5 minutes.

c. Hit 10 forehand and 10 backhand volleys, emphasizing a contact point in front of the body.

d. Rally groundstrokes for 15 minutes from the baseline.

e. Hit 10 forehand and 10 backhand volleys as in 3c.

Pre-Serve Interval

Perform these tasks before Stage 4. Note: This interval can be performed off court and is meant solely to determine readiness for progression into Stage 4 of the interval tennis program.

a. After stretching, with racket in hand, perform serving motion for 10 to 15 repetitions without a ball.

b. Using a foam ball, hit 10 to 15 serves without concern for performance result (focusing only on form, contact point, and the presence or absence of symptoms).

Stage 4

a. Hit 20 minutes of groundstrokes, mixing in volleys using a format of 70% groundstrokes and 30% volleys.

b. Perform 5 to 10 simulated serves without a ball.

c. Perform 5 to 10 serves using a foam ball.

d. Perform 10 to 15 serves using a standard tennis ball at approximately 75% effort.

e. Finish with 5 to 10 minutes of groundstrokes.

Stage 5

a. Hit 30 minutes of groundstrokes, mixing in volleys using a format of 70% groundstrokes and 30% volleys.

b. Perform 5 to 10 serves using a foam ball.

c. Perform 10 to 15 serves using a standard tennis ball at approximately 75% effort.

d. Rest 5 minutes.

e. Perform 10 to 15 additional serves as in 5c.

f. Finish with 15 to 20 minutes of groundstrokes.

Stage 6

a. Repeat Stage 5, increasing the number of serves to 20 to 25 instead of 10 to 15.

b. Before resting between serving sessions, have a partner feed easy, short lobs to attempt a controlled overhead smash.

Stage 7

Before attempting match play, complete steps 1 to 6 without pain or excess fatigue in the upper extremity. Continue to progress the amount of time rallying with groundstrokes and volleys in addition to increasing the number of serves per workout until you can perform 60 to 80 overall serves interspersed throughout a workout. Remember that an average of up to 120 serves can be performed in a tennis match; therefore, be prepared to gradually increase the number of serves in the interval program before engaging in full competitive play.

Baseball Interval Throwing Program: Phase I

Phase I Throwing Guidelines

- All throws should be on an arc with a crow hop.
- Warm-up consists of 10 to 20 throws at approximately 30 feet (90 m).

- The throwing program should be performed every other day, three times per week, unless otherwise specified by your physician or rehabilitation specialist.
- Perform each step two or three times before progressing to the next step.

Distances

45 feet = 13.7 m

60 feet = 18.3 m

90 feet = 27.4 m

120 feet = 36.6 m

150 feet = 45.7 m

180 feet = 54.9 meters

45 ft phase	60 ft phase	90 ft phase	120 ft phase
Step 1	**Step 3**	**Step 5**	**Step 7**
a. Warm-up	a. Warm-up	a. Warm-up	a. Warm-up
b. 45 ft (25 throws)	b. 60 ft (25 throws)	b. 90 ft (25 throws)	b. 120 ft (25 throws)
c. Rest 5-10 min	c. Rest 5-10 min	c. Rest 5-10 min	c. Rest 5-10 min
d. Warm-up	d. Warm-up	d. Warm-up	d. Warm-up
e. 45 ft (25 throws)	e. 60 ft (25 throws)	e. 90 ft (25 throws)	e. 120 ft (25 throws)
Step 2	**Step 4**	**Step 6**	**Step 8**
a. Warm-up	a. Warm-up	a. Warm-up	a. Warm-up
b. 45 ft (25 throws)	b. 60 ft (25 throws)	b. 90 ft (25 throws)	b. 120 ft (25 throws)
c. Rest 5-10 min	c. Rest 5-10 min	c. Rest 5-10 min	c. Rest 5-10 min
d. Warm-up	d. Warm-up	d. Warm-up	d. Warm-up
e. 45 ft (25 throws)	e. 60 ft (25 throws)	e. 90 ft (25 throws)	e. 120 ft (25 throws)
f. Rest 5-10 min	f. Rest 5-10 min	f. Rest 5-10 min	f. Rest 5-10 min
g. Warm-up	g. Warm-up	g. Warm-up	g. Warm-up
h. 45 ft (25 throws)	h. 60 ft (25 throws)	h. 90 ft (25 throws)	h. 120 ft (25 throws)

(continued)

Baseball Interval Throwing Program: Phase I   *(continued)*

150 ft phase	180 ft phase	Flat-ground throwing for baseball pitchers
Step 9 a. Warm-up b. 150 ft (25 throws) c. Rest 5-10 min d. Warm-up e. 150 ft (25 throws) **Step 10** a. Warm-up b. 150 ft (25 throws) c. Rest 5-10 min d. Warm-up e. 150 ft (25 throws) f. Rest 5-10 min g. Warm-up h. 150 ft (25 throws)	**Step 11** a. Warm-up b. 180 ft (25 throws) c. Rest 5-10 min d. Warm-up e. 180 ft (25 throws) **Step 12** a. Warm-up b. 180 ft (25 throws) c. Rest 5-10 min d. Warm-up e. 180 ft (25 throws) f. Rest 5-10 min g. Warm-up h. 180 ft (25 throws) **Step 13** a. Warm-up b. 180 ft (25 throws) c. Rest 5-10 min d. Warm-up e. 180 ft (25 throws) f. Rest 5-10 min g. Warm-up h. 180 ft (20 throws) i. Rest 5-10 min j. Warm-up k. 15 throws progressing from 120 ft → 90 ft ***Return to respective position or progress to step 14***	**Step 14** a. Warm-up b. 60 ft (10-15 throws) c. 90 ft (10 throws) d. 120 ft (10 throws) e. 60 ft (flat ground) using pitching mechanics (20-30 throws) f. 60-90 ft (10-15 throws) g. 60 ft (flat ground) using pitching mechanics (20 throws) **Step 15** a. Warm-up b. 60 ft (10-15 throws) c. 90 ft (10 throws) d. 120 ft (10 throws) e. 60 ft (flat ground) using pitching mechanics (20-30 throws) ***Progress to phase II—throwing off the mound***

Baseball Interval Throwing Program: Phase II—Throwing Off the Mound

Phase II Throwing Guidelines

- All throwing off the mound should be done in the presence of your pitching coach or sport biomechanist to stress proper throwing mechanics.
- Use a speed gun to aid in effort control.
- Values below are expressed as a percentage of maximal effort.

Stage 1: fastballs only

Step 1
a. Interval throwing
b. 15 throws off mound 50%

Step 2
a. Interval throwing
b. 30 throws off mound 50%

Step 3
a. Interval throwing
b. 45 throws off mound 50%
   Use interval throwing

Step 4
a. Interval throwing
b. 60 throws off mound 50%

Step 5
a. Interval throwing
b. 70 throws off mound 50%

Step 6
a. 45 throws off mound 50%
b. 30 throws off mound 75%

Step 7
a. 30 throws off mound 50%
b. 45 throws off mound 75%

Step 8
a. 10 throws off mound 50%
b. 65 throws off mound 75%

Stage 2: fastballs only

Step 9
a. 60 throws off mound 75%
b. 15 throws in batting practice

Step 10
a. 50-60 throws off mound 75%
b. 30 throws in batting practice

Step 11
a. 45-50 throws off mound 75%
b. 45 throws in batting practice

Stage 3

Step 12
a. 30 throws off mound 75% warm-up
b. 15 throws off mound 50%; begin throwing breaking balls
c. 45-60 throws in batting practice (fastballs only)

Step 13
a. 30 throws off mound 75%
b. 30 breaking balls 75%
c. 30 throws in batting practice

Step 14
a. 30 throws off mound 75%
b. 60-90 throws in batting practice (gradually increase breaking balls)

Step 15
Simulated game: progressing by 15 throws per workout (pitch count)

Baseball Little League Interval Throwing Program

Distances

30 feet = 9.1 m
45 feet = 13.7 m
60 feet = 18.3 m
90 feet = 27.4 m

30 ft phase

Step 1

a. Warm-up
b. 30 ft (25 throws)
c. Rest 15 min
d. Warm-up
e. 30 ft (25 throws)

Step 2

a. Warm-up
b. 30 ft (25 throws)
c. Rest 10 min
d. Warm-up
e. 30 ft (25 throws)
f. Rest 10 min
g. Warm-up
h. 30 ft (25 throws)

45 ft phase

Step 3

a. Warm-up
b. 45 ft (25 throws)
c. Rest 15 min
d. Warm-up
e. 45 ft (25 throws)

Step 4

a. Warm-up
b. 45 ft (25 throws)
c. Rest 10 min
d. Warm-up
e. 45 ft (25 throws)
f. Rest 10 min
g. Warm-up
h. 45 ft (25 throws)

60 ft phase

Step 5

a. Warm-up
b. 60 ft (25 throws)
c. Rest 15 min
d. Warm-up
e. 60 ft (25 throws)

90 ft phase

Step 7

a. Warm-up
b. 90 ft (25 throws)
c. Rest 15 min
d. Warm-up
e. 90 ft (25 throws)

60 ft phase	90 ft phase
Step 6	**Step 8**
a. Warm-up	a. Warm-up
b. 60 ft (25 throws)	b. 90 ft (20 throws)
c. Rest 10 min	c. Rest 10 min
d. Warm-up	d. Warm-up
e. 60 ft (25 throws)	e. 60 ft (20 throws)
f. Rest 10 min	f. Rest 10 min
g. Warm-up	g. Warm-up
h. 60 ft (25 throws)	h. 45 ft (20 throws)
	i. Rest 10 min
	j. Warm-up
	k. 45 ft (15 throws)

Reprinted, by permission, from T. Ellenbecker et al., 2006, Use of internal return programs for shoulder rehabilitation. In *Shoulder rehabilitation: Non-operative treatment*, edited by T. Ellenbecker (New York: Thieme Publishers), 152.

Golf Interval Program

Guidelines

- Always emphasize proper golf swing mechanics.
- Allow one day of rest between sessions.
- Perform a thorough complete-body warm-up and active stretching routine before training.
- Perform the program as outlined for each day without complications before advancing to the next step.
- Although minor discomfort is expected intermittently, avoid swinging the golf club through pain. If pain or swelling persists, discontinue the program until examined by a medical professional. Resume the program at the step preceding the offending step.

Key to Golf Program

Chips: pitching wedge

Short irons: W, 9, 8

Medium irons: 7, 6, 5

Long irons: 4, 3, 2

Woods: 3, 5

Drives: driver

	Day 1	Day 2	Day 3
Week 1	10 putts 10 chips Rest 15 chips	15 putts 15 chips Rest 25 chips	20 putts 20 chips Rest 20 putts 20 chips Rest 10 chips 10 short irons
Week 2	20 chips 10 short irons Rest 10 short irons	20 chips 15 short irons Rest 10 short irons 15 chips	15 short irons 10 med irons Rest 20 short irons 15 chips
Week 3	15 short irons 10 med irons Rest 5 long irons 15 short irons Rest 20 chips	15 short irons 10 med irons 10 long irons Rest 10 short irons 10 med irons 5 long irons 5 woods	15 short irons 10 med irons 10 long irons Rest 10 short irons 10 med irons 10 long irons 10 woods
Week 4	15 short irons 10 med irons 10 long irons 10 drives Rest Repeat above	Play 9 holes	Play 9 holes
Week 5	Play 9 holes	Play 9 holes	Play 18 holes

Reprinted, by permission, from T. Ellenbecker et al., 2006, Use of internal return programs for shoulder rehabilitation. In *Shoulder rehabilitation: Non-operative treatment*, edited by T. Ellenbecker (New York: Thieme Publishers), 162.

SUMMARY

This chapter provides anatomical and biomechanical information pertinent to the development and application of functional exercise progressions for the upper extremity. Each exercise progression requires careful monitoring of individual responses to determine optimal progression rates and increases. The subsequent chapters provide similar information using this format to allow the reader to develop functional exercise progression programming for the lower extremities and trunk.

Lower Extremity

Clinical rehabilitation after injury focuses on the restoration of joint range of motion, flexibility, and strength. However, when working with an active population, clinicians must also address more-advanced functional exercises and drills that allow patients to safely progress to their sport activity. Because clinical rehabilitative exercises are like building blocks—simple exercise progressed to advanced activity—functional exercise progressions follow this same concept. Movements begin in the sagittal plane and progress to the coronal plane, gradually building in complexity.

Functional exercises are not only used postinjury but also can be included as part of sport performance programs to enhance and define athletic abilities. Preventive programs specific to the lower extremity have been promoted for injuries such as anterior cruciate ligament (ACL) injuries in the female athlete, focusing on proprioceptive activities as well as jumping and landing techniques.

The purpose of this chapter is to present a brief anatomical overview, delve into basic biomechanical principles of key lower extremity joints, briefly describe the mechanisms and etiologies of specific lower extremity injuries, and guide clinicians as they progress their active patients back to sport activities. We must emphasize the importance of understanding the injury mechanisms and joint mechanics as the patients are advanced from the clinical setting into more-functional activities. As described in chapter 1, the clinician must be aware of the scientific principles of healing, of the need to progress the athlete to activities that require specific movement patterns, and of the need for sport specificity of the functional progression.

ANATOMY OF THE LOWER EXTREMITY

When evaluating and developing treatment programs for patients with knee or ankle pathology, it is important to have a solid foundation of the structural anatomy. A comprehensive understanding of skeletal and soft tissue anatomy through cadaveric advancement and surgical discovery has led to significant improvement in the management of patients with knee and ankle pathology. The anatomy of the lower extremity is presented here in a logical sequence, beginning with skeletal anatomy and progressing through the ligaments, musculature, and menisci.

Bones

This section of the chapter looks at the bones specific to the knee and ankle.

Knee

The osseous structures that make up the bony anatomy of the knee are the femur, the tibia, the fibula, and the patella (figure 4.1).

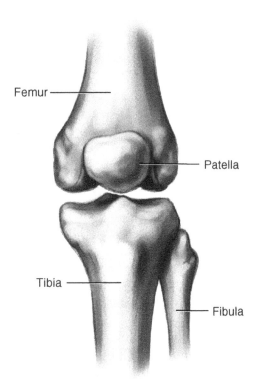

Figure 4.1   Anterior view of the femur, tibia, fibula, and patella.

Femur   The distal aspect of the femur forms the medial and lateral condyles that articulate with the superior aspect of the tibia, including the medial and lateral tibial plateaus. The anterior surface of the femoral condyles articulates with the posterior surface of the patella.

The femoral condyles are convex in shape, with a clear delineation between the structural components of the medial and lateral surfaces. The medial femoral condyle is longer in the anterior–posterior direction, with greater surface area. This increased length allows rolling of the condyle on the tibia with subsequent rotation, contributing to the stability of the tibiofemoral joint in terminal extension. The medial femoral condyle angles away from the longitudinal axis of the femur, accounting for a valgus angulation of approximately 10°. The lateral femoral condyle is wider in the frontal plane and narrower in the sagittal plane as compared with the medial femoral condyle. In line with the longitudinal axis of the femur, the lateral femoral condyle projects anteriorly, providing a bony block to the patella to prevent excessive lateral displacement.

The medial and lateral femoral epicondyles emanate superiorly from the femoral condyles. These bony prominences contribute to medial–lateral stability of the knee by serving as an attachment site on the femur for the collateral ligaments. The highly vascular epicondyles facilitate blood flow to the ligamentous and tendinous structures that originate here. Lying anterior and inferior to the adductor tubercle, the medial epicondyle serves as an attachment site for the medial collateral ligament and the medial head of the gastrocnemius. The lateral femoral epicondyle provides an attachment site for the lateral collateral ligament, popliteus muscle, and lateral head of the gastrocnemius muscle.

The anterior surface of the distal femur is characterized by the trochlea. The central sulcus articulates with the posterior aspect of the patella and forms the patellofemoral joint. This joint incongruence contributes to the inherent risk of patellar subluxation (Tria, Palumbo, and Alicea 1992).

The intercondylar notch divides the medial and lateral femoral condyles. The anterior and posterior cruciate ligaments cross within the intercondylar notch. The lateral wall of the intercondylar notch serves as the proximal attachment site for the anterior cruciate ligament, with the posterior cruciate ligament attaching to the medial wall of the intercondylar notch.

Tibia The tibial plateau is relatively flat with a 9° posterior slope. The medial tibial plateau, the larger of the two, is oval shaped and concave in both the frontal and sagittal planes. The increased length allows the medial femoral condyle to appropriately rotate during terminal knee extension. The lateral tibial plateau is concave in the frontal plane and flat in the sagittal plane. Femoral rotation is facilitated by the circular shape of the lateral tibial plateau. A posterolateral flare off the lateral tibial condyle accommodates articulation with the fibula.

The tibial eminence lies between the medial and lateral tibial plateaus. This roughened, elevated area projects superiorly in a compact linear shape and provides a component of bony stability to the tibiofemoral joint. The anterior–posterior depression in the tibial eminence is the attachment site for the ACL. During knee range of motion, the elevated tibial eminence positions itself in the intercondylar notch of the femur.

The tibial tuberosity lies anterior and inferior to the tibial plateau along the shaft of the tibia. This prominence serves as insertion site for the quadriceps mechanism through the patellar tendon. The lower border of the capsule attaches here.

Fibula The fibula lies posterolateral to the tibia. It has limited function in weight bearing at the knee (Moore 2005). It protects the tibia by withstanding forces during flexion and rotation of the knee (Moore 2005). However, the primary function of the fibular head is to provide an attachment site for muscular and ligamentous structures such as the biceps femoris tendon and lateral collateral ligament.

Patella The patella is a triangle-shaped sesamoid bone that lies within the tendon of the extensor mechanism. By design, it provides protection to the knee joint. Its most important function is to increase the distance of the lever arm of the extensor mechanism from the joint axis, thereby enhancing the force production of the quadriceps by 15 to 30% (Kaufer 1971).

The anterior surface of the patella is widely vascularized, giving it a roughened appearance. The superior pole of the patella is wide and accounts for 75% of the patellar height. It provides protection to the trochlea and femoral condyles from direct impact. Posteriorly, a free section exists at the base of the patella between the patellar tendon and the synovial lining (Fulkerson and Hungerford 1990a). It is often filled with a small peripatellar fat pad. The inferior patellar pole tapers into a V shape, where it attaches to the patellar tendon. The apex of the inferior pole does not articulate with the trochlea during knee flexion.

The patella's posterior articular surface consists of three distinct facets (figure 4.2). A vertical ridge divides the posterior surface into medial and lateral patellar facets. The convex shape of the facet accommodates the concave trochlea. Each facet is subdivided into superior, middle, and inferior zones. The third facet, considered the "odd" facet, lies medially. It is separated from the inferior and medial zones by a small vertical ridge.

The lateral facet is wider to accommodate the shape of the lateral femoral condyle. The medial facet is thicker than its lateral counterpart. The medial and

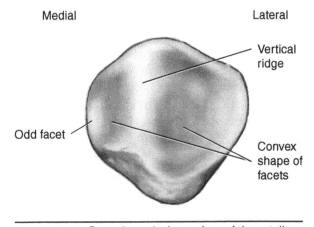

Figure 4.2 Posterior articular surface of the patella.

lateral facets provide attachment for the joint capsule, patellofemoral ligaments, synovium, retinaculum, and vastus medialis and lateralis muscles, respectively. These soft tissue structures contribute to the passive and dynamic stability of the patella.

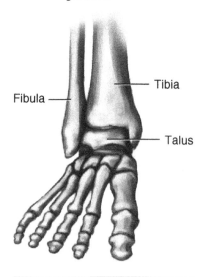

Figure 4.3   Anterior view of the tibia, fibula, and talus.

Ankle

The ankle joint is comprised of three bones: the tibia (medial malleolus), fibula (lateral malleolus), and talus (figure 4.3). The joint is saddle shaped and relies on ligamentous support for stability (Sammarco 1995). It allows locomotion to occur through a series of complex interactions among the bony, ligamentous, and muscular structures that make up the joint. The lateral ankle complex is the focus of this section.

Medial Malleolus   The distal portion of the tibia forms a convex process called the medial malleolus. Laterally, the distal tibia is concave and articulates with the talus. It is an attachment site for the anterior fibers of the deltoid ligament, tibialis posterior, and flexor digitorum longus (Gray 1973). The deltoid ligament has the highest load-to-failure rate in comparison with the lateral ankle ligaments (Conti and Stone 1995).

Lateral Malleolus   Distally, the fibula forms the lateral malleolus and is convex laterally. Medially, it articulates with the lateral portion of the talus. The posterior tibiofibular ligament attaches just posteriorly to the articular surface. The anterior talofibular ligament attaches anteriorly. Peronei longus and brevis course through the shallow posterior sulcus, with the apex of the malleolus providing an attachment site for the calcaneofibular ligament (Gray 1973; Moore 2005).

Talus   The talus has three parts: the body, neck, and head. It articulates with the malleoli and navicular and rests on the superior portion of the calcaneus. It provides attachment for ligamentous structures but not muscular or tendinous structures (Sammarco 1995; Van Dijk 2007). Its function is to transmit forces through the ankle joint and lower extremity (Sammarco 1995), and it is a focal point around which movement occurs (Van Dijk 1994).

Ligaments

In the following subsections, we discuss the ligamentous complexes of the knee and ankle that are involved in sport-related injuries. Specifically, we discuss the following knee and ankle ligaments: anterior cruciate ligament (ACL), posterior cruciate ligament (PCL), medial collateral ligament (MCL), lateral collateral ligament (LCL), anterior talofibular ligament (ATFL), posterior talofibular ligament (PTFL), calcaneofibular ligament (CFL), and deltoid ligament. Their anatomical orientations should be a consideration as clinicians move the athletes from simple to more-complex movement patterns during the functional progression.

Knee

The four main ligaments of the knee provide static stability by means of their tissue characteristics and attachments (see figure 4.4). They protect the knee from excessive tensile loads. The collateral ligaments (MCL and LCL) provide passive restraint to the knee in the frontal plane, while the cruciate ligaments (ACL and PCL) provide passive restraint in the sagittal plane.

To appreciate the structural complexity of the collateral ligaments, a detailed description of the capsular complex is necessary. The capsular complex can be divided into three highly unified levels: the superficial aponeurotic level, the middle tendinous level, and the deep capsular level.

The medial superficial layer is continuous with the fascial tissue of the gastrocnemius and posteriorly with the neurovascular structures and anteriorly with the fascia of the patellar tendon. It also surrounds the semimembranosus and semitendinosus tendons. The medial middle layer is defined by the medial (tibial) collateral ligament (MCL). It is composed of two bundles of fibers, a vertical group and an oblique group.

The deep layer, the actual capsule of the knee, extends from the medial tibial plateau to the medial femoral condyle. The deepest fibers, the meniscofemoral and meniscotibial portions, attach to the medial meniscus. The deep layer of the capsular complex increases in thickness from front to rear. The posteromedial capsule of the knee is made up of the oblique fibers of the MCL and the deep capsular fibers. The posteromedial capsule is reinforced by fibrous extensions of the semimembranosus.

The superficial layer of the lateral capsular complex includes the iliotibial band anteriorly and the biceps tendon posteriorly. The middle layer is formed anteriorly by the lateral retinaculum and posteriorly by the patellofemoral ligaments. The deep lateral layer is similar to that of the deep medial layer in its attachment to the articular borders of the tibia and femur. The lateral collateral ligament (LCL) lies between the superficial and deep lamina of this third layer. The deep lamina of the third layer is continuous with the lateral meniscus (Levy 1994).

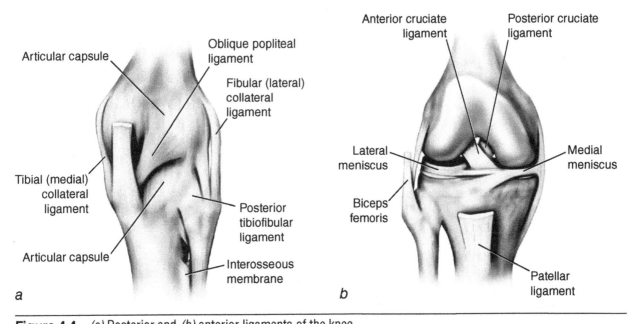

Figure 4.4 *(a)* Posterior and *(b)* anterior ligaments of the knee.

Reprinted from R. Behnke, 2006, *Kinetic anatomy,* 2nd ed. (Champaign, IL: Human Kinetics), 195 and 197.

As mentioned previously, the MCL is actually the middle layer of the medial capsular complex. This forms two distinct bundles, one vertical and one oblique. The vertical fibers arise from the femoral epicondyle and descend to attach on the medial tibial border just posterior to the tendons of the pes anserinus. The oblique fibers lie posterior to the vertical fibers and have common insertion on the femoral epicondyle. However, these fibers insert inferior to the articular surface on the posteromedial aspect of the tibia.

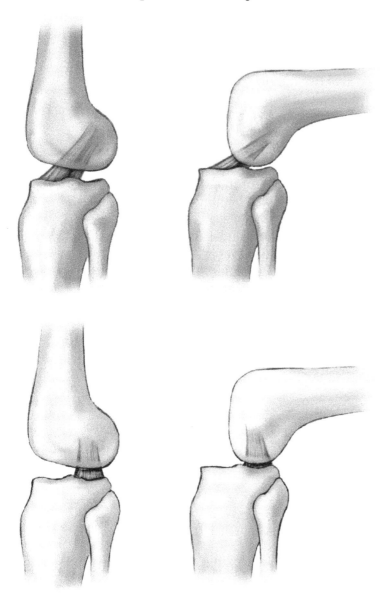

The medial capsular complex protects the knee against excessive valgus forces. The superficial layers of the MCL are the first to sustain injury in a valgus stress. The fibers are taut in extension and relaxed in flexion. Tibial internal rotation positions the fibers in a relaxed vertical manner, whereas in external rotation the fibers are oblique and taut (Levy 1994).

The cruciate ligaments cross through the center of the knee and are named for their attachment sites on the tibia. The ACL travels in an anterior direction from femur to tibia, and the PCL courses posteriorly from the femur to the tibia. The cruciate ligaments, while contained within the joint capsule, are extrasynovial, with the synovial lining passing in front of the ligaments.

The ACL attaches to the lateral femoral condyle and to the anterior medial tibial eminence in an oblique fashion. The tibial insertion is connected to the anterior horn of the medial meniscus. Various portions of this ligament are taut throughout the entire range of knee motion (figure 4.5). The anteromedial bundle is taut in flexion, while the larger posterolateral bundle is taut with the knee in extension (Nogalski and Bach 1994; Gray 1973; Levy 1994). The ligament on average is 4 cm (1.6 inches) in length and 1 cm (0.4 inches) in thickness at the midsection (Watts and Armstrong 2001; Girgis, Marshall, and Monajem 1975). The primary function of the ACL is to minimize anterior tibial translation and internal rotation of the tibia, which is consistent with injury mechanisms to this ligament.

Figure 4.5 Anterior and posterior bundles of the anterior cruciate ligament.

Ankle

The lateral supporting ligaments of the ankle include the anterior talofibular ligament (ATFL), the calcaneofibular ligament (CFL), and the posterior talofibular ligament (PTFL) (figure 4.6). The ATFL originates from the distal anterior portion of the lateral malleolus and inserts into the proximal portion of the lateral articular surface of the talus (Van Dijk 2007). It is the weakest of the three lateral ligaments (Van Dijk 2007). The ligament is relaxed in a neutral position. During plantar flexion, the proximal portion is taut while the distal portion is relaxed.

The origin of the CFL is the anterior portion of the lateral malleolus. It then runs inferiorly and posteriorly to attach to the lateral calcaneus (Van Dijk 2007; Gray 1973). The ligament is only taut in dorsiflexion and remains lax in a neutral or plantar flexed position. The PTFL is the strongest and is located more deeply than the ATFL or CFL (Gray 1973). The ligament courses horizontally from the medial aspect of the lateral malleolus to the posterior surface of the talus. It is taut only in dorsiflexion (Van Dijk 2007).

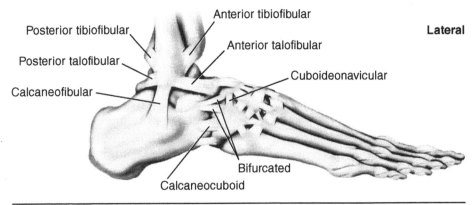

Figure 4.6 The ligaments of the ankle.

Reprinted from R. Behnke, 2006, *Kinetic anatomy,* 2nd ed. (Champaign, IL: Human Kinetics), 213.

MUSCULAR STABILIZATION OF THE LOWER EXTREMITY

The musculoskeletal system provides joint stabilization and allows force production to facilitate locomotion in the lower extremity. The amount of force production is dependent upon the torque generated through the moment arm (Best and Kirkendall 2003).

Knee

The muscular anatomy that provides dynamic stability to the knee is most easily divided into quadrants corresponding to their locations of anterior, posterior, lateral, or medial. These structures enable joint motion to occur and also provide dynamic protection to supporting structures of the tibiofemoral joint, including ligaments and menisci.

Anterior Compartment

The quadriceps muscle group makes up the largest portion of the anterior compartment of the knee and consists of four muscles: rectus femoris, vastus medialis, vastus lateralis, and vastus intermedialis (see figure 4.7). These muscles form a common patellar tendon innervated by the femoral nerve.

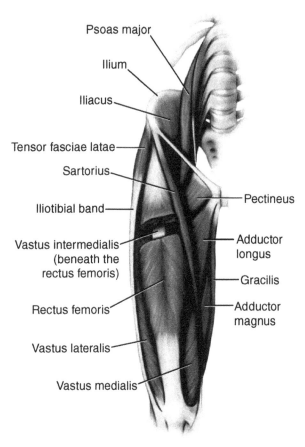

Psoas major

Ilium

Iliacus

Tensor fasciae latae

Sartorius

Iliotibial band

Pectineus

Vastus intermedialis
(beneath the
rectus femoris)

Adductor
longus

Gracilis

Rectus femoris

Adductor
magnus

Vastus lateralis

Vastus medialis

Figure 4.7   Anterior muscles of the knee.

The most anterior of the quadriceps muscles is the rectus femoris, originating from the anterior inferior iliac spine and the superior rim of the acetabulum (Cox and Cooper 1994). The three other heads border the rectus femoris distally. The rectus femoris, as a two-joint muscle, performs both hip flexion and knee extension. Lack of flexibility of the rectus femoris can contribute to abnormal patellar tracking.

The vastus lateralis, the largest head of the quadriceps muscles, originates on the anterior inferior greater trochanter, the intertrochanteric line, the lateral lip of the linea aspera, and the intermuscular septum. The fibers run in a 12 to 15° lateral direction to the femur, with a portion of the distal attachment terminating into the lateral retinaculum (Gray 1973; Lieb and Perry 1968). Dominance of the vastus lateralis along with tightness in the lateral retinaculum can result in excessive lateral displacement of the patella.

The vastus medialis originates at the lower end of the anterior intertrochanteric line. The vastus medialis also originates from the linear aspera and intermuscular septum, with a division that originates from the medial supracondylar line and adductor longus and adductor magnus tendon. The distal portion of the vastus medialis, the vastus medialis oblique (VMO), has fibers that run in a 60 to 65° medial direction to the femur (Gray 1973; Lieb and Perry 1968). Together with the vastus medialis longus, which has a fiber direction 15 to 18° medial to the femur, its primary function is to maintain dynamic patellar alignment. Swelling and pain can occur at the VMO because of its oblique fiber direction, which opposes the Q-angle alignment.

The vastus intermedialis originates on the anterior mediolateral surface of the femoral diaphysis. Its fibers run almost entirely in a vertical direction and contribute to extension of the knee.

The four quadriceps muscles converge into the superior pole of the patella and form the quadriceps tendon. Continuing distally, the patellar tendon extends from the inferior patellar pole to the tibial tuberosity. The tendon is widest at the apex of the patella and tapers slightly as it attaches into the tibial tuberosity. On average, the patellar tendon is 5 to 6 cm (2 to 2.4 in.) long and 7 mm thick (Cox and Cooper 1994; Fulkerson and Hungerford 1990a). However, patellar tendon length is actually a function of the height of the patella itself. The patellar tendon morphology may have ramifications for use as a graft source for ACL reconstruction.

The quadriceps function antagonistically to the hamstrings in an eccentric mode to control knee flexion. In this mode of muscular contraction, the quadriceps absorb compressive forces and decelerate the weighted extremity. The fiber direction of the vastus medialis oblique (VMO) serves to control patellar tracking through varying degrees of knee motion. It is critical to maintain dynamic balance of the quadriceps to limit the dominance of lateral structures.

Posterior Compartment

The hamstrings make up the posterior muscles of the knee. These include the semimembranosus, semitendinosus, and biceps femoris (figure 4.8). All these muscles, with the exception of the short head of the biceps femoris, originate from the ischial tuberosity and extend below the knee. The semimembranosus attaches on the anterior medial aspect of the medial tibia, and the semitendinosus attaches on the proximal medial tibia. The semimembranosus performs flexion and internal rotation of the knee and extension and internal rotation of the hip. It resists excessive hip abduction and external rotation of the tibia as well as provides dynamic support to the posterior capsule. During knee flexion, the semimembranosus, through its attachment to the posterior horn of the medial meniscus, assists with retraction of the medial meniscus. This prevents impingement by the medial femoral condyle and subsequent injury to the medial meniscus during flexion of the knee (Aglietti, Insall, and Cerulli 1983; Wallace, Mangine, and Malone 1997).

The semimembranosus and semitendinosus are innervated by the tibial division of the sciatic nerve. The semimembranosus also shares a branch of the nerve with the posterior section of the adductor magnus muscle.

The semitendinosus arises farther posteriorly from the ischial tuberosity. It inserts inferior to the gracilis and sartorius and with these two muscles forms the pes anserinus. The pes anserine bursa lies directly under these tendons and can be a source of irritation. The semitendinosus provides additional valgus stability to the knee and assists with flexion and internal rotation of the knee and extension of the hip.

The biceps femoris lies opposite to the semimembranosus and semitendinosus on the lateral side. The long head arises from the ischial tuberosity, while the short head originates from the posterior lateral lip of the linea aspera. The tendon of insertion runs distally and anteriorly and splits at the inferior portion of the lateral collateral ligament (LCL). The biceps femoris tendon consists of three

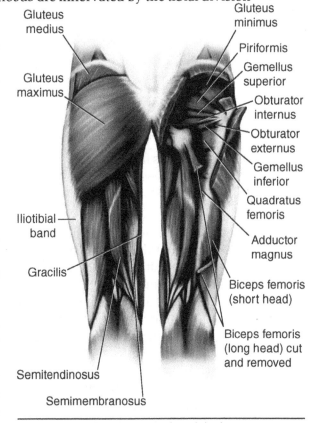

Figure 4.8 Posterior muscles of the knee.

layers: (1) a lateral layer that lies superficial to the LCL, (2) a middle layer that splits around the LCL, and (3) a deep layer that lies medial to the ligament. The superficial layer inserts anteriorly on the crural fascia and Gerdy's tubercle. The middle layer surrounds the LCL to conjoin at the fibular head. The deep layer divides to insert on Gerdy's tubercle anteriorly and the fibular head posteriorly (Terry and LaPrade 1996).

The biceps femoris is an important dynamic stabilizer of the posterolateral compartment of the knee. The multilayered tendon checks rotatory and anteroposterior stresses through its insertion into the posterolateral capsule (Andrews et al. 1994). The long head receives innervation from the tibial branch of the sciatic nerve (L5, S2–S3), while the short head receives a branch from the peroneal division (L5, S2). The biceps femoris prevents excessive adduction of the tibia and excessive anteroposterior displacement of the lateral tibial condyle. It provides dynamic support to the posterolateral knee.

Gastrocnemius

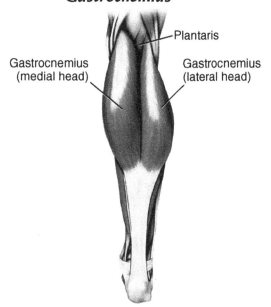

The gastrocnemius has a medial and lateral head that originate from the posterior aspect of the medial and lateral femoral condyle and adjacent femur and joint capsule (figure 4.9). The common tendon of insertion anchors into the posterior calcaneus. Although the gastrocnemius is primarily viewed as an ankle plantar flexor, it also functions as a knee flexor. This muscle plays a vital role in providing dynamic support to the knee during the midstance phase of gait. The gastrocnemius is innervated either by separate branches of the tibial nerve to each head or by a common stem of the nerve.

Figure 4.9   Gastrocnemius musculature.

Reprinted from R. Behnke, 2006, *Kinetic anatomy,* 2nd ed. (Champaign, IL: Human Kinetics), 202.

Lateral Compartment

The lateral muscles that play an important role in knee function arise proximally on the ilium. The tensor fasciae latae originates from the external lip of the iliac crest and outer anterior superior iliac spine and inserts into the iliotibial band (see figure 4.7). The gluteus medius originates from the outer surface between the iliac crest and the anterior and posterior gluteal line (see figure 4.8). Its insertion site is the oblique ridge on the lateral surface of the greater trochanter. Although the tensor fasciae latae flexes, abducts, and internally rotates the hip, the function of the gluteus medius varies depending on which fibers are being activated. The prime action is hip abduction; the anterior fibers also internally rotate and flex the hip, and the posterior fibers also externally rotate and extend the hip. Both muscles are innervated by the superior gluteal nerve.

The gluteus medius acts as a primary stabilizer of the pelvis and influences the biomechanical relationship between the hip, knee, ankle, and subtalar joint. The tensor fasciae latae influences the biomechanics of the hip and patellofemoral joint mainly through relative flexibility of the iliotibial (IT) band. The IT band inserts on the lateral femoral condyle, with fascial attachment to the lateral joint capsule, Gerdy's tubercle on the tibia, and the fibula. A bursa lies between the iliotibial band and lateral femoral condyle and may be a source of irritation secondary to soft tissue imbalances. The iliotibial tract is an active knee extensor in the last 30° of terminal extension. It also serves as an active knee flexor and decelerator of knee extension beyond 30°. A tight IT band, specifically the iliopatellar band, can be associated with excessive lateral patellar compression (Wilk et al. 1998). This can contribute to lateral knee pain in runners and cyclists who function within this short range of motion.

Medial Compartment

Hip adductor muscles are located in the medial compartment of the thigh. The majority of these muscles do not cross the knee joint, and they do not directly influence knee range of motion. However, they contribute to stabilization of the hip and pelvis. The gracilis muscle is the only hip adductor muscle that crosses the joint line by inserting on the proximal tibial diaphysis (see figure 4.8). The gracilis is part of the pes anserinus complex. Its actions include hip adduction and internal rotation, tibial internal rotation, and knee flexion. The obturator nerve supplies innervation to the medial thigh muscles.

Meniscal Anatomy

The menisci are fibrocartilaginous structures that absorb shock and transmit load in the tibiofemoral joint (figure 4.10). The menisci increase the articular surface area during joint contact and provide joint lubrication through forced fluid circulation during weight-bearing and non-weight-bearing activities. In addition, they restrain secondary motion and improve joint stability at the tibiofemoral joint by increasing the concavity of the tibial plateau. The menisci move posteriorly during flexion and anteriorly during extension.

Related Structural Anatomy

The medial and lateral retinacula are defined sections of the anterior capsule of the knee joint. They originate from the patella off the vastus medialis and lateralis, respectively, and extend to the tibia. The medial and lateral retinacula each contribute a slip transversely off the patella to form the medial and lateral patellofemoral ligaments (figure 4.11). The patellofemoral ligaments are generally thin because of the stress relief provided by the dynamic support of the quadriceps. The patellotibial ligaments are thicker bands of tissue because they receive no relief dynamically. The medial patellotibial ligament arises off the medial inferior patella and extends inferiorly to the tibia. The lateral patellotibial ligament connects the iliotibial band distally to the patella proximally (Terry 1989).

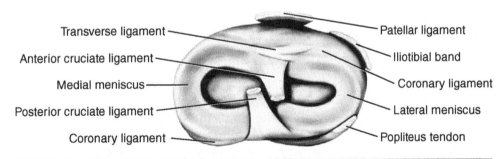

Figure 4.10 Medial and lateral menisci of the knee joint.

Reprinted from R. Behnke, 2006, *Kinetic anatomy,* 2nd ed. (Champaign, IL: Human Kinetics), 194.

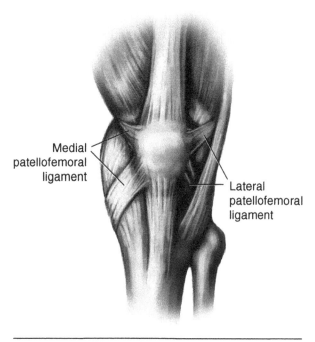

Figure 4.11   The patellofemoral ligaments.

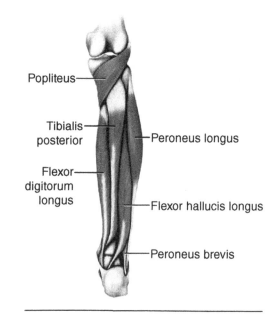

Figure 4.12   Deep view of the posterior muscles of the ankle.

Reprinted from R. Behnke, 2006, *Kinetic anatomy*, 2nd ed. (Champaign, IL: Human Kinetics), 217.

Ankle

Peroneus longus and brevis form the lateral musculature of the ankle joint (figure 4.12). Proximally, peroneus longus originates from the head and lateral body of the fibula. Distally it becomes a long tendon that courses around the posterior portion of the lateral malleolus in the peroneal groove. The tendon runs across the lateral cuboid and plantar surface of the foot, eventually attaching to the lateral aspect of the first metatarsal and medial cuneiform. It functions to pronate and plantar flex the foot and is innervated by the musculotendinous branch of the external popliteal nerve (Gray 1978).

Peroneus brevis is deep to the peroneus longus. Originating from the distal two thirds of the lateral fibula, the tendon runs behind the lateral malleolus, as does the peroneal longus. The peroneus brevis attaches to the base of the fifth metatarsal on its lateral side. It too functions to pronate and plantar flex the foot and is innervated by the musculotendinous branch of the superficial external popliteal nerve (Gray 1978).

BIOMECHANICS OF THE LOWER EXTREMITY

The study of biomechanics, along with functional anatomy, is the cornerstone of the rehabilitation of the lower extremity. A complete understanding of the articulations, kinematics, joint loading, gait cycle, and structures responsible for controlled movement is essential for the clinician to make sound decisions in the treatment of musculoskeletal disorders. The knee and ankle joints are biomechanically fascinating because of the intricacies required to maintain stability as well as allow for mobility. A comprehensive knowledge of the supporting structures and the stress placed on the patellofemoral joint, knee joint, and ankle joint provides the framework for the rehabilitation program and a safe return to sports.

Biomechanical Principles

Arthrokinematics describes the accessory motion that occurs between articulating surfaces. Rolling and gliding are accessory motions that occur in combination during osteokinematics (figure 4.13). This combination allows the articulating surfaces to stay in contact; as one surface rolls, the other glides in the opposite direction (Rosenberg, Mikosz, and Mohler 1994).

At the knee joint, there is large disparity between the femoral condyles and the tibial plateau, which plays a prominent role in the arthrokinematics of sagittal plane movements. During knee flexion, the femur moves on a

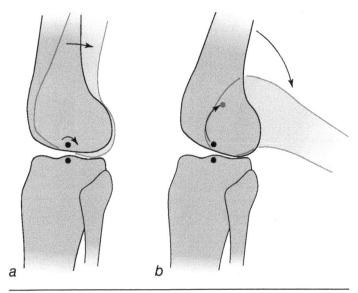

Figure 4.13 Rolling and gliding motion takes place between two joint surfaces.

fixed tibia; thus the femur must glide anteriorly to counteract the posteriorly directed roll that occurs at the tibial plateau. Although rolling and gliding must both occur to keep the tibia and femur in contact, they do not happen simultaneously as the knee flexes. At the initiation of flexion, pure rolling occurs between the joint surfaces, with sliding becoming more prominent at terminal flexion (Rosenberg, Mikosz, and Mohler 1994).

Screw-Home Mechanism

Near terminal extension of the knee, arthrokinematic movement occurs in the transverse plane. Because the medial femoral condyle (MFC) is 1 to 2 cm (0.4 to 0.8 inches) longer than the lateral femoral condyle (LFC), the LFC completes all of its motion when the knee is flexed 30° in a weight-bearing position. As the knee continues to extend and glide on the MFC, it pivots on the fixed LFC, producing medial femoral rotation on the fixed tibia.

Rotation at terminal extension, called the screw-home mechanism, is not produced by muscular forces and is not voluntary (figure 4.14). The screw-home mechanism provides an increase in stability to the knee regardless of position, which would not be possible in a simple hinge joint (Rosenberg, Mikosz, and Mohler 1994). The screw-home mechanism creates knee stability as the tibiofemoral joint becomes "locked" as it moves into a close-packed position. As the femur internally rotates on the fixed tibia, the femoral condyles are in contact with the menisci, the tibial tubercle becomes lodged within the intercondylar notch, and the ligaments are taut. Early flexion occurs as the tibiofemoral joint unlocks from an extended position (Rosenberg, Mikosz, and Mohler 1994).

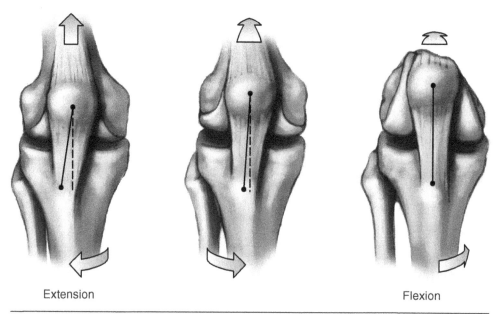

Extension   Flexion

Figure 4.14   The screw-home mechanism.

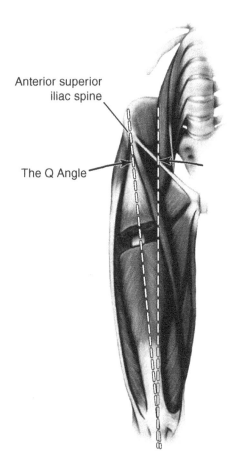

Anterior superior
iliac spine

The Q Angle

Figure 4.15   The Q angle.

Reprinted from R. Behnke, 2006, *Kinetic anatomy,*
2nd ed. (Champaign, IL: Human Kinetics), 200.

Q Angle

The osteomechanic and joint influences on the patellofemoral (PF) joint and the bony structure of the lower extremity combine to form a clinical measure known as the quadriceps (Q) angle. The Q angle is formed by a line connecting the anterior superior iliac spine (ASIS) to the midpoint of the patella and a line that connects the tibial tubercle with the midpoint of the patella (figure 4.15).

A 15° angle formed by these two lines is considered normal (Cox 1985; Aglietti, Insall, and Cerulli 1983). The Q angle may contribute to pathology in the PF joint when it is greater than 20°. A large Q angle can cause displacement of the patella laterally, resulting in a bowstringing effect against the lateral femoral condyle when a quadriceps contraction occurs (Insall, Falvo, and Wise 1976).

There are several concerns when using the Q angle as a diagnostic tool. A large Q angle has not been shown to predispose a knee to PF problems, nor do all patients with PF pain have a large Q angle. The measurement assumes the patella is centered in the trochlea; however, a laterally lying patella can result in a false positive (Grana 1985).

Mechanics Specific to the Patellofemoral Joint

Despite its proximity to the tibiofemoral joint, the PF joint possesses its own unique biomechanical properties. The PF joint facilitates extension of the knee by increasing the distance of the extensor mechanism from the axis of flexion and extension (Fulkerson and Hungerford 1990b). Various portions of the patella contact the trochlea during knee motion. Goodfellow, Hungerford, and Zindel (1976) describe the contact surfaces of the patella at different points of knee flexion during weight-bearing conditions. The patella is free floating without contact with the trochlea in extension and engages with the bony groove between 10 and 20° of flexion. Contact is initiated at the inferior pole and moves superiorly on the retropatellar surface until 90° of flexion, where the major contact point then

becomes the superior pole. The contact of the patella from lateral to medial also varies with knee motion. Patellofemoral contact from 0 to 90° of flexion is exclusively lateral. The contact point moves medially to the odd facet as the knee joint moves beyond 90 degrees (figure 4.16). These contact areas assist the patella in transmission of forces from the quadriceps muscles to the trochlea (Rosenberg, Mikosz, and Mohler 1994).

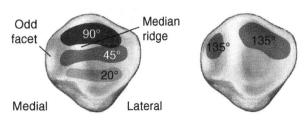

Figure 4.16 Patellofemoral contact points.

Reprinted from *The Knee,* Vol 1, W. Norman Scott, The biomechanics of running and knee injuries, by T.P. Andriacchi, G.M. Kramer, and G.C. Landon, pg. 22, Copyright 1994, with permission from Elsevier.

Dynamic Biomechanics

As motion occurs at a joint, it is important to understand the mechanics that occur and the forces that are being applied throughout a given activity. This section presents explanations of dynamic biomechanics that occur specific to the knee and ankle that will be of benefit to clinicians during both the clinical and functional progressions.

Anterior Cruciate Ligament and Medial Collateral Ligament

The ligaments of the knee are known as the static stabilizers, while the muscles surrounding the knee are called the dynamic stabilizers. The ACL is primarily responsible for controlling anterior displacement of the tibia on the femur. The medial collateral ligament helps stabilize the knee joint from excessive valgus stresses. Rotational stability is achieved through a combination of the collateral and the cruciate ligaments (Fukubayashi, Torzilli, and Sherman 1982).

The anterior cruciate ligament can be divided into two bundles: anteromedial and posterolateral (figure 4.17). According to Amis and Dawkins (1991), the anteromedial fibers become taut when the knee approaches 90° of flexion, while the posterolateral portion is tightened in knee extension. This creates isometry, as some portion of the ACL is taut throughout full knee range

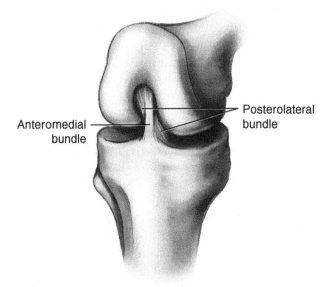

Figure 4.17 Anteromedial and posterolateral bundles of the ACL.

of motion (Amis and Dawkins 1991). With knee flexion, the ACL is the primary stabilizer against excessive anterior tibial translation and is considered a secondary stabilizer for valgus and varus loads placed on the knee (Rosenberg, Mikosz, and Mohler 1994).

Patellofemoral Joint

To apply the biomechanics at the dynamic PF joint, understanding the functions of the joint are crucial. The PF joint is responsible for increasing the effectiveness of the lever arm of the quadriceps and allows quadriceps forces to be transmitted without decreasing force. It also provides functional stability under load by creating an opposing articular surface to the trochlea (Rosenberg, Mikosz, and Mohler 1994).

The amount of force that the posterior surface of the patella encounters with various activities has been well documented. Since the common diagnosis of anterior knee pain results from an abnormal amount of force on the posterior surface of the patella, it is clinically relevant to understand what positions of exercise or function are optimal for patellofemoral joint contact forces. The amount of force the patella encounters does not fully reveal the amount of stress placed on the patella. Joint surface stress is determined by the amount of force placed on a given area of joint surface. Thus the less area to which a force is applied, the greater amount of stress is applied to the joint. The amount of stress placed on a given point of the patella has important clinical implications. It is the amount of stress, not simply the joint reaction force, that can inflict abnormal wear or pain on the posterior surface of the patella (Grelsamer and Klein 1998).

As a result of decreased joint surface area contact as the knee extends in the open chain, the joint stress increases from 90° of flexion to approximately 20° of extension (see figure 4.16). Although it varies among patients, there is typically no contact area at less than 20° of flexion to terminal extension, thus joint stress often does not occur during this range. Patients who maintain some contact experience a greater amount of joint stress because of a small contact area. Joint stress is not an issue during hyperextension because the patella is out of the trochlea (Grelsamer and Klein 1998).

Investigation of joint reaction forces in the closed kinetic chain shows that in contrast to the open chain, the joint reaction force decreases as the knee extends. The joint reaction forces decrease at a lesser rate at less than 30° because of minimal contact between the articulating surfaces of the PF joint (Steinkamp et al. 1993).

The amount of joint reaction force and joint stress encountered in daily tasks can be used to educate patients with anterior knee pain. Seated positions produce a significant degree of force beneath the patella because of the elastic pull of the proximal and distal tendon units (Hungerford and Baumgartl 1979). The increased stress correlates with the patient's subjective complaint of increased anterior knee pain during sitting. Although sitting can impose a low-load, long-duration pressure on the patellofemoral joint, it is the dynamic movements that frequently cause abnormal stress and injury. During gait, the joint reaction force is typically 50% of the body weight as the knee flexes to 10 to 15° during heel strike (Hungerford and Baumgartl 1979). Stair ambulation, which requires increased quadriceps muscle force combined with greater knee flexion, can produce far greater patellofemoral joint reaction force. As the knee reaches 60° during stair ambulation, the force may be as much as 3.3 times the body weight. Deep squatting activities can produce joint reaction forces approaching 7.8 times the body weight as the knee approaches 130° of flexion (Cox and Cooper 1994; Hungerford and Baumgartl 1979).

Ankle Joint

The foot and ankle form a complex joint with great responsibilities. It must provide a sturdy base of support and transform into a rigid structure for toe off during the gait cycle. However, the foot and ankle must be flexible to allow movement, absorb shock, and accommodate changes in position. The ankle joint has large articular surfaces and because of this is able to withstand upwards of 450% of an athlete's body weight during the gait cycle (Stauffer, Chao, and Brewster 1977).

The ankle joint, or talocrural joint, is a simple hinge joint responsible for dorsiflexion and plantar flexion. The talus is wider anteriorly, which can lead to problems when an athlete's ankle is in the extreme ranges of motion. The ankle has both medial and lateral ligamentous stability. The lateral complex is made up of three ligaments, with the weakest and most commonly injured being the anterior talofibular ligament (ATFL). The lateral complex can be disrupted by an ankle inversion injury. Injury to the ATFL is known to result in anterolateral rotatory instability of the ankle (Rasmussen 1982; Rasmussen and Kromann-Anderson 1983; Rasmussen, Tovberg-Jensen, and Hedeboe 1983). The deltoid, or medial, ligament is the less commonly injured of the two complexes, but it can be injured with an extreme eversion moment.

The subtalar joint, or talocalcaneal joint, is more complex and has three articulating surfaces. The subtalar joint allows for inversion and eversion and are a combination of movements from all three articulations (Norkin and Levangie 1992). Pronation and supination are considered the "series of movements of the foot and ankle" (Mann 2003).

Functional Movement Patterns

During gait, running, and lateral movement, different loads and forces are applied to the lower extremity. Specifically, we discuss the effects that patellofemoral pain, ACL tears, and ankle sprains may have during each of these movements so that clinicians can recognize and adjust the rehabilitative plan.

Gait

The gait cycle can be divided into two main phases, the stance phase and the swing phase (figure 4.18). The stance phase consists of heel strike, foot flat, midstance, heel off, and toe off. The swing phase consists of acceleration, midswing, and deceleration. Research shows that 60% of the gait cycle is spent in the stance phase, while the other 40% occurs during the swing phase (Norkin and Levangie 1992). A normal gait pattern requires a person to have full knee extension and at least 60° of knee flexion (Norkin and Levangie 1992).

Running

Forward running applies great forces to the patellofemoral joint and can generate upwards of 5.8 times the amount of force that occurs with normal walking (Rosenberg, Mohler, Mikosz 1994). The hip and knee should be in flexion and the ankle should be in slight dorsiflexion as the heel strikes (figure 4.19). In midstance, the degree of hip and knee flexion and ankle dorsiflexion is even greater

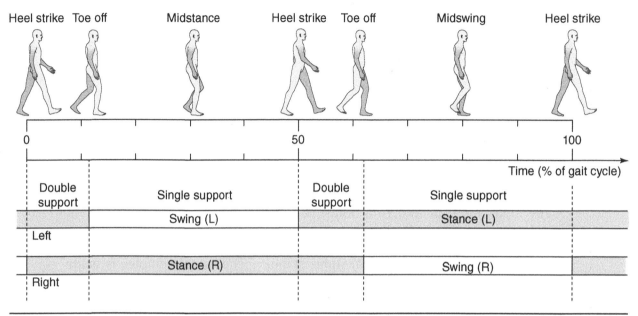

Figure 4.18 Duration of gait phases.

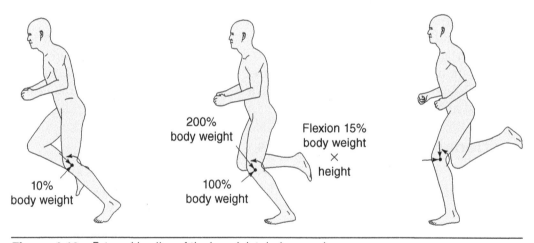

Figure 4.19 External loading of the knee joint during running.

to help absorb forces that can exceed 200% of the runner's body weight. Finally, at preswing, the ankle drops into plantar flexion and the hips and knee move into extension.

An athlete may experience pain specific to the patellofemoral joint with forward running. Contributing factors could be weak gluteus muscles, a tight iliotibial band, an increase in femoral anteversion, and excessive subtalar pronation. A shortened stride length may be noted, as well as a decrease in cadence. With a shortened stride, the athlete may stay in full knee extension longer in order to avoid large joint stresses placed in early knee flexion. By decreasing the cadence, fewer strides will be taken, thus decreasing the amount of stress on the patellofemoral joint. The large external knee flexion moment and the internal moment needed to counteract can lead to excessive forces being placed on the patellofemoral joint (Rosenberg, Mohler, and Mikosz 1994).

Forward running while ACL deficient creates an increase in tibiofemoral internal rotation, and nearly double the amount of external rotation with knee flexion is noted. The degree of knee flexion is greatly decreased in order to avoid quadriceps contraction (Rosenberg, Mohler, and Mikosz 1994). When ACL deficient, there is typically an increase in firing of the hamstrings to control anterior tibial translation (Branch, Hunter, and Donath 1989; Isakov et al. 1986; Kalund et al. 1990).

As an athlete accelerates, the sequence of plantar flexion and dorsiflexion at the ankle joint remains the same. However, the speed at which these motions occur greatly increases. The amount of time spent in stance phases dramatically declines. The muscular activity in the anterior compartment lasts longer and into the first part of the stance phase, whereas the posterior musculature increases its activity, thus providing stability and control to the ankle at heel strike (Delahunt, Monaghan, and Caulfield 2006). These posterior calf muscles also initiate subtalar inversion to assist in creating a platform just before heel strike (Mann 2003).

According to Freeman, Dwan, and Hanham (1965), articular deafferentation occurs after ankle injuries, and the mechanoreceptors in the ankle are damaged. A runner with ankle instability typically lands with the ankle in an inverted position because of the loss of mechanoreceptors. The peroneal muscles fire early at heel strike in anticipation of the inverted ankle position and to help provide dynamic stability (Delahunt, Monaghan, and Caulfield 2006). If the athlete does not have full ankle range of motion, it will limit the amount of shock absorption that can occur as well as limit the rigidity needed for toe off. At heel strike, plantar flexion is needed to help absorb the shock. If the range is limited, the shock cannot be absorbed and distributed appropriately (Mann 2003).

Lateral Movement

At heel strike during a side-step maneuver, there is an anterior force of 10% of the athlete's body weight causing an extension moment at the knee. During the midstance phase, the force is up to 100% of the body weight and is directed posteriorly. The moment changes directions and allows the knee to flex, thus decreasing the stress on the knee. The compressive forces are greatly diminished at preswing.

The posture of an ACL-deficient athlete has an increase in the angle of flexion at both the hips and knees, while the torso tends to be more upright (figure 4.20). With an ACL-deficient patient, the side-step maneuver could be problematic at foot strike because of the large anterior shear force (Rosenberg, Mohler, and Mikosz 1994). An increase in hamstring firing is noted in order to help decrease this anterior tibial translation.

The side-step maneuver places a great deal of stress on the patellofemoral joint. Patellofemoral forces increase as the angle of knee flexion increases. According to Huberti and Hayes (1984), patellofemoral forces increase by 45% when the Q angle is increased by 10°. Maquet (1979) concludes that the amount of patellofemoral

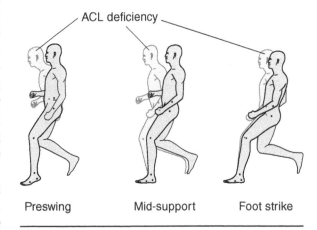

Figure 4.20 Change in body position during a side step cut due to ACL deficiency.

Reprinted from *The Knee,* Vol 1, W. Norman Scott, The biomechanics of running and knee injuries, by T.P. Andriacchi, G.M. Kramer, and G.C. Landon, pg. 22, Copyright 1994, with permission from Elsevier.

force depends on the amount of force in the quadriceps and patellar tendons. Patellofemoral forces increase from 20 to 90° of flexion and then start to decrease through 120°. The greatest increase in patellofemoral pressure occurs between 30 and 60° of flexion. This correlates with the amounts of flexion typically used in running and a side-step maneuver. Patellofemoral pain is typically retropatellar and can be described as an ache but can also be sharp. Many athletes will complain of a sharp pain behind the patella during loaded situations where the knee is flexed greater than 30°. There is less contact surface area and thus greater resultant forces, which causes pain.

Another cause of pain could be a large Q angle, which results in excessive patellofemoral stress. Many times patellofemoral joint pain during high-velocity activities can actually be the result of weak proximal muscles. Weakness in the gluteus medius, gluteus maximus, and iliopsoas muscles can cause an increase in joint forces at the patella, causing pain during higher-velocity activities. Poor flexibility in the hamstrings, quadriceps, soleus, and gastrocnemius can also contribute to patellofemoral symptoms during running and cutting activities.

High-velocity directional changes create excessive forces around the ankle joint (Holt and Hamill 1995). With forward running or side-step maneuvers, an athlete with a history of spraining the ankle tends to land differently than an athlete without prior history. After an ankle sprain, the foot is typically in an inverted position upon heel strike (figure 4.21a). This makes it difficult for the ankle to begin pronating in order to help with shock absorption during foot strike. These athletes often have a loss of kinesthetic awareness, resulting in repeated ankle sprains. With the ankle in an excessive amount of supination, the ankle's ability to adjust to varying surfaces is decreased, thus putting the athlete at risk for yet another lateral ankle sprain. Many times there is a loss of proprioceptive input, and the ankle responds with a quick supinatory movement rather than initiating pronation upon heel strike. Tight Achilles tendons are often seen in conjunction with chronic ankle sprains. This tightness will decrease the amount of time spent at heel strike and foot flat, which can lead to inappropriate shock absorption.

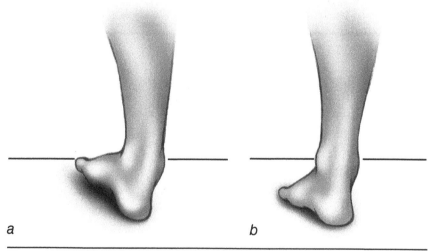

Figure 4.21   *(a)* Supinated and *(b)* normal foot strike.

INJURIES

Injuries to the ACL, MCL, patellofemoral joint, iliotibial band, chondral surface, and ankle ligaments are but a few that can be a challenge for clinicians. These injuries and their mechanisms are briefly described here. Being aware of specific injury mechanisms will not only assist in the development of the rehabilitative program but also be of benefit to the athletes psychologically as they return to their sport activity.

Anterior Cruciate Ligament Injuries

An estimated 1 in 3,000 anterior cruciate ligament (ACL) injuries occurs in the general population per year in the United States (Huston, Greenfield, and Wojtys 2000; Childs 2002). Most ACL injuries occur in athletes (Childs 2002) and are highly publicized in the sports medicine community. Advancements made in both pre- and postoperative rehabilitation as well as in the surgery itself have dramatically changed the way this injury is treated. In spite of recent advancements, there is still knowledge to be gained regarding the long-term outcomes and gender differences after injury to the ACL.

The classic mechanism of an ACL injury involves movements with sudden deceleration or directional changes. Sports such as football, basketball, and team handball have the highest incidence of injury in adolescents (Bahr and Krosshaug 2005). Though ACL injury may seem to be caused by a single event, it has been proposed that the injury occurrence may be multifactorial (Bahr and Krosshaug 2005). Internal factors such as age, gender, and somatotype may predispose the athlete to injury when combined with external factors such as shoe traction or surface friction (Bahr and Krosshaug 2005). The actual injury event may include mechanical factors such as a pivot shift or notch impingement combined with a valgus moment (Bahr and Krosshaug 2005). The internal and external factors in combination with the injury event lead to ACL injury.

ACL injury mechanisms are typically classified as noncontact or contact injuries. There is general agreement in the literature that approximately 70% of ACL injury mechanisms are noncontact (McNair, Marshall, and Matheson 1990; Boden et al. 2000; Krosshaug et al. 2007). Noncontact ACL injuries are frequently defined by lack of body-to-body contact, and contact injuries are defined by a direct blow to the knee. However, neither definition clearly encompasses a perturbation episode where contact is made by another person before the injury. A video analysis of 39 ACL injuries in basketball demonstrated that 11 of 22 female cases involved a perturbation before the time of injury (Krosshaug et al. 2007). Clinically, rehabilitation and prevention programs should include perturbation training that replicates game situations.

Video analysis of ACL injuries has also demonstrated a consistent lower extremity pattern of tibia external rotation near full knee extension with the foot planted during a deceleration maneuver (Boden et al. 2000; Olsen et al. 2004). This position has been termed *valgus collapse*. Most prevention programs are aimed at learning proper landing and cutting mechanics that avoid valgus collapse. A thorough examination of these maneuvers should take place during the agility and functional progression components of rehabilitation before return to play.

Gender also plays a role in ACL injury. Much attention has been given to the female athlete, as numerous authors have reported that ACL injury occurs anywhere from two to eight times more in female versus male athletes (Arendt and Dick 1995; Huston, Greenfield, and Wojtys 2000; Bjordal 1997; Chandy and Grana 1985; Engstrom, Johansson, and Tornkvist 1991; Ferretti 1984; Gray et al. 1985). Multiple sources report similar findings (National Federation of State High School Associations 2002; National Collegiate Athletic Association 2002). Theories have been proposed to explain the disparity of injury by gender. Internal risk factors such as neuromuscular control, valgus loads at the knee joint, ground reaction forces, and hormonal influences and external factors such as playing surfaces, bracing, and contact versus noncontact mechanisms have been discussed (Hewett, Myer, and Ford 2006; Ford et al. 2005; Huston, Greenfield, and Wojtys 2000). Currently, increased risk of noncontact ACL injuries has not been correlated with anatomical variables (Ford et al. 2005).

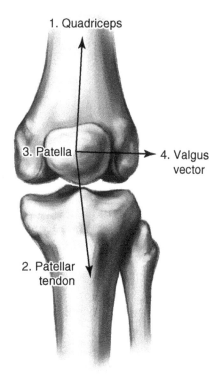

1. Quadriceps
3. Patella
4. Valgus vector
2. Patellar tendon

Figure 4.22   Force that produces valgus stress.

Medial Collateral Ligament Injuries

The medial collateral ligament (MCL) remains the most commonly injured ligament of the knee (Fetto 1978). It is a primary resister of valgus and external rotation forces that occur around the knee joint (Hayes et al. 2000). Medial collateral ligament sprains can be isolated or occur in combination with other soft tissue injury to the knee.

The most common mechanism of injury is direct lateral contact. This occurs when there is a direct force to the outside of the knee, resulting in valgus stress to the medial aspect of the knee (figure 4.22). Injury to the MCL can also occur as a result of indirect abduction or rotational stresses applied to the knee (Indelicato and Linton 2007). A reported history of injury includes a foot planted on the ground that has sustained an indirect rotational force coupled with an increased valgus stress at the knee. It is common during sports that require cutting or pivotal motion.

The incidence of contact versus noncontact mechanisms has been discussed in two individual studies. Hughston (1968) reports that 86% of anteromedial instability injuries and Indelicato and Linton (2007) report that 92% of MCL injuries were sustained as a result of contact mechanism.

Patellofemoral Dysfunction

Patellofemoral (PF) pain has been a challenge for clinicians for years. In the past, the term *chondromalacia* had been used to describe patellofemoral pain. However, it has been recognized that this diagnosis can only be made operatively and does not always correlate with pain (Karlsson, Thomeé, and Swärd 1996; Darracott and Vernon-Roberts 1971; DeHaven and Collins 1975; Hvid, Andersen, and Schmidt 1981; Insall 1982; Leslie and Bentley 1978; Abernethy et al. 1978). *Patellofemoral pain* should be used to refer to general anterior knee pain excluding intra-articular pathology, tendinitis, or bursitis (Karlsson 1996).

Abernethy and colleagues (1978) suggest that the diagnosis "chondromalacia of the patella" be made in those patients without symptoms or transiently symptomatic fibrillation of the articular cartilage of the central medial patellar facet. Persistent patellofemoral pain may be caused by another syndrome. Ambiguity exists in defining terms to describe patellofemoral pain. More recently, the tissue homeostasis theory proposed by Dye and associates may explain the variation of patellofemoral pain among patients better than a structural explanation. Their studies compared age- and activity-matched asymptomatic controls with symptomatic patients. The researchers found no statistical significance between the groups and the resolution of osseous metabolic activity after a nonoperative treatment plan (Dye and Chew 1993; Dye and Boll 1986).

Insall (1979), Fulkerson et al. (1992), and Merchant (1988) have previously proposed classification systems for patellofemoral pain. Their systems were based on the amount of PF cartilage damage, arthralgias, or instabilities, or on etiologies, which were then subcategorized. The systems were difficult to utilize clinically, however.

Holmes and Clancy (1998) have described a classification system for patellar pain and dysfunction based on physical exam, history, and radiographs. Their classifications are as follows:

1. Patellar instability
2. Patellofemoral pain with malalignment
3. Patellofemoral pain without malalignment

The rationale for their categorization is that patients with recurrent instability usually require surgical intervention. Patients with patellofemoral pain with malalignment may require surgery after extensive therapy. Finally, patellofemoral pain without malalignment requires therapy concentrating on the quadriceps musculature. Category three also includes diagnoses of exclusion such as iliotibial band syndrome and patellar tendinitis.

Category One: Patellar Instability

By clinical definition, patellar instability is the partial or complete lateral displacement of the patella from the trochlea of the femur, with associated strain to the medial retinaculum, capsule, and vastus medialis oblique. The amount of displacement varies from patient to patient. Lower extremity biomechanical factors, muscular imbalances, congenital deficiency of the femoral trochlea, and acute injury may cause instability (Wilk et al. 1998). Patellar subluxation can be difficult to diagnose, with the exception of the obvious cases (Noftall 1995). Roentgenograms are often necessary for diagnosis. Hughston (1968) roentgenographically defines a subluxated patella as being displaced laterally to the rim of the lateral femoral condyle, with the "ridge, or apex, of the patella displaced out of, and lateral to, the depth of the intercondylar groove of the femur." Subluxation occurs during the weight-bearing phase of the gait cycle between midstance and takeoff, as described by Hughston (1968) as an injury of acceleration rather than deceleration. Congruence angles are also useful in determining patellar position. Merchant (1988) defines a normal congruence angle as –6 standard deviations $\pm 6°$.

Patellar dislocation occurs as a traumatic, sudden event often accompanied by a torsional component. It is the complete displacement of the patella out of the trochlea (Wilk et al. 1998). Patients realize that the patella has gone out of place. It is often reduced as the patient attempts to extend the leg postinjury. Pain often subsides at that time. Palpation reveals pain at the medial retinaculum and adductor tubercle and is accompanied by an effusion (Holmes and Clancy 1998). Assessment of patella mobility produces apprehension (Wilk et al. 1998).

Category Two: Patellofemoral Pain With Malalignment (Patellofemoral Syndrome)

For our purposes, patellofemoral syndrome is defined as lateral patellar tracking with associated PF joint compression (Dogwood course). Frequently, patients with PF pain present with more-common symptoms such as pain with prolonged sitting, stair climbing, and increased activity as well as a feeling of weakness secondary to quadriceps inhibition (Shelbourne and Adsit 1998). Biomechanical abnormalities such as loss of joint motion, tightness in the lower extremity musculature, and mechanical foot abnormalities all contribute to patellofemoral pain.

Category Three: Patellofemoral Pain Without Malalignment

The iliotibial (IT) band, or iliotibial tract, is a thick band of tissue that extends from the iliac crest to the knee and joins the gluteus maximus to the tibia. The function of the IT band is to lock the knee into extension. At the hip, the IT band contributes to lateral pelvic stabilization (Barber and Sutker 1992). IT band friction syndrome occurs when the IT band becomes inflamed after repeatedly moving across the lateral femoral condyle (Ekman et al. 1994). In a 1994 study, Ekman and associates reviewed MRI scans of seven patients diagnosed with ITB syndrome. The symptomatic knees were found to have fluid deep to the IT band in the area of the lateral femoral epicondyle and significant thickening of the IT band itself. Cadaveric dissection of 10 normal knees found space, possibly a bursa, between the IT band and the knee capsule. This study concluded that IT band syndrome is an inflammation not only of the tendon but of the bursa as well.

Patellar Tendinitis

The patellar tendon, also known as the patellar ligament, attaches the patella to the tibial tubercle (Teitz 1988). The function of the patellar tendon is to transmit force from the quadriceps to the tibial tubercle (Teitz 1988). The patellar tendon is separated from the synovial membrane of the knee by the infrapatellar fat pad (Ferretti et al. 1984).

Patellar tendinitis, or "jumper's knee," is an overuse syndrome associated with eccentric overload during deceleration. Athletes who are involved in repetitive activity such as running, jumping, climbing, or kicking are frequently affected. In a study of 407 high-level volleyball players, Ferretti and colleagues (1984) found that 22.8% experienced patellar tendon pain. The researchers also found frequency of play and floor surface of greater significance in producing symptoms than age, sex, years of play, and type of training. Blazina et al. (1973) describe three phases of patellar tendinitis:

Phase I: Pain after activity, with no functional impairment

Phase II: Pain during and after activity, with difficulty in performance

Phase III: Pain during and after activity, with increasing difficulty in performance

Chondral Injury

Patellofemoral chondral injuries can be caused by trauma, dysplasia, and osteochondral defects (Farr 2005). The articular cartilage has a very limited ability to repair itself because of limited vascularity. The smooth hyaline cartilage is replaced with fibrocartilage (Lewis et al. 2006).

Classification systems such as the Outerbridge scale and that of the International Cartilage Repair Society (ICRS) (table 4.1) are used by physicians to classify the depth, location, and severity of chondral injuries (Lewis et al. 2006; Farr 2005). These systems can be helpful to the clinician during rehabilitation to identify certain ranges of motion and movements that may need to be avoided to allow healing of the defect. Nomura and Inoue (2004) observed 70 consecutive knees with cartilage lesions of the patella after recurrent dislocations. The mean age of the patients was 22 ±7 years (range 13 to 40 years). Dislocation occurred 2 to 10 times in 47 knees and more than 10 times in 23 knees. The authors created their own classification system macroscopically. Sixty-seven (96%) had articular cartilage lesions of the patella, and there was no change in three knees (4%). The medial facet was the site of the most fibrillation or erosion, followed by the central dome (Nomura and Inoue 2004).

Table 4.1   Comparison of the Modified Outerbridge and ICRS Articular Classification Systems

	Modified outerbridge	ICRS
Grade 0	Normal	Normal
Grade 1	Soft blistering	• Soft or superficial openings • Nearly normal
Grade 2	Openings to 50% of cartilage depth	Abnormal lesions to <50% cartilage depth
Grade 3	Openings >50%; palpable but not exposed bone	• Abnormal lesions to >50% of cartilage depth • Down to calcified bone layer but not through the bone
Grade 4	Exposed bone	Severely abnormal; full thickness cartilage loss and bone loss

Ankle Sprains

Ankle sprains are one of the most common injuries in the general population and in athletes, occurring in almost every sport, especially those that require jumping, cutting movements, and sudden stops. In emergency room visits, ankle sprains account for 2 to 6% of all presentations in the United States (Burt and Overpeck 2001) and 3 to 5% of cases at accident and emergency departments in Britain (Watts and Armstrong 2001; Heyworth 2003). A recent report of Dutch national volleyball players showed that 52% of all acute injuries were ankle sprains (Verhagen et al. 2004). In a 3-year prospective study of high school lacrosse players, Hinton et al. (2005) reported that 21% of all girls' injuries and 13% of all boys' injuries during high school play were ankle sprains. In a season-long study of major league soccer in the United States, 18% of all injuries were to the ankle (Morgan 2001), while analysis of four senior soccer divisions in Sweden revealed that 17 to 20% of all injuries were ankle sprains (Ekstrand and Tropp 1990). Messina,

Farney, and DeLee (1999) reported that 30% of all high school basketball injuries were to the ankle. Similarly, in high school cheerleaders, 24% of all injuries were to the ankle (Jacobson et al. 2004).

The basic mechanism of injury for lateral ankle sprains—inversion on a plantar flexed foot—can occur in both contact and noncontact scenarios. Ankle sprains most commonly occur in sports that require high-speed jumping, quick cutting movements, and sudden stops, such as soccer, basketball, and lacrosse. Some sports have a higher propensity for contact injuries, such as the ankle being injured when a jumping athlete lands on another player. In volleyball, a sport where the teams are separated by a net and contact is limited, the majority of ankle sprains occur at the net during contact with a teammate or opponent while landing from a block (Verhagen et al. 2004). A study by Hinton and colleagues (2005) on lacrosse, which involves much more player-to-player contact, showed that the most prevalent injury scenario was an ankle sprain related to indirect force, such as cutting and torsion, rather than contact with another player. Video analysis of foot and ankle injuries in soccer revealed that half of ankle sprains were caused by direct contact owing to the tackling in soccer, with the majority of these injuries being sustained from a tackle force from the side while the athlete remaining weight bearing (Giza et al. 2003).

Several reports outline both intrinsic and extrinsic risk factors for ankle sprains. Gender does not appear to be a risk for ankle sprains as it is for some knee injuries (Beynnon, Murphy, and Alosa 2002). Because disruption of the ligament structures compromises biomechanical stabilizers, previous ankle sprains have been studied as one of the most common risk factors for suffering subsequent ankle sprains. Studies have shown varying results, and as explained by Beynnon et al. (2002), this could be because future injury depends not only on the structures that were damaged but also on compliance with and the appropriateness of the rehabilitation program administered. In a prospective study, Ekstrand and Gillquist (1983) followed soccer players and found an increased risk of ankle injuries in those who had previously suffered a lateral ankle sprain. Similar results have been found more recently in basketball players (McKay et al. 2001) and football players (Tyler et al. 2006; Sitler et al. 1994).

Decreased balance has been found to be predictive of those who sustain a lateral ankle sprain. Trojian and McKeag (2006) used a simple, inexpensive single-leg balance test and found a significant association between a positive test result and athletes sustaining an ankle sprain over the course of a single fall season of high school and college sports. Their study is in agreement with other studies that have shown increased risk for ankle sprain in athletes with proprioceptive deficits (Tropp and Odenrick 1988; Leanderson and Eriksson 1996; McGuine 2000).

FUNCTIONAL TESTING OF THE LOWER EXTREMITY

Functionally, many variables are at work that clinically may be difficult to objectively define, particularly in the areas of neuromuscular control and joint loading. Neuromuscular gender differences have been an area of interest secondary to the increased incidence of ACL injury to females. Neuromuscular control has been shown not to increase in females from prepubescence to adolescence; however, the converse is true for males (Quatman et al. 2006). Neuromuscular imbalances such as ligament dominance, quadriceps dominance, and leg dominance have been seen in females (Myer, Ford, and Hewett 2004; Andrews et al. 1994; Hewett, Paterno, and Myer 2002; Hewett et al. 1996; Ford, Myer, and Hewett 2003; Myer et al. 2004).

Numerous studies have evaluated knee mechanics as well as electromyography (EMG) data during cutting and jumping activities. Sigward and Powers (2006) compared knee position and muscle activation in male and female collegiate soccer players during a side-step cutting maneuver. Their results show a significantly greater knee valgus moment during early deceleration in females. Hewett and colleagues found that female athletes with ACL injury demonstrated significantly increased dynamic lower extremity valgus and knee abduction loads before the injury event (see figure 4.23) (Hewett et al. 2005).

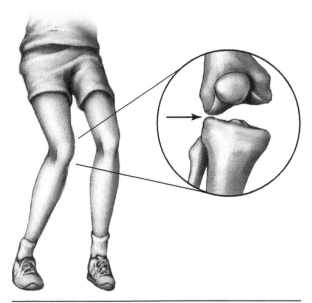

Figure 4.23 Dynamic joint loads prior to ACL injury.

Lack of core stability has recently been suggested as a risk factor for lower extremity injury and particularly ACL injury (Leetun et al. 2004). As a result, the same cohort of male and female soccer players in the Sigward and Powers study (2006) was evaluated during the same side-step cutting maneuver to evaluate hip mechanics (Pollard, Sigward, and Powers 2007). Compared with their male counterparts, females performed the cutting maneuver with significantly greater hip internal rotation and decreased hip flexion. Additionally, females displayed increased hip adduction and decreased hip extension moments. Functionally, the link between hip and knee mechanics is a result of learned movement patterns and a lack of hip extension and abduction control. The clinician must evaluate these differences with a high suspicion in female athletes.

Recently, functional training programs that specifically address jumping, landing, and cutting have been developed to address specific mechanical deficits in athletes. Although most of the current literature addresses female athletes because of the predominance of ACL injuries, their male counterparts are likely to benefit as well. Hewett, Ford, and Myer (2006) performed a meta-analysis to determine the effectiveness of neuromuscular interventions aimed at injury prevention in the female athlete. Anterior cruciate ligament injury was significantly reduced in those who participated in an injury prevention program. However, the authors did recognize that only six studies met the study criteria and that they did not possess enough study power.

This is a relatively new concept at this time that is still being scrutinized. It is our opinion that ACL injuries are multifactorial, although training programs certainly may be beneficial to any athlete.

Isokinetic Considerations

Because of the variability in the literature of the dynamometers used, test speeds, and populations, it is difficult to make specific recommendations in regard to isokinetic criteria for return to functional activity. In our experience, we have found isokinetic quadriceps peak-torque strength deficits of 20% at 180° per second and hamstring deficits of 30% at 180° per second to be acceptable when compared with the noninvolved side. Myer et al. (2006) discussed their criteria-based progression to the return-to-sport phase after ACL reconstruction. They recommend a peak torque for knee flexion and extension within 15% of the noninvolved side at 180° per second and 300° per second. A normative data study by Buchanan and Vardaxis (2003) found average dominant peak torques at 60° per second on a Cybex II dynamometer for 11- to 13-year-old basketball players to be 0.65 (Nm/kg) ± 0.05 for the hamstrings and 1.49 (Nm/kg) ± 0.09 for the quadriceps. Peak torques in 15-to 17-year-olds were 0.89 (Nm/kg) ± 0.07 for the dominant hamstrings and 1.89 (Nm/kg) ± 0.13 for the dominant quadriceps.

The hamstring to quadriceps (H/Q) ratio may be of greater importance in regard to return to activity. The H/Q ratio is functionally significant, as it has been said to potentially reflect predisposition to injury by showing a decrease in antagonistic hamstring coactivation during extension (Rosene, Fogarty, and Mahaffey 2001; Croce et al. 1996; Bennell 1998; Baratta 1988). The conventional method used for the H/Q ratio calculates the maximum knee flexion strength divided by the maximum knee extension strength at specific angular velocities and contractions (Aagaard et al. 1998). The "normal" H/Q ratio has been shown to increase as isokinetic speed increases from 50 to 80% as averaged through the full range of knee motion (Rosene, Fogarty, and Mahaffey 2001).

Aagaard et al. (1998) described a new concept for a functional H/Q ratio that calculates the eccentric hamstring to the concentric quadriceps moment. The results of their study reveal an H/Q ratio of 1.0 or greater at fast speeds, which is two times greater than that of the conventional H/Q ratio. The hamstrings were found to effectively stabilize the knee joint as it reached full knee extension.

Functional Movement Screen

As mentioned briefly in chapter 1, the Functional Movement Screen (FMS) can be used to further define mechanical deficits that could potentially decrease the chance of injury. FMS incorporates principles of proprioceptive neuromuscular facilitation (PNF), muscle synergy, and motor learning (Cook, Burton, and Hoogenboom 2006b; Gray et al. 1985). The screening is objectively scored from 0 to 3, with 3 being the best score. The screen consists of seven specific exercises (see figure 4.24, a-g) to be administered by the clinician to the athlete. The deep squat, hurdle step, and in-line lunge assess the symmetrical mobility and stability of the hip, knee, and ankle joints. The active straight-leg raise assesses hamstring and gastrocnemius–soleus flexibility, while the trunk stability push-up and rotary stability tests assess core stability (Cook, Burton, and Hoogenboom 2006a, 2006b). The equipment used for these tests can be easily duplicated, making this a cost-effective way to address movement deficits.

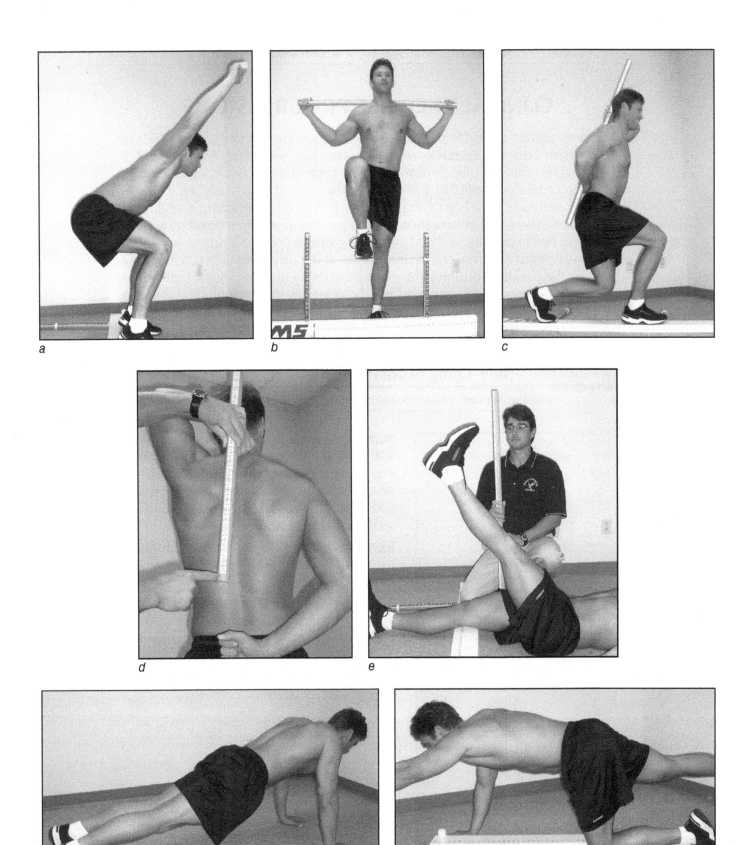

Figure 4.24 Exercises of the FMS: *(a)* deep squat, *(b)* hurdle step, *(c)* in-line lunge, *(d)* shoulder mobility, *(e)* active straight-leg raise, *(f)* trunk stability push-up, and *(g)* rotary stability.

Reprinted by permission from Function Movement Systems.

CLINICAL EXERCISE PROGRESSIONS

Before an athlete advances to a functional progression, he or she must be able to complete a clinical exercise progression that has been part of the rehabilitative program. Once full range of motion has been attained, swelling or effusion has been controlled, flexibility has been addressed, and basic early rehabilitative strength exercises have been completed, then it is time to begin more-difficult strength exercises. The athlete should be able to complete the following exercises with ease before moving to a functional progression specific to his or her sport.

The functional progressions in this section of the text provide detailed instructions for the person performing the exercise. Primary muscle groups, indications, contraindications, and pearls of performance are presented to guide the clinician. Some of the exercise progressions contain stages that provide further progression between groupings of exercises.

Side-Lying Gluteus Medius Exercise

PROGRESSION NAME: Gluteus Medius Strengthening   **STAGE:** Levels I-III

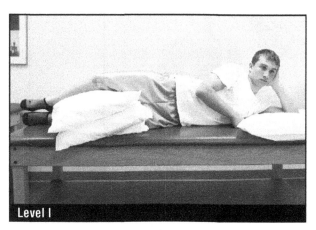

Level I

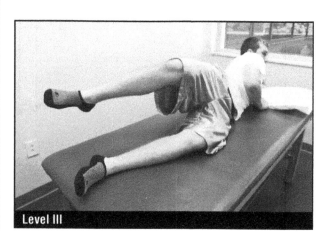

Level III

Starting position: Lie on the unaffected side with two to four pillows between the knees. Knees should be bent approximately 45°. The pelvis should be maintained in a vertical position during the exercise. The trunk should be straight, not bent at the waist.

Exercise action: Level I—Without lifting the leg, rotate at the hip so the knee is positioned toward the ceiling.

Level II—Perform the Level I exercise, and then lift the leg back and slightly upward. Maintain the rotation and lower the leg. Return to the starting position.

Level III—Remove the pillows and complete the exercise as stated in Level II.

Primary muscle groups: Gluteus medius

Indications: Pelvic stabilization

Contraindications: Early post-op rehab after knee or hip surgery

Pearls of performance: The patient's pelvis should remain stable throughout the exercise and not roll backward. The knee should remain in a flexed position.

Quadriceps Straight-Leg Raise

PROGRESSION NAME: Early Quadriceps Strengthening   **STAGE:** Straight-leg raise with hip external rotation

Starting position: Begin in a seated position, with the involved leg extended in front of you and the noninvolved leg bent approximately 110°. Keep the involved leg straight, and rotate at the hip so the foot is turned slightly outward.

Exercise action: Lean forward at the hip and grasp the noninvolved knee. Lock your involved knee by tightening the thigh muscles. Lift your leg off the floor approximately 2 to 3 inches (5 to 8 cm), hold 5 seconds, and slowly lower the leg.

Primary muscle groups: Quadriceps

Indications: Early strengthening once extension has been achieved postoperatively or for patellofemoral diagnoses

Contraindications: early post-op rehab for patellofemoral realignment procedures

Pearls of performance: Ensure the patient maintains the body in upright position, does not allow the trunk to lean backward, and maintains external rotation and leg control throughout the exercise.

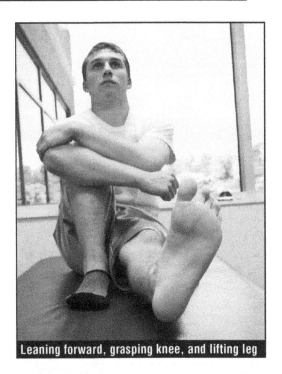

Leaning forward, grasping knee, and lifting leg

Leg Extension Machine

PROGRESSION NAME: Open-Chain Quadriceps Strengthening   **STAGE:** Double- to single-leg extension

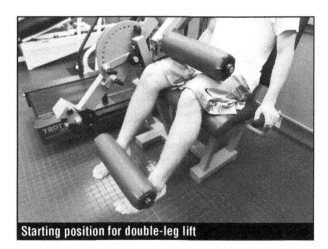
Starting position for double-leg lift

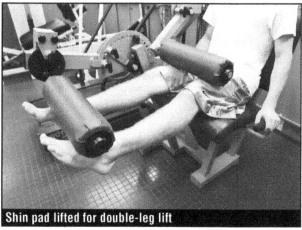
Shin pad lifted for double-leg lift

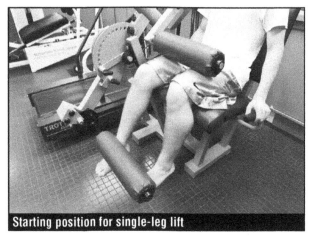
Starting position for single-leg lift

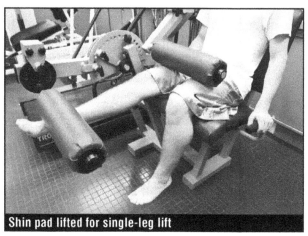
Shin pad lifted for single-leg lift

Starting position: Sit with knees bent and feet placed behind the shin pad.

Exercise action: Lift the shin pad by straightening your legs in front of you, then lower it slowly. Progress from double- to single-leg exercises.

Primary muscle groups: Quadriceps

Indications: Strengthening of the quadriceps muscle group

Contraindications: Patellofemoral pain; less than 90° of knee flexion; early post-op rehab

Pearls of performance: The exercise should not cause patellofemoral pain. The arc of motion may be limited from 90 to 45° to allow a greater dispersion of forces across the patella and therefore limit pain.

Closed-Chain Proprioception With Tubing

PROGRESSION NAME: Proprioceptive Training

STAGE: Advanced proprioception with resistance to hip flexion, extension, abduction, adduction

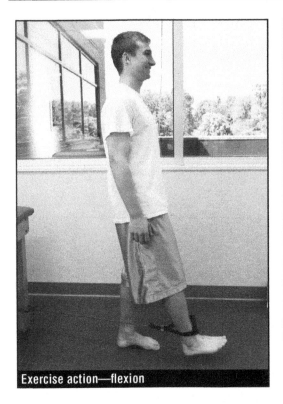

Exercise action—flexion

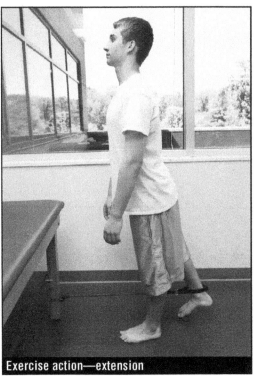

Exercise action—extension

Starting position: Stand far enough from the door to produce some tension in the tubing. Place the tubing around the ankle of the noninvolved leg with the knee slightly bent.

> *Flexion:* Stand with back to the door.
>
> *Extension:* Stand facing the door.
>
> *Abduction:* Stand sideways with the noninvolved leg facing opposite the door.
>
> *Adduction:* Stand sideways with the noninvolved leg toward the door.

Exercise action: Balance on the involved leg, keeping your pelvis level and your torso upright.

> *Flexion:* Pull noninvolved leg with tubing forward.
>
> *Extension:* Pull noninvolved leg with tubing backward.
>
> *Abduction:* Pull noninvolved leg with tubing away from the door.
>
> *Adduction:* Pull noninvolved leg with tubing toward midline of the body.

(continued)

Closed-Chain Proprioception With Tubing   *(continued)*

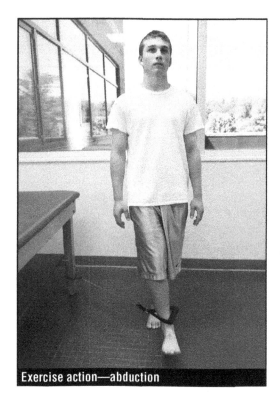

Exercise action—abduction

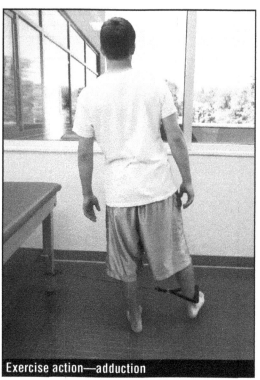

Exercise action—adduction

Primary muscle groups: Lower extremity musculature

Indications: Closed-chain proprioception and limb stabilization of the involved extremity

Contraindications: Resistance should not be added until the patient has achieved normal proprioception in a static position when compared bilaterally.

Pearls of performance: Exercises should be completed slowly and controlled while maintaining pelvic stabilization.

Quarter Squats

PROGRESSION NAME: Closed-Chain Lower Extremity Exercises

STAGE: Double- to single-leg lower extremity strengthening

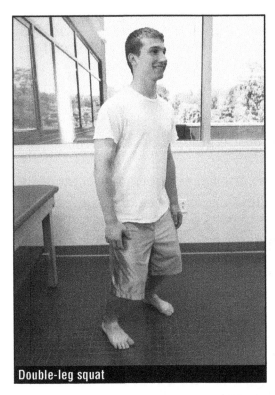
Double-leg squat

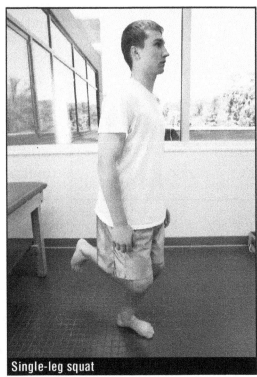
Single-leg squat

Starting position: Stand with feet positioned shoulder-width apart.

Exercise action: Bend the knees until you are not able to see your feet, and return to the starting position. Gradually progress to lifting the noninvolved extremity, and repeat the exercise using only the involved extremity.

Primary muscle groups: Lower extremity musculature

Indications: Strengthening and stabilization of the lower extremity

Contraindications: Limited knee flexion; early post-op rehab

Pearls of performance: During the bilateral exercise, the patient's weight should be equally distributed through the lower extremities. Pelvic stabilization should be maintained when completing the unilateral exercise.

Step-Downs

PROGRESSION NAME: Closed-Chain Lower Extremity Exercises

STAGE: Height progression of step box from 2 inches (5 cm), 4 inches (10 cm), and 6 inches (15 cm)

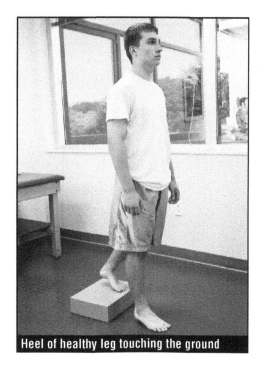

Heel of healthy leg touching the ground

Starting position: Begin with a 2-inch (5 cm) step, and progress in height as tolerated to 6 inches (15 cm). Stand on the involved leg, and extend the noninvolved leg to the front of the box.

Exercise action: Bend the involved leg until the heel of the noninvolved leg touches the ground, and return to the starting position.

Primary muscle groups: Lower extremity musculature

Indications: Strengthening of the lower extremity

Contraindications: Patellofemoral pain; poor leg control; early post-op rehab

Pearls of performance: The patient should not quickly drop the heel to the ground. The motion should be controlled while maintaining pelvic stabilization and should not cause patellofemoral pain.

Forward Lunge

PROGRESSION NAME: Closed-Chain Lower Extremity Exercises

STAGE: Progression to adding weight to the exercise

Starting position: Stand with feet shoulder-width apart and hands on hips.

Exercise action: Step forward with the involved leg until the knee bends to 90°. Return to the starting position.

Primary muscle groups: Lower extremity musculature

Indications: Strengthening and stabilization of the lower extremity

Contraindications: Limited knee range of motion; patellofemoral pain

Pearls of performance: Ensure the patient maintains the body in an upright position as a step is taken forward, does not bend the involved extremity to more than 90° when performing the exercise, or steps so far forward that it is necessary to lean backward to return to the starting position.

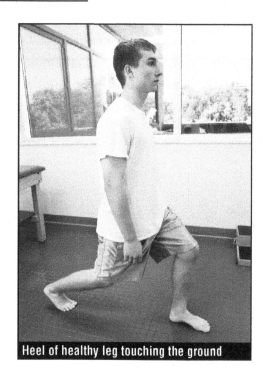

Heel of healthy leg touching the ground

Leg Press

PROGRESSION NAME: Closed-Chain Lower Extremity Exercises

STAGE: Progression from double to single leg and progression of weight

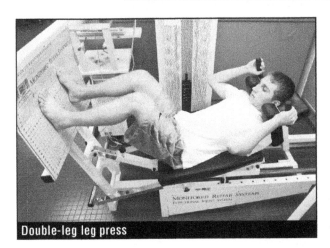
Double-leg leg press

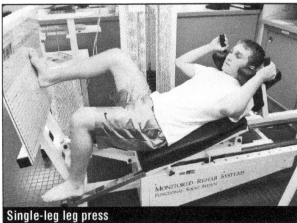
Single-leg leg press

Starting position: Either sit or recline depending on the type of machine, with feet placed shoulder-width apart on the platform or foot pads.

Exercise action: Push against the weight, bending the knees to 90° of flexion.

Primary muscle groups: Lower extremity musculature

Indications: Strengthening of the lower extremity

Contraindications: Limited knee range of motion; patellofemoral pain

Pearls of performance: Movement should be slow and controlled, with equal weight distribution when performed bilaterally.

Aggressive Peroneal Exercise

PROGRESSION NAME: Peroneal Strengthening   **STAGE:** Aggressive side-lying with and without weight

Starting position: Lie on your side, with opposite leg supporting involved calf. Have involved foot off the end of a table or bed. Foot should be in a dorsiflexed and inverted position.

Exercise action: Plantar flex and evert your foot in one smooth motion. Return to the starting position and then repeat.

Primary muscle groups: Peroneals

Indications: Strengthens peroneal muscles

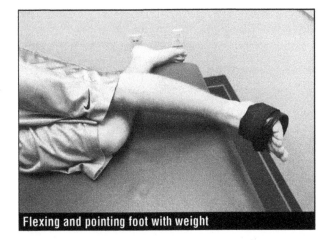
Flexing and pointing foot with weight

Contraindications: Posterior tibialis tendon repair patients until at least 2 months postoperative

Pearls of performance: Monitor patient to ensure the ankle is moving into plantar flexion and eversion. Add weight to increase difficulty of exercise.

Posterior Tibialis Exercise

PROGRESSION NAME: Posterior Tibialis Strengthening   **STAGE:** Thera-Tubing seated and standing

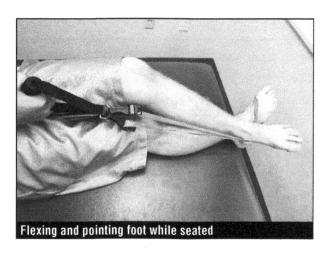

Flexing and pointing foot while seated

Starting position: Sit with Thera-Tubing around forefoot, with noninvolved foot crossed over top. Foot should be off the end of the table.

Exercise action: Plantar flex and invert your foot in one smooth motion. Return to the starting position, and then repeat.

Primary muscle groups: Posterior tibialis

Indications: Strengthens posterior tibialis

Contraindications: Peroneal tendon repair patients until at least 2 months postoperative

Pearls of performance: Monitor patient to ensure the ankle is moving into plantar flexion and inversion without hip internal rotation. To increase difficulty, tie the tubing to an object and have the standing patient pull into inversion and plantar flexion.

Calf Raises

PROGRESSION NAME: Calf Strengthening   **STAGE:** Double- to single-leg calf raises

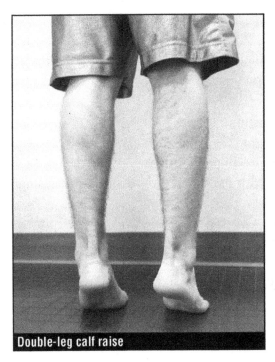
Double-leg calf raise

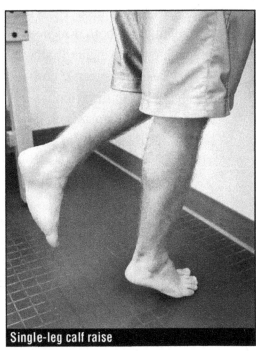
Single-leg calf raise

Starting position: Stand with feet shoulder-width apart, with weight evenly distributed.

Exercise action: Rise up on toes as far as tolerated. Slowly lower and repeat.

Primary muscle groups: Gastrocnemius and soleus

Indications: Strengthens gastrocnemius and soleus

Contraindications: none

Pearls of performance: Limiting upper extremity support will increase proprioceptive training. To advance the exercise, have the patient gradually increase weight onto involved foot until a single-leg calf raise is tolerated.

FUNCTIONAL EXERCISE PROGRESSIONS

Once the athlete has been clinically assessed for functional deficits, it is time to progress to the functional movements necessary to return the athlete to his or her sport. At this point, full range of motion, a normal gait pattern, symmetrical flexibility, strength, proprioception, and balance should be close to their preoperative levels. As previously discussed, the clinician should be cognizant of the basic injury mechanisms and biomechanics while moving the athlete through the functional progression. Athletes should not experience pain or altered gait mechanics as they attempt each movement. Supervision by the clinician or coach is imperative to ensure that each movement is mechanically correct. Braces or tape can be worn if needed during the functional progression.

Wrestling

1. Jumping on both legs: 5 times
2. Jumping on injured leg: 5 times
3. Jogging laps: both directions
4. Jogging figure eights (half, three quarter, full speed): 10 yards (10 m)
5. Cariocas (crossovers): both directions
6. Circling: both directions
7. Stand-up sequence from down position: 5 times
8. Spin drills, partner in down position (wrestler uses hands for balance, chest on opponent's back), both directions: 5 times
9. Shooting from standing position, with opponent progressively increasing speeds
10. Circling, with tying-up opponent
11. Shoot and sprawl: wrestler balances on injured leg while working against unanticipated maneuvers of opponent
12. Down position sequence: opponent applies resistance as injured wrestler attempts to get up
13. Live wrestling

Court Sports

1. Heel raises, injured leg: 10 times
2. Walking at fast pace: 50 yards (50 m)
3. Jumping on both legs: 10 times
4. Jumping on injured leg: 10 times
5. Jogging straight: full court
6. Jogging straight and curves: 2 laps
7. Sprinting (half, three quarter, full speed): full court
8. Running figure eights (half, three quarter, full speed): baseline to quarter court
9. Triangle drills: sprint baseline to half court, backward run back to baseline, defensive slides along baseline; repeat in opposite direction
10. Cariocas (crossovers): half, three quarter, full speed
11. Cutting: half, three quarter, full speed
12. Position drills

Baseball and Softball

1. Heel raises, injured leg: 10 times
2. Walking at fast pace: first base
3. Jumping on both legs: 10 times
4. Jumping on injured leg: 10 times
5. Jogging straight: first base
6. Jogging straight and curves: 2 laps around bases
7. Sprinting (half, three quarter, full speed): first base
8. Sprinting (half, three quarter, full speed): rounding first base
9. Running figure eights: home plate to pitcher's mound
10. Backward running: simulate fielding fly ball
11. Throwing: short toss to long toss
12. Hitting: tee to batting cage to live
13. Position drills

Field Sports

1. Heel raises, injured leg: 10 times
2. Walking at fast pace: 50 yards (50 m)
3. Jumping on both legs: 10 times
4. Jumping on injured leg: 10 times
5. Jogging straight: 50 yards (50 m)
6. Jogging straight and curves: 2 laps
7. Sprinting (half, three quarter, full speed): 40 yards (40 m)
8. Running figure eights (half, three quarter, full speed): 15 yards (15 m)
9. Cariocas (crossovers), both directions: 40 yards (40 m)
10. Backward running: 40 yards (40 m)
11. Cutting (half, three quarter, full speed)
12. Position drills

Distance Running: Distance

When an athlete is able to begin running again, it is necessary to return to previous mileage gradually. Provide the following guidelines to help ensure a safe return to the road.

- Make sure you stretch before and after running.
- Keep the running surface as soft, smooth, and level as possible.
- Emphasize form.
- Ice the involved area until numb after running.
- Follow these mileage guidelines. Do not progress to the next step if the previous one caused pain.

Previously Running 20 to 30 Miles per Week

Week	DAY							Total miles
	1	2	3	4	5	6	7	
1	1	0	1	0	1	0	2	5
2	0	2	0	2	0	3	0	7
3	3	2	0	3	2	0	3	13
4	3	0	4	3	0	4	4	18
5	0	5	4	0	5	5	5	24

Previously Running 30 to 40 Miles per Week

Week	DAY							Total miles
	1	2	3	4	5	6	7	
1	2	0	2	0	2	0	3	9
2	0	3	0	3	0	4	3	13
3	0	4	4	0	5	4	0	17
4	5	4	0	5	5	0	6	25
5	5	0	6	5	5	0	6	27

Distance Running: Time

When an athlete is able to begin running again, it is necessary to return to previous mileage gradually. Provide the following guidelines to help ensure a safe return to the road.

- Make sure you stretch before and after running.
- Keep the running surface as soft, smooth, and level as possible.
- Emphasize form.
- Ice the involved area until numb after running.
- Follow these mileage guidelines. Do not progress to the next step if the previous one caused pain

Previously Running 30 to 45 Minutes per Day

Week	DAY							Total minutes
	1	2	3	4	5	6	7	
1	10	0	10	0	12	0	14	46
2	0	16	0	18	0	20	0	54
3	25	20	0	25	25	0	30	125
4	30	0	30	35	0	35	40	170
5	0	40	35	0	45	40	45	205

Previously Running 45 Minutes per Day

Week	DAY							Total minutes
	1	2	3	4	5	6	7	
1	10	0	12	0	15	0	17	54
2	0	20	0	20	0	22	0	62
3	25	20	0	30	25	0	35	135
4	30	0	35	35	0	40	35	175
5	0	40	40	35	0	45	40	200
6	40	0	45	45	40	0	50	220
7	45	45	50	0	55	50	50	295

Gymnastics: Jumping and Skills Progression

A major component of the functional progression for full return to gymnastics participation is jumping. The gymnast should be able to jog pain free before beginning the jumping activities. Jogging should be initiated by having the gymnast run the length of the vaulting run. This provides a firm surface (versus the floor exercise mat) and sufficient length to run. Increase until the gymnast can jog the length three times, pain free.

Guidelines

- These progressions should be performed on a firm surface such as panel mats.
- The gymnast should be able to perform three sets of 10 of each activity before proceeding to the next jump.
- Each jump should be performed both forward and backward to simulate front and back tumbling.
- Proper form should be emphasized when performing each jump: When squatting and landing the patella should be aligned forward. When jumping, the gymnast should push through the toes, and as she leaves the floor her feet should be fully pointed.

1. Jumping
    a. Hop in place on two feet
    b. Jump **up** on two legs: 6 to 8 inches (15 to 20 cm)
2. Skills
    a. Start cartwheels, front and back walkovers on floor mat
3. Jumping
    a. Jump **up** on two legs: 12 to 14 inches (30 to 35 cm)
    b. Jump **down** on two legs: 6 to 8 inches (15 to 20 cm)
    c. Jump **up** on two legs: 18 to 20 inches (45 to 50 cm)
    d. Jump **down** on two legs: 12 to 14 inches (30 to 35 cm)
    e. Jump **up** on one leg: 6 to 8 inches (15 to 20 cm)
4. Skills
    a. Start leaps and jumps in place on the tumble track; start basic jump rope drills on the tumble track
5. Jumping
    a. Jump **up** on two legs: 24 inches (60 cm)
    b. Jump **down** on two legs: 18 to 20 inches (45 to 50 cm)
    c. Jump **down** on one leg: 6 to 8 inches (15 to 20 cm)
6. Skills
    a. Start round-offs, front and back handsprings with two-foot landings on the tumble track

7. Jumping
   a. Jump **down** on two legs: 24 inches (60 cm)
   b. Jump **up** on one leg: 12 inches (30 cm)

8. Skills
   a. Start individual skills such as round-offs, front and back handsprings with step-out on the floor exercise mat
   b. Start combinations on the tumble track: round-off back handspring step-out

9. Jumping
   a. Jump **down** on two legs: 36 inches (90 cm)
   b. Jump **down** on one leg: 12 inches (30 cm)
   c. Jump **up** on one leg: 18 inches (45 cm)

10. Skills
   a. Start combinations on floor exercise mat: round-off back handspring step-out, front handspring step-out round-off
   b. Increase force of tumbling combinations on tumble track, and practice rebound for final skill in series

11. Jumping
   a. Jump **down** on two legs: 48 inches (120 cm)
   b. Jump **down** on one leg: 18 inches (45 cm)

12. Skills
   a. Increase force of tumbling combinations on floor exercise mat, and practice rebound for final skill in series
   b. Start back and front tucks, and progress to full tumbling once tucks are pain free and have good form

SPORT-SPECIFIC PROGRESSIONS

Athletes who have passed the field and court functional progressions should move to positional drills. The following drills are only examples. Collaboration with coaches will assist with the proper drill choices.

Football: Skilled Positions

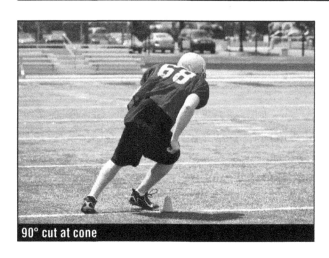

90° cut at cone

Square Drill: Place four cones in a square 3 to 5 yards (3 to 5 m) apart. The player runs as fast as he can under control and makes a quick 90° cut at each cone. He should stay low and push off on the outside extremity. ◀

Spin Drill: The player runs full speed for approximately 10 yards (10 m), spins in one direction, and then repeats, spinning in the opposite direction. ▶

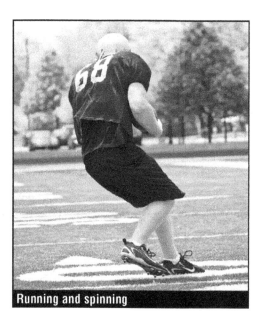

Running and spinning

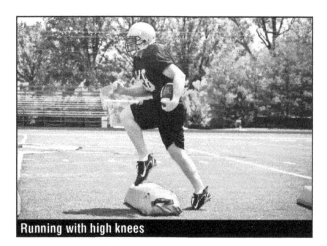

Running with high knees

High-Knees Drill: Place five square bags an equal distance apart. The player must run full speed with the knees high and head up, looking downfield. ◀

Football: Lineman

Mirror Dodge Drill: Set up two cones, 5 yards (5 m) apart. One other player will be needed for this drill. The injured player shuffle-steps, keeping his head up and shoulders square, mirroring his opponent's motions. ➡

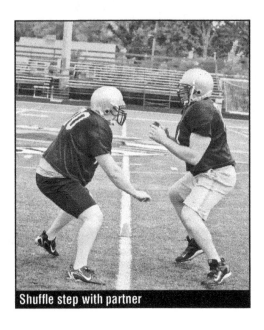

Shuffle step with partner

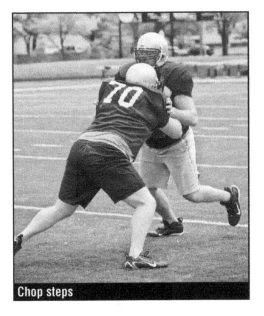

Chop steps

Partner Drill: The injured player fits up with a partner, and while doing chop steps, moves ⬅ the partner 10 yards (10 m).

Chutes Drill: The player begins in the proper three-point stance at the start of the chute. He should concentrate on using the proper foot technique while staying low, keeping his head up and feet wide. ➡

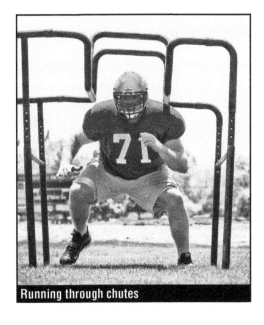

Running through chutes

Soccer: Skilled Positions

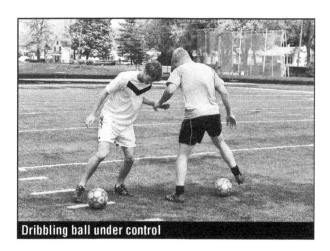

Dribbling ball under control

Defensive Ball Drill: Set up four markers in a diamond fashion approximately 15 to 20 yards (15 to 20 m) from a 20- × 20-yard (20 × 20 m) square. The player dribbles the ball under control inside the area while trying to tackle and knock another player's ball out of the area.

Triangle Drill: Three players each stand at a different cone; only one player has a ball at her feet. The cones are approximately 15 to 20 yards (15 to 20 m) away from each other in a wide-angled triangle. There are also three markers forming a bigger triangle a further 15 to 20 yards (15 to 20 m) away. On the signal, the player with the ball passes it to either of the first players positioned at the other two cones, follows the ball past the player who is receiving the pass, and approaches the static player at the marker, who plays a one-two pass with the first player. Each player must control the ball to face another line before passing and following it for a one-two with the player at the marker.

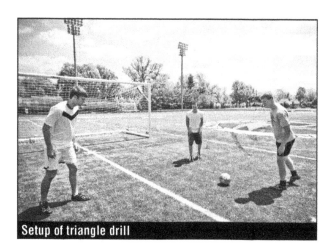

Setup of triangle drill

Soccer: Goalies

Diving Drill: The goalkeeper positions himself in the center of his goal a few yards in advance of his goal line, with the coach facing him several yards away. The coach or a partner serves him a set number of balls (6 to 12). The server should deliver a certain type of ball in a set routine as follows:

A slow rolling ball

A bouncing or medium-height ball

A slow high ball

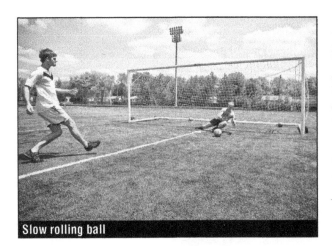

Slow rolling ball

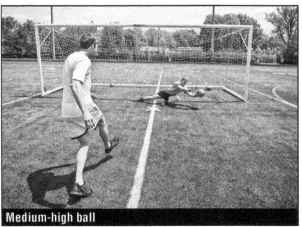

Medium-high ball

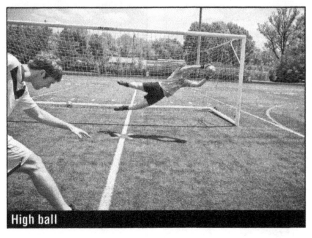

High ball

(continued)

Soccer: Goalies   *(continued)*

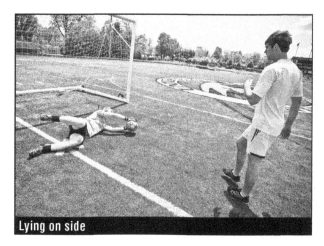

Lying on side

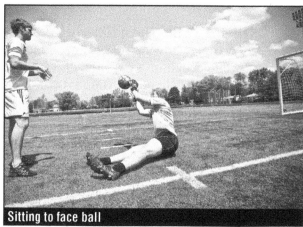

Sitting to face ball

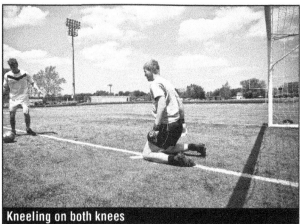

Kneeling on both knees

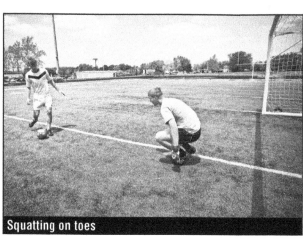

Squatting on toes

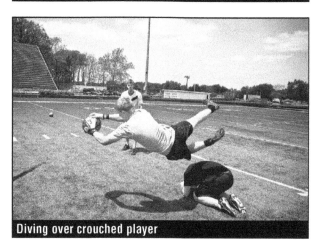

Diving over crouched player

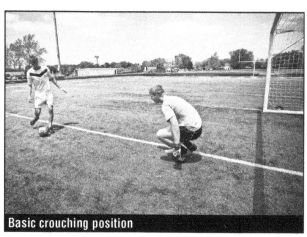

Basic crouching position

Serving the ball farther away each time gradually stretches the goalkeeper (remember to serve the ball to both sides). The goalkeeper should be made to use a set sequence of defense techniques that progressively gets more difficult. Here is an example: (a) lying on his side; (b) sitting to face the ball; (c) kneeling on one or both knees; (d) squatting down on his toes; (e) diving over a ball or crouching player; (f) assuming a basic crouching position.

Hit-the-Target Drill: Target areas are marked on realistic parts of the field; the goalkeeper, who should have a good supply of balls, distributes the balls and tries to hit the target areas where retrievers are positioned. ➡

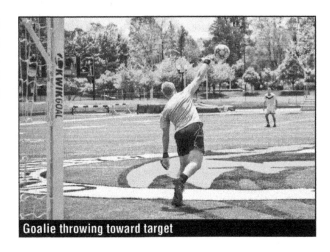
Goalie throwing toward target

Basketball: Inside Players

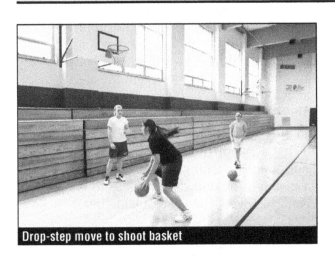
Drop-step move to shoot basket

Drop-Step Drill: Three people start in the drill. One ball is placed at the first line above the block on one side and the same on the other block. One player starts as the post player while each of the other two players is assigned a ball to put back at the same spot after every shot. The player who starts as the post player jump-stops to the first ball, picks it up, chins the ball, checks inside, then makes a drop-step move to score. The player ⬅ does the same thing on the other side.

Post-Up Hook Shot: The player posts up, gets to the middle of the paint, fakes to the opposite direction that she is going to shoot, brings the ball up, and turns to the rim, extends, and shoots. ➡

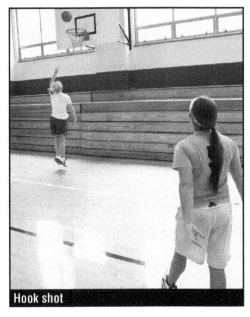
Hook shot

Volleyball: Net Players

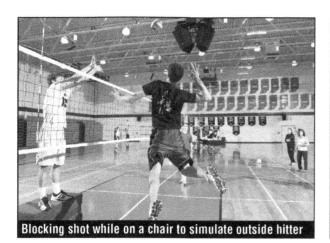

Blocking shot while on a chair to simulate outside hitter

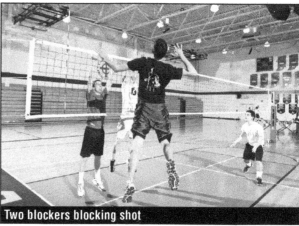

Two blockers blocking shot

Blocking Drills: One player stands on a chair on the opposite side of the net, simulating an outside hitter. The injured player (blocker) lines up on the opposite side of the net. The blocker jumps (keeping good form), and the opposing player hits a ball into the block. Then alternate and have two blockers, both lining up 2 feet (0.6 m) away from the opposing player. They must shuffle-step 2 feet (0.6 m) to get to the angle of approach and jump to block. This works the team concept of blocking as well as the shuffle step.

Burn: A coach tosses a ball high outside, and the outside hitter takes an approach to the net. A defender decides whether to charge the tip or stay deep and cover deep tips. A third person helps the outside hitter by telling him whether the defender is deep or short. If the defender is short, the outside hitter has to tip over the head of the defender. If the defender is deep, then the outside hitter must tip short.

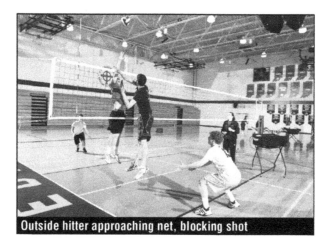

Outside hitter approaching net, blocking shot

Volleyball: Back Row Players

Clubhouse Drill: A coach or second player stands on the same side of the net in the setter's position, midcourt. The injured player stands in the ready position, near middle back. The coach or player hits the ball hard or tips it to the injured player. The player needs to return the ball in a controlled manner back to the coach. This drill should be done at a fast tempo.➡

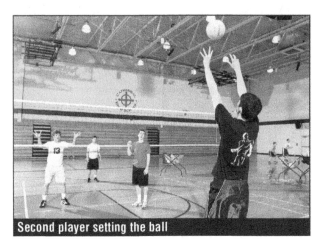

Second player setting the ball

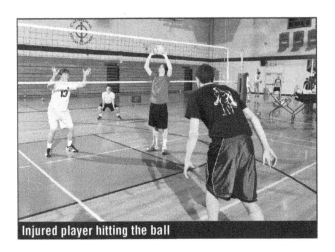

Injured player hitting the ball

Hit and Recover: One coach or player is positioned on each side of the net with a ball. One coach or player tosses a ball to the injured player for an attack on an opposing player (player position can vary). As soon as the injured player hits the ball, the coach or player on the opposite ⬅ side of the net drops her ball over.

SUMMARY

Successfully implementing a functional progression requires the clinician to have a detailed understanding of the functional anatomy and biomechanics of the lower extremity. The specific pathomechanics behind lower extremity injuries will ultimately direct the rehabilitation program and specific activities within the functional progression. Before starting a functional progression, the patient must demonstrate appropriate levels of strength as well as normalized functional movement patterns. Finally, the functional progression must be tailored to meet the specific demands of each person.

C·H·A·P·T·E·R
5

Trunk

Rehabilitation for mechanical spine pain has undergone significant change over the past decade. From a model that emphasized pain modulation and pain relief as the primary intended outcome has evolved today's model, which emphasizes measurable improvement in function. The intended outcomes of functional training for the trunk are to enhance neuromuscular efficiency, strength, power, endurance, coordination, and control. The control role of the trunk is based on the principle that the optimal function of the trunk and pelvis is dependent on the precise timing and interplay between the trunk muscles. Thus it is not only the capacity of the muscles to perform but also the integration of afferent sensory information received by the central nervous system, such as the instantaneous change of forces experienced by the body at a moment in time, perturbations, and the momentary status of the stability of the body, that results in the CNS planning and initiating a sequence of efferent outputs to the muscles.

Concurrent with the paradigm shift for patients with mechanical spine pain has been a simultaneous increase in attention to the role of the trunk in sport. Numerous strategies to improve sport performance by emphasizing an improvement in the neuromuscular efficiency of the trunk have emerged. Sometimes loosely referred to as "core stability" of the trunk, it actually encompasses much more than that as it combines elements of strength training, endurance training, coordination development, and ultimately motor learning. Training programs for nearly every professional sport now include attention to optimizing neuromotor function of the trunk. Thus high-level athletes as diverse as professional golfers, football players, baseball pitchers, soccer players, and swimmers have all come to realize that optimal functioning of the trunk is the necessary keystone for precise functioning and explosive motion of the extremities for many of the complex and coordinated activities seen in sport. No matter where on the continuum one might be—from a worker in industry to an elite athlete—the health of the trunk musculature and the integration of the nervous and muscle systems are critical not only for optimal performance but also for avoiding injury, especially injuries to the important specialized connective tissues of the spine.

The purpose of this chapter is to provide the reader with contemporary information and ideas regarding training of the trunk, using a framework of anatomy and biomechanics. When discussed in this manner, a more-logical and scientific rationale for the different exercises is better appreciated and modifications that might be necessary as a result of injury can be more-easily integrated into exercise programs. In addition, any innovative or unique exercise progression that might be developed will ultimately be measured by its potential to safely load the spine.

The chapter begins with an examination of the key anatomical and biomechanical aspects of the lumbopelvic region that must be considered when designing functional testing and exercise progressions for the trunk. To reinforce the anatomy, some of the more-common injuries seen in this region are then presented, which allows for a meaningful discussion regarding functional testing and prescribing functional activities. The spine is a multisegmental, multiaxial structure, so there is great overlap between functional tests and functional progressions as they relate to the spine.

Because most of the functional tests and progressions for activities of daily living and sport emphasize the trunk, particularly the lumbopelvic region, the section discussing anatomy and biomechanics primarily pertains to this region. In addition, attention is focused on the lumbopelvic region because of the preponderance of low back injuries that can occur with poor exercise technique or poorly designed programs. However, when specific functional progressions are discussed at the end of the chapter, the contributions of head and neck positioning as well as scapulothoracic motion are included when these are considered essential aspects of the technique.

ANATOMY OF THE TRUNK

The lumbopelvic complex consists of the five lumbar vertebrae, the sacrum and coccyx, paired innominate bones, and articulating femurs, with intervening soft tissues including the intervertebral discs, ligaments, and muscles. This chapter also describes how the shoulder girdle musculature is linked to the lumbopelvic system, which is essential to understand when developing comprehensive functional progressions for the trunk.

Bones

The trunk, or core, consists of the vertebrae, sacrum, and innominate bones. However, no description of functional exercises for the trunk is complete without reference to the scapulae and femurs because musculature associated with these bones directly tie into the spine. These bones are addressed in chapters 3 and 4, respectively.

Lumbar Vertebrae

The lumbar spine is composed of five individually segmented vertebrae. Occasionally the caudal region varies in segmentation. This variation results in either the first sacral vertebra failing to fuse with the rest of the sacrum (lumbarization of the first sacral vertebra) or fusion of the fifth lumbar vertebra to the sacrum (sacralization of the fifth lumbar vertebra).

The components of the lumbar vertebrae are shown in figure 5.1. The anteriorly placed vertebral body consists of spongy bone covered by a thin shell of cortical bone. The size of the vertebral bodies increases from the first lumbar vertebra to the fifth. The posterior aspect of the vertebral body, which helps form the anterior limitation of the spinal canal, is generally concave in the upper lumbar segments and slightly convex in the lower. The posterior aspect also features several small openings, referred to as nutrient foramina, that serve as the ingress and egress of blood vessels feeding the vertebral body. From a sport and exercise perspective, it is important to note that the spongy bone is subject to compression fracture if the force exceeds bone tolerance.

The pedicles are two short, stout bony projections from the posterolateral aspects of the vertebral body. The region under the inferior aspect of the pedicle is referred to as the subpedicular recess, and its relationship is important because the nerve root complex traverses this region as it makes its exit through the intervertebral foramen. Sports and exercises that place excessive extension loads on the lumbar spine can result in bony changes in this region, thereby affecting the nerve root and leading to radicular signs or symptoms. Because most of the musculature of the lumbar spine attaches to the various posterior processes of the vertebrae, such as the transverse and spinous processes, the force of muscle contraction is ultimately transmitted to the vertebral body–intervertebral disc interface through the pedicles via these processes.

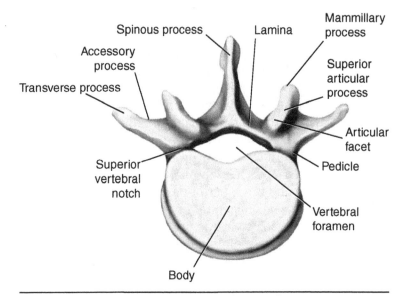

Figure 5.1 Components of typical lumbar vertebrae.

The paired laminae originate from the posterior aspect of the pedicles. Above and below the pedicles of the vertebrae are the superior and inferior notches. When two lumbar vertebrae are placed together, the superior and inferior notches of the articulating vertebrae come together to form the intervertebral foramen, through which the spinal nerve exits and begins to divide into the anterior and posterior rami. This region is also the area in which the dorsal root ganglion lies. Any instability between two segments alters the architecture of the intervertebral foramen, potentially irritating the nerve root. One of the philosophical foundations of core stabilization exercises for the lumbar spine is based on this anatomical construct: Teaching a patient how to contract muscles in order to maintain stability between segments may minimize stress on supporting ligaments and the adjacent nerve root complex.

Each lumbar vertebra has two superior facets, which face superiorly and medially, and two inferior facets, which face anteriorly and laterally (figure 5.2). The inferior articulating process lies medial to the superior articulating process. Understanding this anatomical relationship helps the clinician visualize the forces generated into and through this joint as movement analysis is carried out during the examination process as well as during assessment of the proper and safe lumbar mechanics for a particular sport. In many ways, the facet relationship of adjacent vertebrae is the foundation of exercise program design for the trunk.

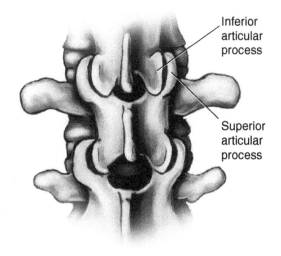

Figure 5.2 Facet orientation of the lumbar spine.

The facet is the portion of the articular process that meets the facet of its joint partner and is covered with hyaline cartilage. The correct anatomical term for the synovial joint formed as the two facets approximate each other is the *zygapophyseal* joint, although the term *facet* or *apophyseal joint* is used quite often. On the posterior surface of the superior articulating process is the mammillary process, which serves as an attachment for the multifidus muscle, one of the key muscles involved in most lumbar strengthening programs.

An important part of the posterior arch in the region, lying between the superior and inferior articular processes, is the pars interarticularis. A pars defect, often referred to as a spondylolysis, is a gap between the inferior aspect of the facet above and the superior part of the facet below (figure 5.3). A pars interarticularis gap can be congenital or traumatic, such as with repeated stresses to the bone, which leads to a fracture resulting in bony separation. Fractures in this region resulting in spondylolisthesis, a translation of one vertebrae upon an adjacent vertebrae, are very common in sports that require a high rate of flexion–extension cycles of the lumbar spine. These sports include gymnastics, diving, weightlifting, and football (in particular, the position of offensive lineman). Note that when developing functional progressions for athletes suspected of having a spondylolisthesis, the clinician must be cognizant of the number of flexion–extension cycles of the activity. Often this critical point is not understood, and instead of carefully prescribing the number of flexion–extension cycles when developing functional progressions, the clinician becomes focused on the compressive loading conditions over the lumbar spine.

Just anterior to the facets are the laterally projecting transverse processes, which serve as attachments for muscles. The lumbar transverse processes are quite stout when compared with the cervical and thoracic spinous processes but are very difficult to definitively palpate because of the mass of the erector spinae group lying on their posterior surfaces.

The spinous processes of the lumbar vertebrae project directly posterior. Generally, the spinous processes of the third and fourth lumbar vertebrae are larger than those of the fifth, which makes the fifth lumbar spinous process difficult to palpate. The spinous processes serve as attachments for the multifidus muscles, erector spinae aponeurosis, posterior layer of thoracolumbar fascia, interspinous

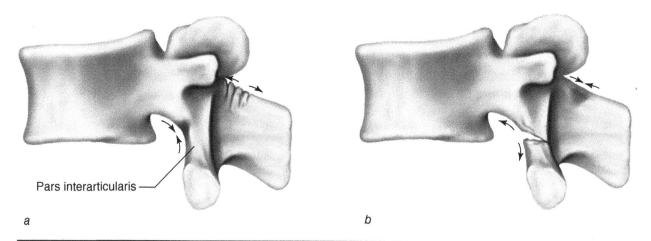

Pars interarticularis

a   *b*

Figure 5.3   Location of the pars interarticularis and the site of fracture potentially resulting in spondylolisthesis.

ligaments, and supraspinous ligaments. Thus major muscle generators of force are attached to the spinous processes, which give such generators an excellent lever arm over the lumbar spine.

Several examination techniques use the spinous process as the bony lever through which different forces can be applied. It is important to note, however, that palpating spinous process position in order to draw conclusions about malposition of the vertebra has extremely poor reliability and validity (Troyanovich, Harrison, and Harrison 1998; McCombe et al. 1989).

Sacrum

The sacrum consists of five fused vertebrae that lie interpositioned between the two ilia and under the fifth lumbar vertebra. The coccyx is attached to the inferior aspect of the sacrum at the sacrococcygeal junction. Ground reaction forces, such as the force at heel strike, traverse the lower extremities through the ilia and to the sacrum, then ultimately through the spine. Conversely, trunk forces travel through the spine to the sacrum, which then dissipates the forces laterally through the ilium and to the lower extremity. The sacrum thus serves as a hub through which ground and trunk forces converge. The sacroiliac joint—described in more detail later in the chapter—serves to attenuate this confluence of forces.

For the most part, the sacrum is wider superiorly and anteriorly than it is inferiorly. When seen alone, it typically resembles a truncated pyramid. From a superior to inferior perspective, the anterior aspect of the sacrum is concave and the posterior aspect is convex. The lateral aspect of the sacrum, which serves as the articulating surface for the ilium, has numerous ridges and indentations, with one of the more-prominent indentations occurring at the level of S2. This indentation is the "seat" for the prominence of the ilium referred to as Bonnaire's tubercle. The lamina of the fifth sacral vertebra does not usually fuse during development, and the sacral hiatus is formed. This hiatus is continuous with the epidural space and can serve as a portal of entry for epidural injections.

The sacrum articulates with the fifth lumbar vertebra via the linkage between the superior facets of the sacrum and the inferior facets of the fifth lumbar vertebra. This is referred to as the lumbosacral junction. The angle formed between the intersection of a line running parallel to the superior aspect of the first sacral vertebral body and a line parallel to the horizontal is referred to as the lumbosacral angle (figure 5.4). The wedge-shaped L5–S1 intervertebral disc also serves as an articulating link between the body of the fifth lumbar vertebra and the cranial aspect of the sacral surface. The sacrum also articulates with the ilium, forming the sacroiliac joint.

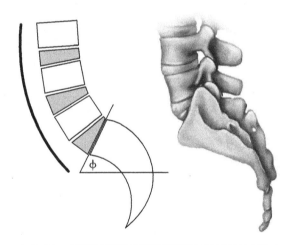

Figure 5.4 The lumbosacral angle. This angle is important because the higher the angle degree, the greater the shear force at the lumbosacral junction.

Innominate Bone

The innominate bone is formed by the fusion of the ilium, ischium, and pubis. It contributes to the formation of the sacroiliac joint, pubic symphysis, and hip joints. The ring formed by the articulation of the paired innominates with the sacrum is called the pelvis, and thus the posterior wall of the pelvis is the sacrum.

The pelvis serves as an attachment for many trunk and lower extremity muscles, while the sacrum has minimal muscle attachments. Contraction of these muscles while the foot is fixed to the ground in the upright standing posture can alter the relationship of the pelvis to the lumbar spine and hence the weight-bearing characteristics of the lumbar spine. In addition, contraction of the lower extremity muscles that are attached to the innominate with the foot fixed to the ground introduces different forces to the sacroiliac joint and pubic symphysis.

It is important to note that the hip joints are the primary location for rotation when a person is standing. Many sports have a higher incidence of low back injuries because the hips are not rotating adequately and instead the rotation occurs at the lumbar spine. Failure to rotate through the hips results in abnormal loading of the lumbar facet joints in compression and is a common etiological factor in low back injuries seen in golf, bowling, and hitting in baseball.

Specialized Connective Tissues: Intervertebral Disc

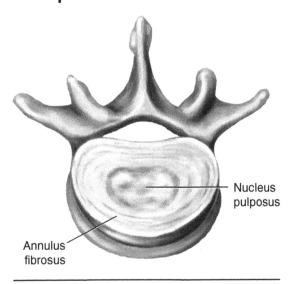

Nucleus pulposus

Annulus fibrosus

Figure 5.5 The components of the intervertebral disc.

Two vertebral bodies are linked by an intervertebral disc. Typically the intervertebral disc consists of an outer annulus fibrosus and inner nucleus pulposus, although it is difficult to distinguish the outermost aspect of the nucleus pulposus from the innermost aspect of the annulus fibrosus. From a histologic perspective, the cartilaginous end plate can also be considered part of the intervertebral disc because of the intimate relationship between the collagen framework of the vertebral end plate and the annulus fibrosus (figure 5.5).

The shape of the lumbar intervertebral discs is roughly elliptic. Generally, the anterior height of the last two lumbar discs is nearly twice their posterior height. This 2:1 relationship, resulting in a wedge shape for the disc, is nearly always present in the L5–S1 disc. Although the anterior inclination of the sacrum is a contributing factor, the wedge shape of the disc contributes greatly to the development of lumbar lordosis.

Approximately 12 to 20 concentric rings of fibrocartilage, referred to as lamellae, form the annulus fibrosus (Taylor 1990) (see figure 5.5). The term *ring* is a bit of a misnomer, however, because not every lamella completely encircles the complete disc (Tsuji et al. 1993). Each layer of fibers is obliquely offset from the next layer, with the fibers forming an approximately 30° angle with the horizontal (White and Panjabi 1978). In the anterior annulus, the lamellae are thick and fairly distinguishable. In contrast, the posterior annulus is thinner, and the lamellae tend to be compressed and merged together. The proportion of collagen increases from the inner to outer annulus, and there is also a variation of the type of collagen within the intervertebral disc. Type I collagen, the type that is structured to counter tensile forces, is found mainly in the annulus. Type II collagen, which counters compressive forces, is in the nucleus (Buckwalter, Einhorn, and Simon 2000; Buckwalter 1995). In degenerating intervertebral discs, type II collagen is replaced with the more-fibrous type I collagen. Nicotine leads not only to a reduction in viable cell numbers in the disc but also to a change in the type of collagen synthesis from type II to type I in the nucleus pulposus (Akmal et al. 2004).

The nucleus pulposus is primarily a hydrated gel of proteoglycans consisting of sulfated glycosaminoglycans bound to a protein core, with a small number of cells of collagen present. Water typically accounts for more than 80% of the weight of the nucleus. Because of the presence of negatively charged sulfate groups, water is attracted to the proteoglycan macromolecule, hence the term *hydrophilic*. One of the most striking age-related changes of the nucleus pulposus is loss of water. This loss is generally attributed to changes in the glycosaminoglycan type and content of the nucleus pulposus.

The major components of the intervertebral disc are collagen fibers, proteoglycans, and water. The histochemistry changes from the periphery to the center. A more densely arranged collagen framework is evident in the peripheral annulus, whereas a greater concentration of proteoglycans and less collagen are found in the central nucleus pulposus. Because the water content depends on the water-binding properties of the proteoglycans, there is a greater amount of water in the nucleus pulposus. It is beyond the scope of this text to discuss in detail the types and behavioral characteristics of the specific types of collagen and proteoglycans, and the reader is encouraged to review sources providing this information (Buckwalter et al. 1985; Bushell et al. 1977; McDevitt 1988). As the intervertebral disc ages, it is increasingly difficult to distinguish the nucleus pulposus from the annulus fibrosus.

The cartilaginous end plates consist of hyaline cartilage over the subchondral bone plates of the vertebral body. The cartilage is approximately 0.6 mm thick and is generally thicker peripherally and thinner toward the center (Roberts, Menage, and Urban 1989). The vertebral end plates are connected directly to the lamellae that form the inner one third of the annulus fibrosus. Thus the end plates completely cover the nucleus pulposus but cover only the inner portion of the annulus fibrosus. From a sport and exercise perpective, it is important to note that the cartilaginous end plate, not the intervertebral disc, is the "weak link" if compression loads are too great for the vertebral segment.

The cartilage resembles the intervertebral disc in that it has a higher concentration of proteoglycans and water than collagen toward the center and more collagen than proteoglycans peripherally. Multiple perforations in the cartilage end plate permit contact with the vascular buds from the marrow of the cancellous bone of the vertebral body. This vascular communication plays an important role in the nutrition of the intervertebral disc. Because of these vascular contacts and the thinness of the cartilage, diffusion of nutrients such as oxygen and glucose is facilitated. Since the intervertebral discs are essentially avascular structures, this source of nutrition and the blood vessels that enter the periphery of the annulus fibrosus are the primary sources of nutrition for the disc. The central aspect is the most metabolically active region of the cartilaginous end plate, and the vascular channels in this region are the most numerous and complex (Fagan, Moore, and Vernon Roberts 2003).

Because collagen fibers reinforce a tissue, provided that the applied stress is in the axial direction of the fiber, it should be apparent that the orientation of the collagen fibers of the annulus fibrosus allows restraint to nearly all motions of the spine. For example, twisting (torsion), anterior shear forces that accompany weight bearing, or forward bending of the spine results in tension being applied to specific regions of the annulus fibrosus. The increase in tension to the annular fibers minimizes motions between the two adjacent vertebrae. Any motion of the lumbar spine places at least a portion of the annulus fibrosus under tension, and thus the annulus serves as the key ligamentous restraint of the vertebral column.

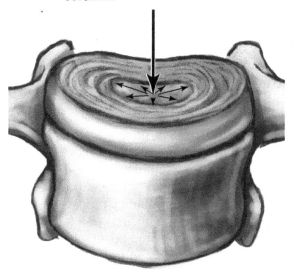

Figure 5.6 An increase in pressure of the nucleus pulposus results in the force being applied tangentially, thus increasing the tension of the annular rings. The increase in tension of the annulus results in enhanced stability between the adjacent bony segments.

The annulus fibrosus and the nucleus pulposus work in concert to resist compressive loads. The proteoglycan–water component of the nucleus provides a hydrostatic mechanism that helps distribute compressive forces tangentially toward the annulus. This increases the tension of the annular rings, further stabilizing the intervertebral disc (figure 5.6). Increased compressive loads to the disc raise the pressure within the nucleus, which further increases tension of the collagen fibers of the inner annular lamellae. Attraction and binding of water by the proteoglycans result in a swelling pressure that ultimately allows the intervertebral discs to support compressive loads.

It is not simply trunk forces and ground forces that increase compression between adjacent vertebrae. Note also that contraction of the muscles of the spine, in particular the erector spinae group, multifidus, and psoas major, also increases vertebral compression as a result of the muscle fiber direction. In fact, intervertebral compressive forces that ultimately increase intradiscal pressure are dependent on, in probable decreasing order of influence, muscle contraction, preload by the ligaments spanning the vertebral segment, and superincumbent weight. The synergistic action of the annulus and nucleus stabilizes the disc complex and distributes forces properly to restrict movement, maintain the size and shape of the neuroforamen, and ensure that the apophyseal joint maintains an invulnerable loading position during weight bearing.

The lumbar intervertebral disc has meager innervation. This is concentrated in the periannular connective tissue and the central end plate. Although receptor threshold appears closely related to nociceptive function, innervation density suggests consideration of mechanoreceptor contributions via this nerve supply as well (Fagan, Moore, and Vernon Roberts 2003). Noxious stimulation of the intervertebral disc appears to result in low back pain and distally referred symptoms, including symptoms below the knee, with the distal extent of the referral being dependent on the intensity of the stimulus (O'Neil et al. 2002). The innervation density of the periannular connective tissue and the central end plate is suggestive of proprioceptive as well as nociceptive functions (Fagan, Moore, and Vernon Roberts 2003).

Joints

The joints that are especially important to detail are the zygapophyseal joints of the lumbar spine, the sacroiliac joints of the pelvis, and the pubic symphysis. These joints guide motion of the lumbopelvic region while simultaneously attenuating ground forces. Disruption of the delicate interplay of force attenuation, load bearing, and motion direction is one of the fundamental reasons for joint injuries of the low back in sport and functional activities. There is a very precise amount and specific direction of movement available at these joints, and this precision influences the exercise prescription. Motions or loading conditions that exceed the limits or that do not precisely follow the joint planes result in injury or accelerate the breakdown of the articulating elements. Low back injuries of this sort result in major limitations in activity and can often preclude a return to activity.

Zygapophyseal (Facet) Joints

The superior facet of the subjacent vertebra lies lateral to the inferior facet of the vertebra above it and is slightly concave, while the inferior facet lies medial to the superior facet of the subjacent vertebra and has a slightly convex orientation. As a result of these two planes, the joints are oriented to limit both anterior shear and torsional stresses. The frontal plane of the facets provides a bony "check" to anterior shear, while the sagittal plane of the facets provides a "check" to torsion, or rotary motion between each lumbar vertebra. It is essential to be able to visualize this relationship because a rotary force applied to the lumbar spine during exercise results in compression between the facet surfaces on one side and decompression between the facets of the contralateral side (Porterfield and DeRosa 1998). Excessive compression between the facet surfaces has the potential to injure the articular cartilage. Furthermore, if a degree of cartilage degeneration is already present, the increased compressive load cannot be properly attenuated by the articular cartilage and instead must be borne by the subchondral bone.

As a consequence of lumbar lordosis, a continuous anterior shear stress results from the force of gravity, especially at the lumbosacral junction and the L4–L5 articulation. Because of the multiple planar arrangement of the joint structure, the cartilaginous surface of the facet oriented in the frontal plane is the first region of the joint to show early signs of degeneration (Taylor and Twomey 1985; Twomey and Taylor 1985).

The zygapophyseal joints are the only true diarthrodial joints in the lumbar spine and are typical of synovial joints that contain a fibrous joint capsule with a synovial lining. Motions allowed between the lumbar facets are largely flexion and extension motions. As a result of the sagittal orientation of the lumbar facets, minimal lateral bending or rotation occurs at the lumbar joints. Only 2.5° of rotation is available between lumbar segments because almost immediately the facets of the lumbar spine impact each other (Pearcy and Tibrewal 1984; Farfan et al. 1970). In contrast, the average range of flexion and extension at each segment is 15°, with the majority of flexion and extension occurring between the L4–L5 and L5–S1 segments (Adams and Dolan 1995). Thus the reader will appreciate that many of the exercises described later in this chapter take advantage of the safety of sagittal plane motion of the lumbar spine.

The articular cartilage of the facet is aneural, and thus pain does not arise directly from that structure. However, the apophyseal joint is innervated by the medial branch of the dorsal ramus, and thus other aspects of the joint may be the source of pain. Possible sources of pain from pathology associated with the zygapophyseal joints include the following:

- Overloading of the subchondral bone trabeculae (Lemperg and Arnoldi 1978)
- Microfractures of bone trabeculae (Lemperg and Arnoldi 1978)

- Mechanical deformation or chemical irritation of joint capsule nociceptors (Mooney and Robertson 1976; Schwarzer et al. 1994; Schwarzer et al. 1995)
- Internal derangements from joint loose bodies (Bogduk and Engel 1984)
- Meniscoid synovial folds (Bogduk and Engel 1984)
- Vascular disturbances in the bone or soft tissues (Lemperg and Arnoldi 1978)
- Joint inflammation (Mooney and Robertson 1976; Schwarzer et al. 1994; Schwarzer et al. 1995)

Overloading of the articular cartilage is recognized as potentially accelerating the degenerative process. Underloading of articular cartilage also results in degenerative changes because of cartilage softening and decreased proteoglycan synthesis of the chondrocyte (Palmoski and Brandt 1980). It should be recognized that the apophyseal joint is under a constant variety of loads because of its position in the weight-bearing chain and muscular contraction. Adams and Hutton (1980) have noted that in the upright posture, compressive force on the lumbar vertebrae is distributed in such a way that 86% of the force is borne by the bone–disc complex and 14% by zygapophyseal joints. The degree of lumbar flexion or extension alters the magnitude of this compressive force. When the lumbar spine is more in flexion, the zygapophyseal joints have less compressive force while there is more compression between the vertebral body–intervertebral disc interface. Extension of the lumbar spine increases the compressive force between the articulating facets and compresses the posterior aspect of the disc, creating an anterior shear of the vertebra above on the vertebra below. Each of these factors is critical to consider in the design and ultimate execution of any exercise program incorporating the trunk.

Sacroiliac Joint

The sacroiliac (SI) joint is formed by the articulation between the sacrum and the ilium. The iliac surface is composed of thin fibrocartilage, and the articular surface of the sacrum is formed by hyaline cartilage that is 1.7 to 5 times thicker than the iliac cartilage (Porterfield and DeRosa 1990; Beal 1982; Bowan and Cassidy 1981). As a person ages, the topography of the joint surface changes from being relatively smooth to having reciprocal elevations and depressions. The fit of the various curvatures into corresponding depressions contributes to the inherent stability of the joint. In general, only the first three sacral vertebrae contribute to the formation of the sacroiliac joint.

Much controversy has surrounded the types, amounts, and relevance of sacroiliac joint movements. The axis of motion has been described as occurring at the junction of the cranial and caudal aspects of the sacral surface (Kapandji 1974), as well as just posterior to the pubic symphysis (Lavignolle et al. 1983). Most likely, these two fixed-axis theories represent points on a continuum of instantaneous axes of motion at the sacroiliac joint (DeRosa and Porterfield 1989).

With the axis of motion located at the sacrum, the iliac motion at the sacrum is typically described as anterior or posterior torsion, whereas sacral motion on the ilium is described as nutation (flexion) or counternutation (extension). In reality, this articulation is under constant load, and the joint structure permits deformation of the two cartilaginous surfaces, allowing a combination of rotary and shear stresses to be attenuated simultaneously. Thus, the main function of the sacroiliac joint is one of force attenuation; the SI joint is a deformable structure that allows the closed ring of the pelvis to absorb and dissipate the stresses—torsional and translational—that reach it. The connective tissues of the SI joint contain both paciniform and nonpaciniform mechanoreceptors and are therefore assumed to carry both pain and proprioceptive impulses to the central nervous system (Vilensky et al. 2002).

The amount of motion is minimal because of the joint topography and reinforcing ligaments, and the evidence is very weak suggesting that palpation of bony positions of either the sacrum or ilium withstands the tests of reliability and validity. Sturesson, Selvik, and Uden (1989) found 1 to 2° of movement at the sacroiliac joint. On average, there are approximately 3° of flexion, 0.8° of lateral bending, and 1.5° of axial rotation (Miller, Schultz, and Andersson 1987; Vleeming et al. 1992). Many purported sacroiliac joint tests are neither sensitive nor specific. Manual stresses to the joint complex that are designed to provoke symptoms are considered more reliable than tests deemed to assess joint mobility (Laslett and Williams 1994). Later in the chapter it is suggested that such tests quickly performed by the examiner provide an idea as to how cautious or aggressive an exercise program design might be in the presence of low back pain.

Pubic Symphysis

The articulation between the medial aspects of the pubic bones forms a cartilaginous joint. The complete articular surface of each bone is covered by hyaline cartilage. Between the two articulating surfaces is a fibrocartilaginous interpubic disc that is generally thicker in females than males. The superior pubic ligament, arcuate pubic ligament, and decussations of the rectus sheath help reinforce the joint.

The pubic symphysis does not normally allow significant movement (Gamble, Simmons, and Freedman 1986). However, during pregnancy the ligaments associated with the joint soften and allow some degree of separation between the joint surfaces (Golighty 1982; Weiss, Nagelschmidt, and Struck 1979). This separation is approximately 2 mm and allows for more space to be created for passage of the infant through the birth canal. These mechanics are essential to understand in the design of functional progression exercises for the postpartum female.

Ligaments

The ligaments of the spinal column (figure 5.7) contribute greatly to the stability of the spine by providing restraint to specific spinal motions. In addition, the position of the ligaments allows for reinforcement of the intervertebral discs. Ligaments are pain-sensitive structures and consequently serve as a source of pain if injured or placed under excessive strain.

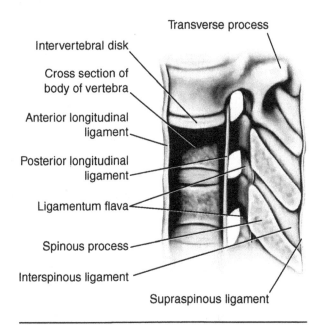

Transverse process

Intervertebral disk

Cross section of body of vertebra

Anterior longitudinal ligament

Posterior longitudinal ligament

Ligamentum flava

Spinous process

Interspinous ligament

Supraspinous ligament

Figure 5.7 Ligaments of the spinal column.

Reprinted from R. Behnke, 2006, *Kinetic anatomy,* 2nd ed. (Champaign, IL: Human Kinetics), 126.

The anterior longitudinal ligament is a very strong structure in the lumbar spine. It runs the entire length of the spine, being widest and most stout in the lumbar region, and typically is fixed firmly to the annulus fibrosus and more loosely blended with the periosteum of the vertebral bodies.

The posterior longitudinal ligament runs the entire length of the spine. It has an hourglass arrangement because of the location of the pedicles on the posterior aspect of the vertebral body. It fans out over the posterior aspect of the intervertebral disc to which it is connected. Note that since the ligament lies posterior to the axis of motion for the lumbar spine, it is subject to increased tension during lumbar flexion. All the spinal ligaments contain free nerve endings and complex unencapsulated endings; however, the posterior longitudinal ligament appears to have the greatest density of nerve endings (Weinstein et al. 1989).

The paired ligamenta flava run from one lamina to the adjacent one. Each is attached to the front of the lower border of the lamina above and passes downward and backward to the back of the upper border of the lamina below. Because the ligament has a high elastin fiber content, it is more yellow than other spinal ligaments. The different histochemistry allows greater elastic properties, as it contains more than 75% elastin (Yahia et al. 1990). This larger portion of elastic fibers prevents the ligament from buckling into the spinal canal when the spine is extended. As mentioned earlier, the lateral extent of the ligament forms the anterior limitation of the zygapophyseal joint capsule.

The interspinous ligaments are present in the entire spine but are most completely developed in the lumbar region, where they consist of ventral, middle, and dorsal parts (Heylings 1978). These ligaments run in an oblique fashion superiorly and posteriorly from one spinous process to the next. The ligaments occupy the space between the supraspinous ligament and the ligamentum flavum.

The supraspinous ligaments attach to the tips of the spinous processes, terminate at approximately the third lumbar segment, and are reinforced in the lower lumbar region by the decussation of the posterior layer of thoracolumbar fascia. In general, the supraspinous ligament is continuous with the posterior edge of the interspinous ligaments.

The iliolumbar ligaments connect the fifth and occasionally the fourth lumbar transverse processes with the ilium. The ligament is broad and stout and typically continues to reinforce the anterosuperior aspect of the sacroiliac joint (Gray 2000). The ligament is a major stabilizer of the L5 vertebra on the sacrum. The iliolumbar ligament is present only in adults. In children it is represented by muscle tissue. Luk and colleagues (Luk, Ho, and Leong 1987) suggest that the iliolumbar ligament is an example of metaplasia because age-related changes of the quadratus lumborum result in a replacement of the lower muscle fibers of the quadratus lumborum with thick connective tissue of the iliolumbar ligament, perhaps as a result of the gravitational forces on the lumbar lordosis in the upright posture.

The posterior sacroiliac ligaments lie just anterior to the multifidus muscle and course in two directions to counter the inferior and anterior components of the inferiorly directed trunk force. The posterior sacroiliac ligaments are separated from the next layer, the interosseus ligament, by the dorsal rami of the sacral spinal nerves and the blood vessels that course between the two ligaments. The interosseus ligament is the major stabilizer of the sacroiliac joint and forms the chief bond between the two bones (figure 5.8). Any potential movement between the sacrum and ilium must deform this ligament, which is one of the strongest ligaments in the human body, further illustrating the limited motion available at this joint.

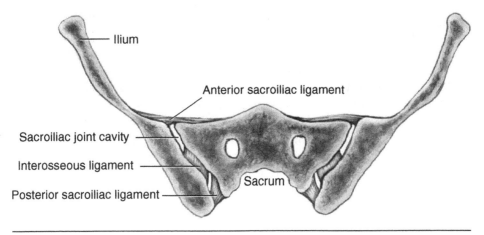

Ilium

Anterior sacroiliac ligament

Sacroiliac joint cavity

Interosseous ligament

Posterior sacroiliac ligament

Sacrum

Figure 5.8 Cross section of the sacroiliac joint, illustrating the location of the interosseous ligament and the joint space.

Adapted from J.A. Porterfield and C. De Rosa, 1998, *Mechanical low back pain,* 2nd ed. (New York: W.B. Saunders).

The sacrotuberous and sacrospinous ligaments are attached to the sacrum and the ischial tuberosity and ischial spine, respectively. Their attachments allow extrinsic stability of the sacrum as it is wedged between the ilia, especially in the upright standing posture. The gluteus maximus takes part of its origin from the sacrotuberous ligament, and the biceps femoris can be seen to blend in with the ligament at the ischial tuberosity. Thus the force of contraction from these strong muscles results in increased tension being imparted to the ligament, which has been suggested as a possible means of dynamic stabilization for the sacroiliac articulation (Porterfield and DeRosa 1998).

Vleeming and colleagues have described the long dorsal sacroiliac ligament and its potential relationship to various low back pain syndromes, including peripartum low back pain (Vleeming et al. 1996; Vleeming et al. 2002). The ligament is anatomically related to the thoracolumbar fascia, erector spinae aponeurosis, and sacrotuberous ligament. It connects the posterior superior iliac spine and a small portion of the iliac crest to the lateral aspect of the sacrum at approximately the S3 and S4 regions, where it is covered by the extensive aponeurosis of the gluteus maximus muscle, which can increase tension in the ligament via contraction. Tension is also increased in the ligament when an extension (counternutation) force is introduced to the sacrum.

MUSCULAR STABILIZATION OF THE TRUNK

It is important to be able to relate trunk muscle activity to the disc and joint mechanics just discussed. Understanding the role of the trunk muscles, and their connections to the key fascial elements linking them to the skeletal framework, allows clinicians to develop scientifically based exercise programs. What follows is a description of the key aspects of the muscle structure, spatial relationships, and function associated with the trunk.

Thoracolumbar Fascia

Most of the muscles of the low back are covered and encased by the thoracolumbar fascia, which is thick and extremely well developed in the low back (Bogduk and Macintosh 1984). The posterior layer of the fascia attaches to the spinous processes and features a superficial and deep lamina coursing in different directions. Besides covering and serving as the posterior wall of the erector spinae and multifidus muscles, the superficial layer serves as the anatomical and biomechanical link between the latissimus dorsi and gluteus maximus muscles (Vleeming et al. 1995). From this attachment the thoracolumbar fascia (TLF) courses laterally and then anteriorly to surround the erector spinae and multifidus muscles of the lumbar spine. Anteriorly it attaches to the lumbar transverse processes (figure 5.9).

The juncture of the posterior layer of thoracolumbar fascia with the relative anterior layer attached to the transverse processes occurs at the lateral aspect of the erector spinae. This juncture is referred to as the lateral raphe. The lateral raphe is attached inferiorly to the iliac crest and laterally blends in with the aponeuroses of the latissimus dorsi, transversus abdominis, and occasionally the internal abdominal oblique.

Considerable attention has been given to the biomechanics of the thoracolumbar fascia. Its attachment to the spinous processes affords it the longest lever arm at the lumbar spine, and it has been suggested that the fascia contributes greatly to the stability of the lumbar spine from the flexed posture (Gracovetsky, Farfan, and Lamy 1981). The attachments of the internal abdominal oblique and transversus abdominis potentially exert a pull on the fascia, increasing its tension and providing stability of the lumbar spine (Gracovetsky, Farfan, and Helleur 1985; Barker, Briggs, and Bogeski 2004). This is one of the key aspects of muscle training for the internal oblique and, in particular, the transversus abdominis. One of the intended outcomes of training is enhancing the ability of the abdominal mechanism to exert a pull on the thoracolumbar fascia, increasing its tension and thus increasing stability between the adjacent bony segments.

The erector spinae and multifidus muscles are encased within the thoracolumbar fascia. It has been suggested that the broadening of the muscles during a contraction can help fill the fascial envelope and further provide an increase in spinal stability through enhanced tension within the thoracolumbar fascia (Farfan 1973; Gracovetsky, Farfan, and Lamy 1981). Finally, the potential of the latissimus dorsi muscle and the gluteus maximus to exert a tensile force on the fascia and thus contribute to stability of the lumbar spine has also been proposed (McGill and Norman 1988).

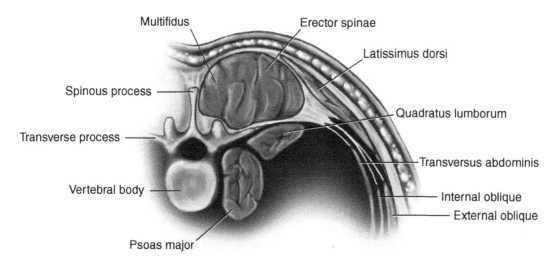

Figure 5.9   Cross section of the lumbar spine showing the attachments of the thoracolumbar fascia. Note how the fascia encases muscles as well as serves as an attachment point for muscles.

It is readily apparent that the thoracolumbar fascia has the potential to contribute to both passive and active stabilization of the lumbar spine by virtue of its bone and muscle attachments. The fascia is a strong tissue with a well-developed latticework of collagen fibers, whose function may be described broadly as that of a type of extensor muscle retinaculum. Exercises focused on training the latissimus dorsi muscle, thus taking advantage of this connection, are shown in table 5.1. Exercises that take advantage of the linkage between the gluteus maximus and thoracolumbar fascia (from easy to more difficult) are shown in table 5.2.

Again, with each of these exercises, the position of the lumbar spine needs to be carefully monitored according to the anatomical principles previously described. Finally, to complete the review of muscles that pull on the thoracolumbar fascia, exercises that take advantage of the linkage between the abdominal obliques and

Table 5.1   Exercises That Train the Latissimus Dorsi Muscle

Exercise	Illustration
Latissimus pull-down	
Seated rowing exercise	
One-arm row	
Overhead pull-over	

Table 5.2 Exercises That Promote the Linkage of the Gluteus Maximus and Thoracolumbar Fascia

Exercise	Illustration	
Simple bridging		
Standing hip extension with selectorized machines providing the overload		
Leg press		
Ball squat		
Back squat		

the transversus abdominis include the abdomen drawing-in maneuver (a prerequisite for all exercises) and the prone and lateral plank exercises (described later in the text).

Erector Spinae

Studies of the erector spinae have clearly demonstrated that these muscles can be divided into two separate anatomical and functional components in the low back: the superficial (thoracic) and deep (lumbar) components (Macintosh and Bogduk 1987). The superficial erector spinae attach to the pelvis and sacrum via the erector spinae aponeurosis and course superiorly to attach to the ribs. The superficial erector spinae can be further subdivided into a lateral iliocostalis lumborum and a medial longissimus thoracis. These two divisions of the superficial erector spinae act over the thoracic vertebrae and ribs, which results in indirect action over the lumbar spine. The lever arm afforded by these two divisions allows the muscles to increase the lumbar lordosis actively. With the trunk nearly completely bent forward, the superficial erector spinae become electromyographically silent as stabilization of the trunk occurs via connective tissue structures such as the fascia and joint capsules (Kippers and Parker 1984).

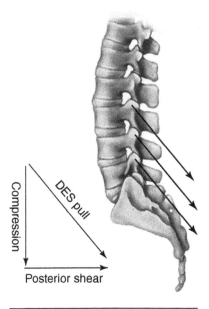

The deep erector spinae can also be subdivided into the lumbar iliocostalis and the lumbar longissimus (Macintosh and Bogduk 1987). These names are chosen because these divisions, which originate on the ilium and lateral aspect of the sacrum, attach directly to the transverse processes of the lumbar vertebrae. Thus, these muscles travel superiorly from the pelvis and course anteriorly and medially (figure 5.10). Because the muscles are attached to the transverse processes, the lever arm for extension is not as great as that of the superficial erector spinae or multifidus muscles. The posterior-to-anterior inclination of the deep erector spinae allows the muscles to exert a posterior shear force over the lumbar vertebrae, providing dynamic stabilization in the form of countering anterior shear in the sagittal plane. Muscular stabilization via an anterior–posterior guy-wire effect is suggested by analysis of the vectors of the psoas major and deep erector spinae (Porterfield and DeRosa 1998). Both divisions of the erector spinae are innervated by branches of the posterior rami.

Figure 5.10 Orientation of the deep erector spinae of the lumbar spine. Note how the muscle vector can be resolved into a compression force over the lumbar spine and a posterior shear force.

Multifidus

The multifidus muscles course the complete length of the spine but are most completely developed in the lumbar spine. These muscles arise from the dorsal surface of the sacrum and, in fact, are the largest soft tissue structures between the skin and the sacrum. The muscles also attach to the mammillary processes and joint capsules of the lumbar vertebrae. From these origins, the muscles insert two to four levels above into the spinous processes. The attachments to the spinous processes give the muscles an excellent lever arm for lumbar extension in addition to their role as stabilizing muscles by increasing the compressive load between

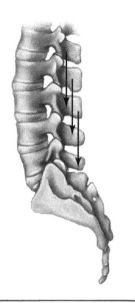

Figure 5.11   Orientation of the multifidus muscle of the lumbar spine. Because of its attachment to the lumbar spinous processes, the muscle has a good lever arm for lumbar extension.

adjacent lumbar segments (figure 5.11). As such, they are exceptional dynamic stabilizers of the lumbar spine as well as the sacroiliac joint and play an important role in the development of the exercise prescription for patients with low back pain (Hungerford, Gilleard, and Hodges 2003; Niemisto and Lahtinen-Suopanki 2003). Retraining of the multifidus muscles is considered an essential part of the rehabilitation process for patients undergoing surgery of the lumbar spine (Hides, Richardson, and Jull 1996).

Although typically described in anatomy textbooks as a rotator of the spine, the multifidus does not have an appreciable lever arm or muscle fiber orientation to be effective in this action. It has also been speculated that the capsular attachment of the muscle allows active retraction of the joint capsule to avoid impingement between the facet surfaces. All the fascicles of the multifidus are innervated by the medial branch of the dorsal ramus.

Extensor Compartment and Its Relationship to Exercise

Because the superficial erector spinae, deep erector spinae, and multifidus muscles are housed within the thoracolumbar fascia, contraction of these muscles results in a broadening effect that increases tension to the fascial network. In addition, relative hypertrophy of these muscles maintains tension on the thoracolumbar fascia via this "pushing" effect, and thus training these large extensor muscles is extremely important, not only in rehabilitation but for sport as well. Exercises (from easy to more difficult) that place an overload on these key lumbar extensors are shown in table 5.3. It is important to note that the pelvis should be supported during lumbar back extension exercises. When the support is placed more distally over the proximal aspect of the femur, the resultant exercise is more pelvis rotation over the hips (action of the hip extensors and hamstrings) instead of motion of the lumbar spine over the pelvis (action of the spinal extensors).

Quadratus Lumborum

Although typically studied with muscles of the posterior abdominal wall, the quadratus lumborum is an important muscle of the low back. From its attachment to the pelvis the muscle courses superiorly, anteriorly, and medially to gain attachments to the 12th rib (iliocostal division) and lumbar transverse processes (iliotransverse division). Occasionally, a 3rd division courses from the 12th rib to the lumbar transverse processes (costotransverse division).

The orientation of the muscle allows it to contribute to stabilization of the lumbar spine in the frontal plane. Stabilization in the frontal plane is important in the lumbar spine because of the coupled axial torsion that occurs with lateral bending. Excessive torsional stresses on the lumbar joints adversely affect the intervertebral discs and the facets of the zygapophyseal joints. Working with such structures as the iliolumbar ligament, psoas major, and lateral abdominal muscles, the quadratus lumborum contributes to lumbar stabilization. The innervation of the muscle is from the 12th thoracic and 1st lumbar nerves.

Table 5.3   Exercises That Place Overload on Key Lumbar Extensors

Exercise	Illustration
Bilateral row over a gymnastics ball	
Lumbar back extension	
Squat	
Variations of the deadlift	

Psoas Major

The psoas major muscles are attached to the anteromedial aspect of the transverse processes, the anterolateral aspect of the bodies of the lumbar vertebrae, and the intervertebral discs. From this attachment the muscle courses inferiorly and descends to join the tendon of the iliac muscle, and together they travel inferiorly and laterally over the pelvic brim to attach to the lesser trochanter. In close relation to the psoas major are the abdominal aorta, inferior vena cava, and most of the large intestine and colon. All these structures are in turn covered by the greater omentum and muscles and fascia of the abdominal wall. The psoas major is obviously a very deeply placed muscle, with numerous visceral structures completely covering its anterior and lateral surfaces.

In addition to being a strong flexor and external rotator of the hip joint, the muscle fiber orientation of the psoas major suggests that it has the potential to exert many different forces on the lumbar spine and indirectly on the pelvis. If the fixed end of the muscle is considered to be the lesser trochanter, psoas major contraction exerts an anterior translational stress on the lumbar vertebrae that is most likely countered by the posteriorly directed vector of the deep erector spinae, causing a check and balance to the lumbar spine in the sagittal plane. The muscle can also cause a resultant anterior torsional moment of the innominate bone at the sacroiliac joint because it descends over the pelvic brim and dives posteriorly to attach to the lesser trochanter.

Furthermore, contraction of the psoas major muscles from a supine position exerts a pull on the lumbar spine, and through indirect action the pelvis can be flexed at the hip joints toward the sitting position. It has already been noted that the psoas major can also contribute to sagittal and frontal plane stability of the lumbar spine. The psoas major is electromyographically active in nearly all postures and movements of the lumbar spine and is innervated by directed branches from the lumbar plexus.

Abdominal Muscles

Because of the many misconceptions about training and strengthening the abdominal muscles, a greater degree of detail in regard to these muscles is provided to give the reader a better three-dimensional appreciation of the anatomy of this important region in order to safely and more effectively develop functional exercise progressions.

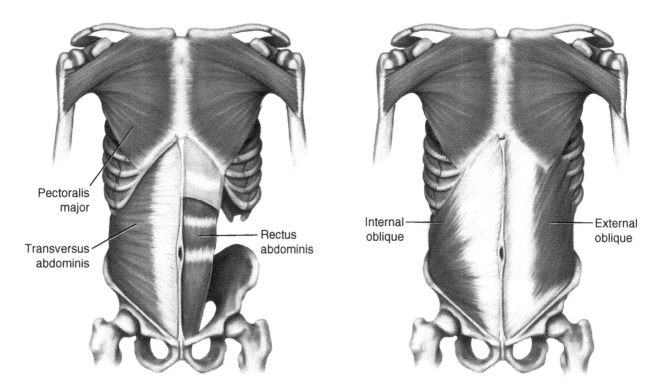

Figure 5.12   The abdominal fascial system. Note how the external abdominal oblique is attached to the lateral aspect of the abdominal fascia. This is the same area of attachment for the internal abdominal oblique and transversus abdominis. The rectus abdominis muscles are encased within the abdominal fascial system. Note also how the pectoralis major muscles are attached to the superolateral aspects of the abdominal fascia.

Abdominal Fascial System

Like the thoracolumbar fascial system of the posterior aspect of the trunk and the fascia lata system associated with the lower extremity, the abdominal fascial system consists of muscles encased within the fascial network (the paired rectus abdominis muscles) and muscles that are attached to the fascial network (the transversus abdominis, internal abdominal oblique, and external abdominal oblique) (figure 5.12). Contraction of the external oblique, internal oblique, and transversus abdominis increases tension to the abdominal fascia, much the same as how the latissimus dorsi and gluteus maximus increase tension to the thoracolumbar fascia.

Just as a powerful shoulder muscle, the latissimus dorsi, exerts a strong pull on the posteriorly placed thoracolumbar fascia in the back, the anteriorly placed pectoralis major exerts a pull on the abdominal fascia via its linkage to the abdominal fascia. Furthermore, another key shoulder girdle muscle, the serratus anterior, interdigitates with the serrated posterior aspect of the external abdominal oblique muscle. These important connections effectively link the powerful shoulder girdle muscles to the abdominal mechanism through the abdominal fascial system. An exercise that takes advantage of the linkage between the pectoralis major and oblique muscles is the cable crossover (see figure 5.13). The motion should include strong shoulder horizontal adduction and protraction, coupled with a safe rotary motion against resistance.

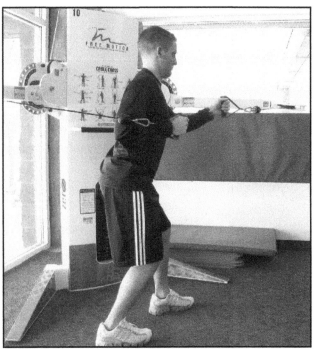

Figure 5.13 The cable crossover exercise illustrates the linkage between the pectoralis major and the oblique muscles.

Rectus Abdominis

The rectus abdominis muscle extends vertically from the pubic tubercles to attach to the lower rib cage on either side of the sternum and features intermuscular connective tissue bands. It is surrounded by its own fascial layer (the rectus sheath), formed by the individual aponeurotic contributions of the transversus abdominis, external oblique, and internal oblique muscles as they converge toward the linea alba. The oblique muscles attach to the rectus sheath at the level of these tendinous intersections, thereby exerting a laterally directed force to the rectus sheath and anchoring these tendinous intersections (figure 5.14). A lateral pull at the intermuscular septa stabilizes the rectus attachments and in essence results in the rectus abdominis functioning segmentally rather than simply as one long strap muscle.

External Abdominal Oblique, Pectoralis Major, and Serratus Anterior

The abdominal muscles are extremely important in regard to stability of the lumbar spine and pelvis. The most superficial muscles contributing to the anterior and anterolateral abdominal wall include the external oblique, the pectoralis major, and

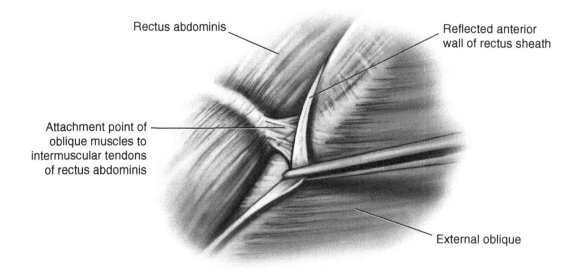

Rectus abdominis

Reflected anterior wall of rectus sheath

Attachment point of oblique muscles to intermuscular tendons of rectus abdominis

External oblique

Figure 5.14   The rectus abdominis muscle has tendons strategically placed within the body of the muscle. Note how the lateral edges of these tendons are effectively "anchored" via the pull of the external abdominal oblique, the internal abdominal oblique, and the transversus abdominis.

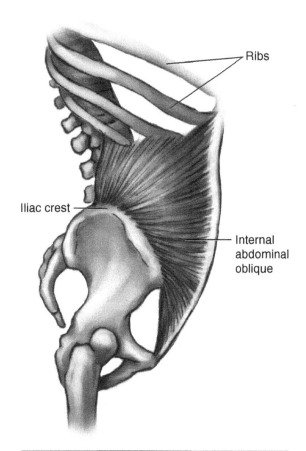

Ribs

Iliac crest

Internal abdominal oblique

Figure 5.15   The internal abdominal oblique courses from the iliac crest toward the ribs. The muscle fiber direction is such that the pull of the muscle brings the pelvis up and forward, such as in running and bounding exercises.

the serratus anterior. The line of pull on the abdominal fascia of the external oblique muscle is cranialward and posterior (figure 5.15). In addition, close inspection of the pectoralis major muscle reveals that its lower attachment is also to the abdominal fascia, and contraction of the pectoralis major also increases the tension to the upper aspect of the abdominal fascia. The pull on the abdominal fascia helps serve as a dynamic check to the anterior shear over the lumbar spine in the upright posture. This is especially important to understand in order to properly perform resistance exercises in the standing position or during compound movements from the upright position. It is important to utilize strong shoulder action during such exercises, in particular, scapular protraction.

Internal Abdominal Oblique

The internal abdominal oblique is a substantial muscle, often thicker than the transversus abdominis or the external oblique. As can be seen in figure 5.15, it has a large attachment to the iliac crest and the thoracolumbar fascia. The more inferiorly placed portion of the muscle exerts a pull on the pelvis, a motion that is medially directed, effectively increasing compression of the pubic symphysis. The superior and middle extent of this muscle can exert a powerful forward and elevation movement of the pelvis, a motion that is essential in sprinting (figure 5.16), for example, or during high-step, bounding types of exercise. The internal oblique powerfully brings the pelvis up and forward, accelerating the swinging leg under the body.

Transversus Abdominis

The transversus abdominis is a key stabilizer of the lumbar spine (Richardson et al. 2002; Hodges 1999; Porterfield and DeRosa 1998). The muscle is optimally aligned for a posterior pull on the abdominal fascial complex (figure 5.17). This posteriorly directed pull, especially around the slightly pressurized abdominal cylinder, complements the more-angled pulls of the external and internal abdominal oblique muscles. This posterior pull combined with the contraction of the diaphragm and the pelvic floor increases intra-abdominal pressure, further assisting in stabilization of the lumbar spine.

Linkage of the Shoulder Girdle and Abdominal Mechanism

Like the linkage of the lower extremity to the trunk muscles, the shoulder girdle is also intimately linked to the abdominal mechanism. On the posterior aspect of the spine, the rhomboid major and minor muscles angle inferiorly and laterally from their origin on the thoracic spinous processes to reach the medial border of the scapula. This region of the scapula also serves as the attachment point for the serratus anterior. As noted already, the serratus interdigitates and is often fused with the external abdominal oblique. If the line of muscle fiber direction of the external abdominal oblique is followed across the midline of the body, it can be seen to lie parallel to the muscle

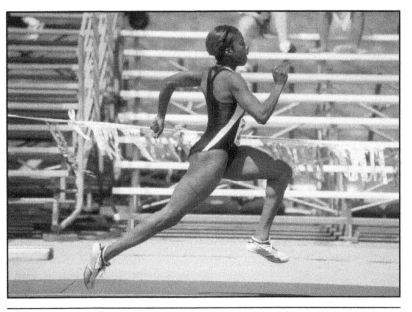

Figure 5.16 When the pelvis is drawn upward and forward vigorously as in running, bounding, or running against a resistance, a strong contraction of the internal abdominal oblique is required owing to its orientation on the swing-side limb.

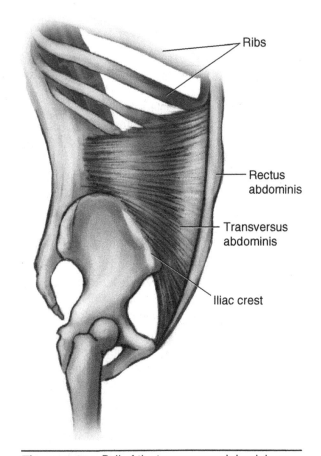

Figure 5.17 Pull of the transversus abdominis on the abdominal fasical network is primarily in a lateral direction, which minimizes the anterior shear over the lumbar spine.

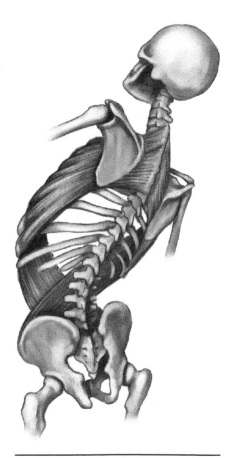

Figure 5.18 Muscle fiber orientation of the rhomboids, serratus anterior, external oblique, and internal oblique. The muscles form a "wrap" around the body much like a shawl draped over the trunk, hence the name "serape" effect. Understanding this line of muscle force helps the clinician appreciate the linkage between the shoulder girdle and the abdominal mechanism.

fiber direction of the contralateral internal abdominal oblique, thus forming a continuous line of muscle fiber orientation from the shoulder girdle to the abdominal wall (figure 5.18).

Most functional anatomy textbooks describe the abdominal muscles as flexors and rotators of the trunk, with the exception of the rectus abdominis, which only flexes the trunk. It is intuitively obvious that in the standing position these muscles do not contribute significantly to this action, because it is the eccentric muscle activity of the spinal and hip extensors that controls the descent of the trunk by decelerating it as gravitational forces cause it to flex forward.

The abdominal muscles are extremely important in controlling the manner in which forces traverse the lumbar spine. Because the abdominal muscles also control the abdominal contents and regulate pelvic position, they directly influence the amount of flexion or extension in the spine. It was noted earlier that compression forces are shared by the vertebral body–disc complex (86%) and the posterior joints (14%). When the line of gravity of the trunk falls too far anterior to the transverse axis of motion of the spine, the resultant forward bending moment must be countered by increasing the amount of lumbar extension. As a postural habit, whether it be a static posture or a dynamic one required for occupation or sport, this has the potential to load the posterior joints excessively. The abdominal muscles offer a dynamic means of controlling the position of the line of gravity of the trunk as well as the sagittal plane position of the lumbar spine, thus helping reduce vulnerability of the lumbar spine. In addition, the abdominal muscles, in particular the transversus abdominis, are extremely important stabilizers of the lumbar spine and pelvis and as such provide the stable base from which the upper and lower extremities function (Richardson et al. 2002; Hodges 1999). The timing of their contraction is carefully sequenced with upper and lower extremity muscle function (Hodges and Richardson 1996).

In summary, there are several key functional roles of the abdominal muscles. These include acting in concert with the pelvic diaphragm, and spinal extensors to form a trunk cylinder; increasing tension to the thoracolumbar and abdominal fascial networks; influencing anterior shear of the lumbar spine by controlling the sagittal plane position of the pelvis; controlling the rate and amplitude of lumbar spine torsion; controlling the frontal plane position of the pelvis during gait; controlling the relationship between the thorax and the abdominal wall; and increasing compression between the sacroiliac and pubic symphysis articulations (Porterfield and DeRosa 1998).

BIOMECHANICS OF THE TRUNK

Several key aspects of spinal mechanics are discussed in the section on anatomy of the trunk, but to better illustrate the function of the spinal components, this section briefly summarizes several biomechanical aspects to consider when developing exercise and functional progression programs related to the spine.

The sacroiliac joint is designed to attenuate the forces of compression, torsion, and shear. Many injuries seen in sport or in activities of daily living are combinations of torque and shear at the joint. Torque is a rotary force of the ilium on the sacrum or the sacrum within the ilia, while shear is a force that is parallel to the joint surfaces. When someone steps into a small hole while running or slips and lands on the ischial tuberosity, an excessive torsional and shear force occurs, potentially resulting in injury to the support ligaments. When this is the injury mechanism, the clinician must carefully monitor exercises, especially those exercises that move the hip joint to end-range positions. When that happen, the resultant tightening of the hip's capsular and muscle tissues results in a transference of the force to the sacroiliac joint—often resulting in further torsional and shear stress to the already injured joint.

The lumbar apophyseal joints are oriented primarily in the sagittal plane and thus primarily resist lumbar rotation. In contrast, this joint plane allows more freedom of motion in flexion and extension. Consequently, the design of exercise and functional progression programs must be such that the rate and amplitude of lumbar torsion are controlled. Unchecked rotary stresses increase the compressive load to the facet joint contralateral to the side rotated, resulting in a potential compression injury to these joints. When guiding an athlete or patient through exercise from the standing position, the clinician must be sure that the primary rotary movement is via the pelvis over the femurs rather than between the lumbar vertebrae or between the fifth lumbar vertebrae and the sacrum. One of the functions of the oblique muscles is to help control the rate and amplitude of lumbar torsion.

Extension of the lumbar spine also increases facet joint compression; as noted earlier in the discussion about fracture of the pars interarticularis, this can result in lumbar spondylolisthesis. Extension and rotation compound the loading to the lumbar facets, with the rotated facet joint on the contralateral side having the greatest compressive load. While the bone–disc interface is built to withstand compressive loads, the facet joints are not. Care must be taken in exercise positions or movements that adversely load these facet joints in compression.

The review of the intervertebral disc in the first section of the chapter delineates the role of the annulus fibrosus and the nucleus pulposus. The biomechanics of the disc are such that the annulus is particularly vulnerable to excessive tensile loads. Therefore, flexion and rotation of the lumbar spine place an increased tensile load on the annular rings, potentially exceeding their viscoelastic capacity. Like any other ligament of the body that is subject to a tensile load it cannot attenuate, the result can be tearing or overstretching of the collagen framework.

In the case of the annulus fibrosus, the resultant problem is twofold. First, there is a loss of stability between adjacent vertebral bodies because of the damage to the annulus. Second, and perhaps slightly more critical, the altered annulus cannot exert an equal and opposite force against the pressure of the nucleus pulposus.

As a result, the nucleus pulposus may "leak" through defects in the annulus and into the spinal canal, irritating the thecal sac and nerve root complex and resulting in signs and symptoms of nerve root irritation. The nucleus pulposus material can also exert pressure against the annulus, causing it to bulge into the spinal canal and mechanically distort structures such as the posterior longitudinal ligament, thecal sac, or lumbosacral nerve roots. These cases can then present with signs and symptoms of either nerve root irritation or nerve root compression. Intradiscal pressure is typically higher when in the sitting position, lower when standing, and even lower when lying down. Since the erector spinae group and the psoas major span the lumbar column, contraction of these muscles further increases intradiscal pressure.

Movement of the trunk is tightly integrated with movement of the extremities. In fact, there is evidence that contraction of trunk muscles occurs even before movement of the extremities begins (Hodges and Richardson 1997a, 1997b; Moseley, Hodges, and Gandevia 2002). This certainly results in a unique perspective regarding the spine when the subject of functional movement patterns is considered. There is often no observable movement pattern of the trunk; instead there is a coordinated contraction of trunk muscles, allowing the axial skeleton to serve as the stable platform from which the upper and lower extremities can act. The central nervous system programs trunk muscle activity, resulting in anticipatory postural adjustments allowing the body to counter the perturbations encountered with throwing, running, jumping, kicking, and so on.

Conversely, there are functional movement patterns in which the trunk moves powerfully in order to allow the distal segment to move effectively. A proximal (from the trunk) to distal development of force occurs, much like the speed and force felt when standing on the peripheral edge of a merry-go-round while it is spinning rapidly as compared with standing closer to the center. Torque generated through the trunk is passed through the proximal bony levers to the distal bony levers of the extremities in much the same manner.

Thus the functional movement patterns of the trunk can be arbitrarily divided into two broad patterns: (1) those patterns that are focused on coordination and precision of trunk muscle activity in order to optimally position the spine and pelvis and (2) those patterns in which the strength, endurance, and power of the trunk muscles are used to generate torque in order to allow for optimal torques and forces to be applied though the extremity levers. Each is trained in a different way, but often both elements are combined when teaching functional movement patterns.

The first pattern—muscle activity designed to optimally position the spine and pelvis—is often a first step in managing the person who has spine pain or is returning to activity after injury to the spine. The key aspects of determining the optimal position of the spine for exercise is described in the section on functional progressions. This aspect of functional movement patterns is largely a motor control phenomenon. Feedforward and feedback information to the central nervous system readies the spinal system to attenuate loads. The normal functional movement pattern of the spine is smooth, coordinated, and sequential. A forward bending motion, for example, involves controlled eccentric muscle activity to allow the pelvis to rotate over the femurs, the last lumbar vertebra to rotate over the sacrum, and the lumbar and thoracic spine to rotate over their subjacent segments. Ultimately, control and balance of the forward bending position are passed from active muscle activity to the connective tissues that support end-range positions of the spinal segments.

Figure 5.18 illustrates this orientation of the muscles from the shoulder girdle, through the trunk, and down to the pelvis. The clinician can appreciate from this perspective the spiral-diagonal muscle fiber orientation. Furthermore, it is easy to recognize that the total spine is geared to multiplanar dynamic movement (i.e., movement simultaneously through the sagittal, frontal, and horizontal planes). In functional training, such combined planar movement must be incorporated instead of uniplanar movement. Throwing is an excellent example of the multiplanar motion of the trunk, as it simultaneously moves from a position of extension, side bending, and lateral flexion to a completed throw position of flexion, rotation to the opposite direction, and lateral flexion to the opposite direction. This winding up and then unwinding via the lengthening and subsequent shortening of the musculature allow the muscles to serve as prime movers over several spinal joints simultaneously, ultimately producing force at the trunk and transfering the force and motion to the distal terminal segment (in this case, the upper extremity).

INJURIES

In most injuries to the spine, the precise anatomical structure involved cannot be identified. Nerve root conditions, however, do have a much greater chance of being identified because the signs and symptoms of nerve root irritation and nerve root compression are fairly well understood. When a person has leg pain greater than spine pain, when a straight-leg raise reproduces leg pain, when the pain pattern is clearly demarcated over lower extremity dermatomes, and when pain results in excessive radiation into the lower extremities with gentle spinal motion, the clincian can reasonably assume that a radicular disorder—inflammation of the nerve root—is the problem. When there is even greater compromise of the nerve root, signs such as muscle weakness in the related myotome, sensory loss in the related dermatome, reflex changes, or muscle atrophy are all strong indicators of nerve root injury. Thus, one of the first issues to clarify in the examination is whether the case is presenting as a radicular disorder or a nonradicular disorder.

Nerve root injuries are typically caused by chemical or mechanical irritation of the root complex within the spinal canal. There are several mechanisms. Perhaps the most common is intervertebral disc injury. As noted already, the intervertebral disc is often injured by excessive flexion and rotation of the spine. This potentially damages the posterior annulus, allowing the nucleus pulposus to cause an inflammatory response in the nerve root.

Another sequelae of disc injury is instability. Just as the loss of the capsular restraints of the glenohumeral joint result in excessive translation of the humerus and glenoid, so too can damage to the annulus fibrosus result in excessive translation of the adjacent vertebral segments. When instability of the spine results, the architecture of the spinal canal and intervertebral foramen change, potentially resulting in nerve root compromise.

The apophyseal joints can also be sources of pain in the low back as well as referred pain into the lower extremities. As noted earlier in the chapter, the apsophyseal joints can be involved with pain syndromes such as overloading of the subchondral bone trabeculae, microfractures of bone trabeculae, mechanical deformation or chemical irritation of joint capsule nociceptors, internal derangements from joint loose bodies, vascular disturbances in the bone or soft tissues, and joint inflammation. Referred pain such as that from involvement of the apopshyseal joints is different from radicular pain in that it is characterized by spine pain being worse than leg pain, while radicular pain is characterized by leg pain being greater than spine pain. Apophyseal joint injury can occur with extension rotary stresses or end-range flexion and rotary stresses. These joints are quite small, and they cannot tolerate large compression loads. Injury can result in subchondral bone fracture or articular cartilage fissuring. This typically results in a decreased capability of the joints to tolerate loading—a condition resulting in early-onset degenerative joint changes. Besides being a source of pain themselves, degenerative changes of the joint can result in altered architecture of the intervertebral foramen and the lateral recess of the spinal canal. Both these conditions can result in compromise to the nerve root complex or the vasculature supplying the nerve root complex.

Trauma directly to the spine or trauma resulting in excessive motion of the spine can result in bony fracture. Particularly susceptible areas of fracture include the vertebral body, pars interarticularis, facet, and pedicle. Since the pars, facet, and pedicle are all part of the posterior neural arch, and the major muscles acting to stabilize the spine are attached to the neural arch, spinal mechanics are compromised with any fracture. Most important, however, fracture of the spine can result in compromise of the neural tissues within the spinal canal and the intervertebral foramen.

Spondylolisthesis, one of the most common injuries to the spine in athletics, has already been detailed in preceding sections. This injury to the pars interarticularis potentially results in an instability between adjacent spinal segments. Spondylolisthesis alters the shape and volume of the intervertebral foramen, thus potentially compromising the thecal sac, the nerve root, or the dorsal root ganglion at that segmental level.

The disc itself can also be a source of pain and should be suspected when pain is primarily centrally located but has a history of shifting to left of center and right of center. Facet joint pain and muscle pain will typically present as unilateral pain, which makes their presentations subtly different from discogenic pain. The disc is a central structure of the spine, and its pain is typically related as such. Imaging studies and invasive disc testing such as discography, however, are typically needed to confirm disc involvement.

Muscles can also be a source of pain and can also refer pain into the lower extremities. Unfortunately, the diagnosis of muscle strain is often given when the clinical presentation is unclear. Advances in imaging technology will no doubt increase the accuracy of muscle strain diagnoses in spinal conditions. Muscle spasm and muscle guarding are very common sequelae with many back injuries, and it is difficult to discern true muscle injury from the protective muscle guarding that often occurs with joint, disc, or nerve root injury.

FUNCTIONAL TESTING OF THE TRUNK

This section considers how to assess trunk function in order to develop exercise progressions, keeping the previous detail of the specialized lumbopelvic connective tissues, muscle anatomy, and biomechanics in mind. Many factors come into play when considering testing of the trunk. To develop a training program as specific as possible for the required need, the clinician must not only consider the activity to be performed but also understand and account for the biological factors.

The normal attenuation of loads through the lumbar spine must be such that the load does not exceed the physiological capacity of the tissues. If the load exceeds the physiological capacity of any of the specialized connective tissue elements, such as the articular cartilage of the facet or the collagenous framework of the annulus fibrosus, then injury results—in particular, damage to the specialized connective tissues associated with the lumbopelvic region. Load attenuation is determined by many factors, but two of the most important to consider are age and injury. Both decrease the ability of the tissues to attenuate loads. Injured or aged tissue does not have the same capacity to attenuate loads, and exercise programs and functional progressions must take this into account.

One of the main reasons that people drop out of individualized exercise programs is simply because the program made their particular musculoskeletal problem worse rather than better. This is especially true with the low back, as the wrong exercise or faulty exercise technique can load the spinal segment excessively, beyond its physiological loading capacity, resulting in pain or—worse—exacerbation of previous injury. Therefore, understanding the mechanics of the lumbar spine and pelvis, especially when prescribing or implementing resistance exercises, is paramount to success.

A functional exercise progression for someone who does not have a history of low back pain should still take into account the previously described biomechanics. However, it is rare for a person to never have a course of back pain in his or her life. Low back discomfort is common and indeed in many ways can be considered normal for humans. So at least a screening process before developing an exercise progression is warranted for most people. One of the major differences in the examination of the low back as compared with the examination of the extremities is that in more than 85% of all cases, the precise anatomical cause of low back pain cannot be identified. Therefore, when examining a person who has a history of back pain, the clinician should focus primarily on identifying the motions, positions, and mechanical stresses that reproduce familiar pain.

The scope of this text is not to detail a complete low back physical examination, and the reader is referred to other resources for that information (Porterfield and DeRosa 1998). However, if a client has a history of back pain or a previous injury to the low back, it behooves the health care professional to perform an examination of the low back that attempts to identify the pathomechanics of the syndrome. In the absence of any history of low back pain, exercise prescription and functional progressions must still follow the principles outlined in regard to lumbopelvic biomechanics.

With all this in mind, the clinician can perform region-specific and functional testing of the lumbopelvic area. Region-specific testing involves localized testing, primarily through the introduction of manual stresses, and the region can be tested with specific tasks and movements. The first level of screening primarily tests the ability to attenuate loads rather than performance capabilities. Therefore, the first step in designing functional progressions for the lumbopelvic region is to determine its ability to attenuate loads, thus allowing for the development of safe and effective progression to functional training.

Specific testing of the lumbopelvic region helps the clinician determine how rigorous an exercise program can be and perhaps what exercises might be contraindicated because of their potential to exacerbate a condition. This is true whether the person is a high-level athlete or a patient in the clinic presenting with low back pain. The assumption from this point on is that the reader has completed the necessary history, and if needed, appropriate diagnostic testing has been completed in order to rule in or rule out lumbopelvic pathology. A suggested battery of tests to quickly screen for any pathomechanical problems associated with the lumbopelvic region is included in table 5.4. A positive finding for pain, unexplained pain, unexplained limitations of motion, or excessive or aberrant motion warrant a complete examination of the lumbopelvic region.

Table 5.4   Pathomechanical Tests for Examination of the Lumbopelvic Region

Position	Test
Supine	Hip range of motion Shear stress to sacroiliac joint Straight-leg raise
Sitting	Slump test Lumbar extension and flexion Lumbar rotation
Prone	Posterior–anterior lumbar spring Sacral spring Hip range of motion
Standing	Forward bending in all quadrants Backward bending in all quadrants Forward and backward bending with overpressure

Functional testing is important because it assesses the lumbopelvic region's ability to simultaneously meet the demands of mobility and stability. The specialized connective tissues such as cartilage of the facet joints, the supporting ligaments, and the intervertebral discs must attenuate the loads they are subjected to as a result of movement and muscle contraction. Muscle contraction is essential because it creates a stiffening effect over the spine, thereby increasing its stability. Simply stated, a spine devoid of musculature has little inherent stability and collapses. In the broadest and most practical sense, stability refers to the neuromotoric control of the trunk that allows it to serve as a stable yet constantly adjusting platform from which extremity motions occur.

The key muscles of the trunk include the abdominal muscles, the superficial and deep spinal extensor mechanism, and the multifidus muscles, all collectively referred to as "the core." The functional progressions described in the latter part of this chapter focus primarily on these muscle groups. The importance of spinal, or core, stabilization has not only received a great deal of attention in the therapeutic exercise literature but permeates the lay literature as well. Indeed, numerous infomercials and fitness magazines tout exercise programs designed to maximize core strength.

Some advocates of core strengthening programs attempt to isolate muscles locally and globally based on Bergmark's classic mechanical engineering model (Bergmark 1989). Local muscles refer to the smaller muscles such as interspinales, segmental multifidi, and intertransversarii, while the global muscles refer to the more-superficial trunk muscles that have longer lever arms and are thus able to generate greater amounts of torque. Although some batteries of tests and resultant exercise programs purport to specifically assess or train the local or global muscles, it is far more likely that the more-complex functional progressions, and the exercise programs that subsequently develop, place demands on both groups of muscles simultaneously. Cholewicki and McGill note that no single muscle, either global or local, predominates in terms of stability of the lumbar spine; instead, a combination of trunk muscles is responsible for core strength and thus spinal stability (Cholewicki and McGill 1996). Therefore, instead of focusing on training individual small muscles, trunk and core assessment and strengthening are more a function of analyzing movement and then developing and training motor patterns that utilize well-coordinated, synchronous activation of axial and appendicular skeletal muscles (Kavic, Grenier, and McGill 2004).

Similarly, there is no single abdominal exercise that places a maximal challenge simultaneously on all components of the abdominal mechanism. Ultimately, as with any other region of the musculoskeletal system, ideal exercises are those that overload the neuromuscular system in order to stimulate the necessary anatomical and biochemical changes while at the same time placing minimal joint loads over the region in order to spare the articular cartilage and other specialized connective tissues.

Forces converge on the lumbar spine from activities as simple as coughing to those as complex as the Olympic clean and jerk. Thus there are nearly infinite combinations of motions and activities that can be used as functional tests. Many of the higher-level tests require a coordinated effort between the axial skeletal muscles (abdominal mechanism and trunk extensors) and the appendicular skeletal muscles (muscles of the lower and upper extremity). Since the combination of tests is so extensive, it is often important to consider the sport or work activity in question and then design specific functional tests that mimic the required activity. Many of the functional tests used can then be incorporated as a component of an exercise and functional progression program.

Although functional testing and functional progression often overlap in regard to training to optimize trunk function, for the purposes of this chapter, functional testing is largely the building blocks, or key components, of the more-complex tasks. For example, lying supine over a gymnastics ball and attempting to maintain a stable position of the lumbar spine while simultaneously extending one hip and flexing the contralateral upper extremity may serve as a functional test to assess the coordination and strength capabilities of the axial–appendicular linkage because such integration is an essential element for numerous sport movements. It is "functional" because it asks for a motor activity that requires coordination of numerous muscles. However, even though coordination of the trunk and appendicular muscles is essential for nearly all activities, the functional test itself is not an activity that is commonly performed in daily living or in sport. Despite such limitations, it is often prescribed as an exercise regimen or part of a functional progression in and of itself.

This should be distinguished from functional training, which is largely repetition of an actual skill activity. An example might help illustrate the continuum. The complete process for developing, implementing, reassessing, and further improving one's ability to perform the Olympic clean and jerk might be seen as follows:

- Pathomechanical screen of the relevant musculoskeletal regions associated with the Olympic clean and jerk
- Breakdown of the activity into essential components (pull from the floor, pushing through the heels, strong shrug, fast split, and so on)
- Functional testing of individual components (the building blocks) of the activity (ability to do a proper squat; lumbar extension strength; ability to reach necessary shoulder girdle, spine, and hip ROM; speed one can drop into a split; and so on)
- Incorporation of specific exercises based on results of functional testing that repeat those tests (they now become exercises), with gradually increasing neuromotoric challenges, as well as supplementation with additional exercises that provide overload to the same muscle groups required for the activity;

for example, modified deadlifts (strengthening of the hamstrings and hip extensors), back extensions (strengthening of the spinal extensors), and plank exercises (strengthening of the abdominal mechanism) now become part of the exercise program

- Functional training, which is the specific activity of the Olympic clean and jerk in which adjustments to form and posture are continually made to improve the precision of the activity, in addition to gradually applying overload to the lift itself to improve the level of performance
- Using the Olympic clean and jerk as a functional test and part of a functional progression in and of itself (e.g., for a football player who is attempting to improve explosive power, gain strength, and so on), even though the Olympic clean and jerk may qualify as functional training because the established goal is to improve the lift itself

The clinician can thus see how overlap between the terminology might occur depending on the end goal. This is especially true with the trunk since it serves as the foundation for functional progressions of the upper and lower extremity.

This section provides examples of tests and related exercises focused on trunk activity that can be used anywhere along the continuum, from rehabilitation to improvement of high-level athletic performance. The clinician will notice that with many tests and exercises, it is not possible to isolate the trunk. Instead, since the trunk serves as a stable yet dynamic platform for extremity motion, attention to spine posture and motion during extremity motion, particularly when overload is applied, becomes the focus.

A prerequisite for training the trunk is to be assured that the person can contract the abdominal mechanism satisfactorily and that proper breathing patterns are maintained regardless of the activity. The first point—contracting the abdominal mechanism satisfactorily—is a logical place to begin trunk training. With an understanding of the muscle fiber orientation of the transversus abdominis, it becomes clear that concentric contraction of this muscle results in a "hollowing" of the abdominal wall. We teach the patient as well as the athlete the same preliminary maneuver—pull the abdomen in away from one's belt line. This is not an action that should result in flexion or extension of the spine. The abdomen drawing-in maneuver increases tension to the thoracolumbar fascia and together with the pelvic diaphragm muscles provides a more stable lumbopelvic platform.

In many ways, this preliminary training is similar to the core awareness concept of many of the adjunct training programs such as Pilates and yoga. The center of gravity of the body is located in the lower aspect of the lumbopelvic region (approximately S2 level), and the ability to contract and then fully relax within this region builds proprioceptive awareness of trunk position. Competitive lifters for example, are first taught this lower abdominal postural awareness exercise, and then it is incorporated into their training and their competitive lifting by having them properly "set the abdominal muscles" before performing their explosive lifts.

Breathing during various trunk exercises is often subjected to a wide range of interpretation and misinterpretations. From an anatomical perspective, the contraction of the abdominal muscles results in an increase in intra-abdominal pressure, which is part of the expiratory phase of respiration. In contrast, relaxation of the abdominal mechanism better allows for descent of the thoracic diaphragm, which is part of the inspiratory phase of respiration. Therefore, when observing an exercise, the clinician would typically encourage expiration during the most active phase of abdominal muscle contraction. For example, during a classic curl-up, the exhalation phase is most logical during the curl-up (concentric contraction of the abdominal muscles) because that is the period when abdominal muscle contraction is at its peak.

Combining these two elements—drawing in the abdomen while simultaneously exhaling—is a very good first step in teaching lower abdominal and lumbopelvic awareness. It contributes to the development of motor control over the region and serves as an essential relaxation exercise through a rhythmical and anatomically based breathing pattern. This technique is often very difficult for a person who is hurried in his exercise program or who is rushing to increase the resistance of the exercise too quickly without understanding the importance of proper technique and posture to render the activity safe and maximally effective.

Typically, exercise programs progress from simple to complex and from minimal weight-bearing postures to full weight-bearing, dynamic activities. This is one of the important aspects of functional progression to consider with the trunk. The lumbar spine is least loaded in compression in the supine, prone, and side-lying position. In addition, there is typically less shear stress over the lumbar spine in these positions than in the upright antigravity postures. However, the clinician should ultimately progress the activity to the antigravity postures and begin to experiment with increasing loading conditions in order to best prepare the person for sport and activities of daily living.

FUNCTIONAL EXERCISE TESTS AND PROGRESSIONS

Several components of the functional progressions for the spine serve as building blocks for more-advanced and demanding exercises. They help develop a sense of proprioceptive and kinesthetic awareness of the lumbopelvic region. Although some of these exercises are prescribed with the instruction to maintain the spine in a particular position, that instruction is a bit misleading to the client or the athlete. The spine is built for movement, and in the sagittal plane, that movement is extensive—approximately 25° at the lumbosacral junction and 20° at the L4–L5 interface. That is a significant amount of motion just between those two segments. The goal of exercise prescription for the trunk is ultimately to develop neuromotoric control over motion velocity and position of the spine and to maintain invulnerable positions of the spine during functional activity.

From this basic core, the more-functional and sport-specific progressions can be built on. Many require a higher level of trunk muscle control, and because they challenge the lumbopelvic region at a higher level, they are often incorporated as functional exercises within functional training programs. It is extremely important that the clinician keep the essential biomechanical principles in mind because the potential for injury to the spine is greater with this level of testing and exercise progression than in the previous group. Of particular note is the potential for excessive torsional loading to the lumbar spine, excessive shear stress to the lumbar spine, and excessive torsional loading of the sacroiliac joint.

An overview of the tests makes it apparent that many require coordinated activity between the trunk and the extremities and thus cross over as functional tests for these regions. A key consideration is determining the weak link if difficulty with the test occurs. The experienced observer must carefully assess the complete motion pattern of the functional test and analyze whether failure to perform the test (or the exercise) is because of deficits associated with the trunk, the lower extremity, or a combination of both. From that point, the examiner must determine the actual deficit itself (e.g., motion, strength, endurance, proprioception, coordination), further break down the functional test to a smaller component level (one of the building blocks of the complex task), and then retest and train according to those examination findings.

The functional progressions in this section of the text provide detailed instructions for the person performing the exercise. Primary muscle groups, indications, contraindications, and pearls of performance are presented to guide the clinician. Some of the exercise progressions contain stages that provide further progression between groupings of exercises.

Quadruped Lumbar Range of Motion

PROGRESSION NAME: Lumbopelvic Flexion and Extension

STAGE: Initial stages of return to activity and kinesthetic awareness training of lumbar spine and hip positions

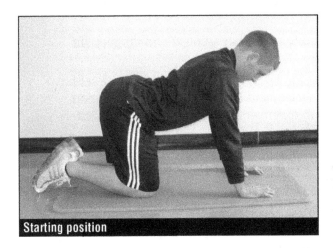

Starting position

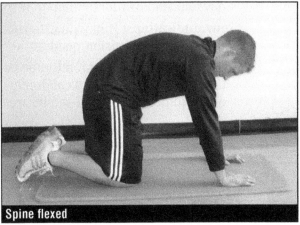

Spine flexed

Starting position: Begin in the quadruped position, with equal support on the hands and knees. The lumbar spine is extended.

Exercise action: Move the lumbar spine toward full flexion and simultaneously rotate the pelvis around the hips.

Primary muscle groups: Abdominal mechanism, trunk extensors, hip flexors, hip extensors

Indications: Teaches safe range of flexion and extension for the lumbar spine

Contraindications: Reproduction of pain at end ranges

Pearls of performance: Ensure the patient maintains sagittal plane motion and does not rotate the lumbar spine during movement.

Crossed Extremity Stability Strengthening

PROGRESSION NAME: Trunk Stability Training With Dynamic Extremity Motion

STAGE: Initial stages of trunk training to develop kinesthetic awareness of trunk position

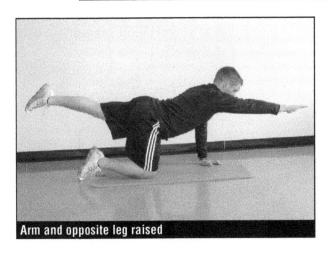

Arm and opposite leg raised

Starting position: Begin in the quadruped position, with equal support on the hands and knees. The lumbar spine is at midrange between lumbar flexion and extension.

Exercise action: Lift one arm and then return to starting position. Extend one hip and then return to starting position. Raise contralateral arm and leg and then return to starting position.

(continued)

Crossed Extremity Stability Strengthening   *(continued)*

Primary muscle groups: Shoulder flexors, scapulothoracic retractors, spine extensors, deep spine stabilizers, abdominal obliques, hip extensors, hamstrings

Indications: Improves coordination of trunk–extremity synergy, especially to develop stabilization potential of trunk musculature

Contraindications: Pain with extension testing of lumbar spine at end range; pain with lumbar extension quadrant testing

Pearls of performance: Monitor the patient for correct form. Watch for rotation of the spine (caused by weak abdominal muscles) and hyperextension and rotation of the lumbar spine (caused by weak hip extensors); both should be avoided.

Prone Plank

PROGRESSION NAME: Plank positions

STAGE: Beginning to intermediate

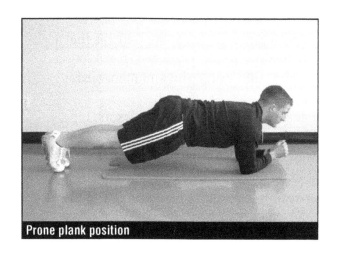

Prone plank position

Starting position: Start in the prone position supported by the elbows and feet, your body off the ground.

Exercise action: Hold this position isometrically. The starting positions can be varied from flexion of the lumbar spine to extension of the lumbar spine. From any starting position, the action is to hold the position until fatigue results in loss of position.

Primary muscle groups: Shoulder girdle, abdominal mechanism, spine extensors and stabilizers, hip flexors and extensors

Indications: Strengthens the trunk musculature; improves ability to maintain spine or scapula positioning

Contraindications: Shoulder instability

Pearls of performance: As with most isometric strengthening activities, the starting position should be varied in order to train muscles at several joint ranges.

Side Plank

PROGRESSION NAME: Plank Positions

STAGE: Beginning to intermediate

Starting position: Start in the side position supported by the elbow and feet, your body off the ground.

Exercise action: Hold this position isometrically. The starting positions can be varied from right or left lateral flexion of the lumbar spine. From any starting position, the action is to hold the position until fatigue results in loss of position.

Primary muscle groups: Shoulder girdle, abdominal mechanism, spine extensors and stabilizers, hip flexors and extensors

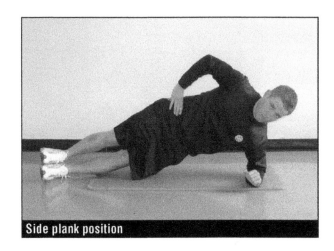

Side plank position

Indications: Strengthens the trunk musculature; improves ability to maintain spine or scapula positioning

Contraindications: Shoulder instability

Pearls of performance: As with most isometric strengthening activities, the starting position should be varied in order to train muscles at several joint ranges.

Active Trunk Extension I

PROGRESSION NAME: Dynamic Trunk Extension

STAGE: Beginning to intermediate

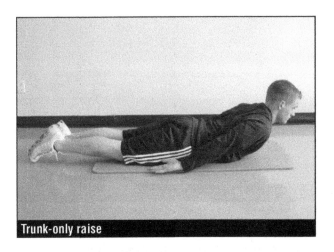

Trunk-only raise

Starting position: Start in the prone position, your arms at your sides.

Exercise action: Retract the scapulae and lift your head, neck, and thoracic cage.

Primary muscle groups: Scapula retractors, spine extensors for scapula and spinal motion , hip extensors for stabilizing pelvis

Indications: Strengthens the trunk extensors

Contraindications: Pain with extension testing of lumbar spine at end range; radicular pain with lumbar extension testing

Pearls of performance: A strong scapular retraction motion is a key to initiating spine extensor muscle contraction.

Active Trunk Extension II

PROGRESSION NAME: Dynamic Trunk Extension

STAGE: Beginning to intermediate

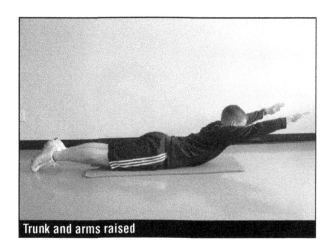

Trunk and arms raised

Starting position: Start in the prone position, your arms overhead.

Exercise action: Retract the scapulae and lift your head, neck, arms, and thoracic cage.

Primary muscle groups: Scapula retractors, spine extensors for scapula and spinal motion, hip extensors for stabilizing pelvis

Indications: Strengthens the trunk extensors

Contraindications: Pain with extension testing of lumbar spine at end range; radicular pain with lumbar extension testing

Pearls of performance: Arms overhead results in a longer lever arm over the lumbar spine, thus increasing the demand of the lumbar extensors to complete the action.

Active Trunk Extension III

PROGRESSION NAME: Dynamic Trunk Extension

STAGE: Beginning to intermediate

Starting position: Start in the prone position, your arms overhead.

Exercise action: Retract the scapulae and lift your head, neck, shoulders, thoracic cage, and lower extremities.

Primary muscle groups: Scapula retractors, spine extensors for scapula and spinal motion; hip extensors for hip motion

Indications: Strengthens the trunk extensors

Contraindications: Pain with extension testing of lumbar spine at end range; radicular pain with lumbar extension testing

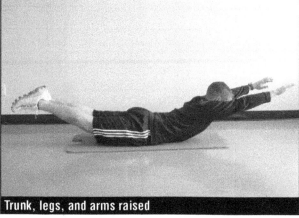

Trunk, legs, and arms raised

Pearls of performance: Monitor the patient for correct form. The spine should move in the saggital plane; extension and lumbar rotation should be avoided.

Supine Bilateral Hip and Trunk Extension

PROGRESSION NAME: Dynamic Trunk Extension

STAGE: Beginning

Starting position: Start in the supine position, with your hips and knees flexed and supported over a support apparatus such as a bolster or gymnastics ball.

Exercise action: Pushing through the legs, raise your hips, thereby extending them and moving the lumbar spine from the starting position of flexion to a neutral or slightly extended end position.

Primary muscle groups: Hip extensors, abdominal muscles to control trunk rotation, spine extensors

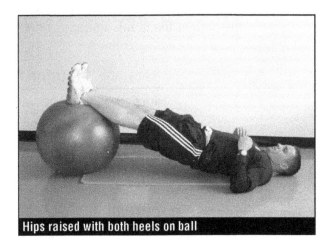

Hips raised with both heels on ball

Indications: Initial training of trunk and hip extensors when the lumbar spine is too painful to be trained from a weight-bearing position and when lumbar spine compression should be avoided

Contraindications: Pain at end-range flexion of the lumbar spine

Pearls of performance: Monitor the patient for correct form. The spine should move in the sagittal plane; lumbar rotation should be avoided.

Supine Unilateral Hip and Trunk Extension

PROGRESSION NAME: Dynamic Trunk Extension

STAGE: Beginning to intermediate

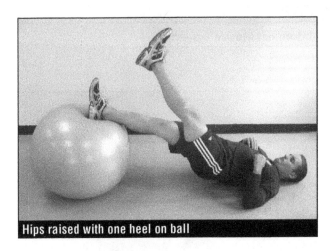

Hips raised with one heel on ball

Starting position: Start in the supine position, with your hips and knees flexed and supported over a support apparatus such as a bolster or gymnastics ball.

Exercise action: Pushing through one leg, raise your hips, thereby extending them and moving the lumbar spine from the start position of flexion to a neutral or slightly extended end position.

Primary muscle groups: Hip extensors, abdominal muscles to control trunk rotation, spine extensors

Indications: Initial training of trunk and hip extensors when the lumbar spine is too painful to be trained from a weight-bearing position and when lumbar spine compression should be avoided

(continued)

Supine Unilateral Hip and Trunk Extension   *(continued)*

Contraindications: Pain at end-range flexion of the lumbar spine

Pearls of performance: The unilateral push places torque over the lumbar spine, which must be countered by strong abdominal muscle contraction. Watch that the patient maintains motion in the sagittal plane and avoids lumbar rotation.

Supine Trunk Curl

PROGRESSION NAME: Dynamic Abdominal Muscle Training

STAGE: Beginning

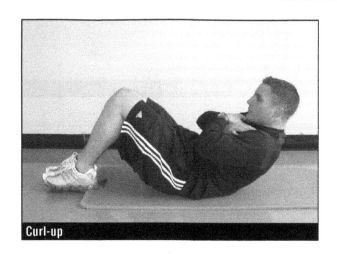

Curl-up

Starting position: Start in the supine position, with your hips and knees flexed.

Exercise action: Lift your head, neck, and thoracic cage from the floor so that the thoracic cage moves toward the pelvis.

Primary muscle groups: Abdominal muscles, especially the rectus abdominis

Indications: initial training of abdominal mechanism

Contraindications: Discogenic pain; radicular pain; compression injuries of the lumbar vertebral body

Pearls of performance: Monitor the motion of the thoracic cage as it moves toward the pelvis to ensure contraction of the rectus abdominis muscles.

Supine Trunk Curl With Active Straight-Leg Raise

PROGRESSION NAME: Dynamic Abdominal Muscle Training

STAGE: Intermediate

Starting position: Start in the supine position, with your hips and knees flexed.

Exercise action: Lift your head, neck, and thoracic cage from the floor so that the thoracic cage moves toward the pelvis. Perform a straight-leg raise to maintain complete knee extension and active ankle dorsiflexion.

Primary muscle groups: Abdominal muscles, especially the rectus abdominis; hip flexors, knee extensors, ankle dorsiflexors

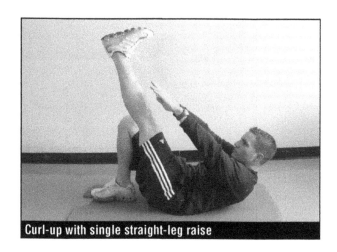

Curl-up with single straight-leg raise

Indications: Training abdominal mechanism to stabilize lumbar spine during lower extremity motion; an active neural mobilization maneuver

Contraindications: Discogenic pain; radicular pain; compression injuries of the lumbar vertebral body

Pearls of performance: If the patient feels radiating pain in the lower extremity at any point of the leg raise, the progression should be avoided.

Diagonal Bilateral Leg Lowering

PROGRESSION NAME: Dynamic Abdominal Muscle Training

STAGE: Intermediate to advanced

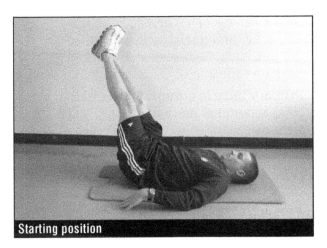
Starting position

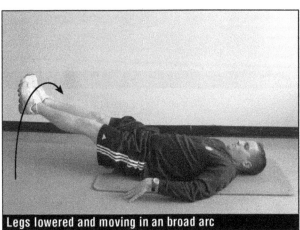
Legs lowered and moving in an broad arc

Starting position: Start in the supine position with the hips flexed, keeping a straight-leg raise position bilaterally, arms out in abduction and shoulders externally rotated in order to place the latissimus dorsi and thoracolumbar fascia in a more-elongated position.

Exercise action: Lower your legs diagonally toward the floor, moving the legs toward one side and then in a broad arc toward the opposite side.

Primary muscle groups: Abdominal muscles to stabilize pelvis, hip flexors, abductors, adductors, extensors to control rate and descent of lower extremities

Indications: Strengthens the abdominal muscles

Contraindications: Discogenic pain; compression injuries of the lumbar vertebral body; pain with lumbar extension or rotation overpressure in pathomechanical exam

Pearls of performance: This maneuver further develops the isometric capacities of the abdominal mechanism.

Walking Lunge

PROGRESSION NAME: Core and Extremity Functional Strength Training

STAGE: Intermediate to advanced

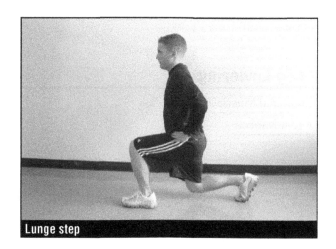

Lunge step

Starting position: Stand with the lumbar spine in a neutral position.

Exercise action: Step out with one leg, keeping the spine upright and shoulders retracted. The lunge foot should strike the ground with the heel. Upon striking with the heel, immediately move your foot to the foot-flat position. At foot flat, the pelvis descends straight down by simultaneous extension of the low back, flexion of the hip, and flexion of the knee.

Primary muscle groups: Spine extensors, abdominal mechanism, hip and knee extensors

Indications: Improves strength and coordination of the trunk and lower extremities

Contraindications: Sacroiliac injuries

Pearls of performance: Monitor the patient for correct form. The trunk pitching forward during the descent indicates weakness of the spinal extensors.

Walking Push Press With Free Weight

PROGRESSION NAME: Core and Extremity Functional Strength Training

STAGE: Advanced

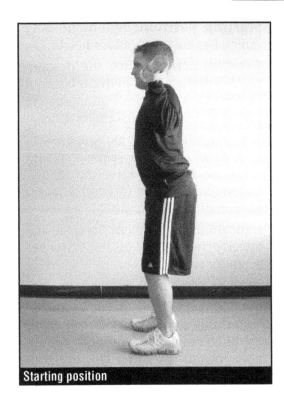

Starting position

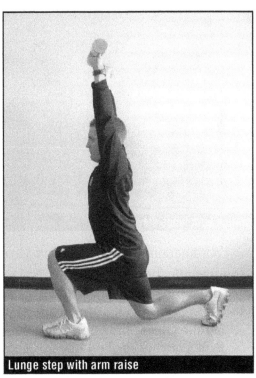

Lunge step with arm raise

Starting position: Stand, holding weights at shoulder height.

Exercise action: With the descent portion of the lunge, press the weight directly overhead.

Primary muscle groups: Spinal extensors, shoulder flexors, scapula upward rotators, hip and knee extensors, abdominal muscles to control rotary motion of lumbar spine

Indications: Strengthens the spine and lower extremity extensors; improves coordination between trunk and lower extremity extensors

Contraindications: Sacroiliac pain; lumbar extension quadrant testing pain; limitation in lumbar extension range of motion

Pearls of performance: This exercise requires a strong spine extensor contraction and the ability of the lumbar spine to move to end range of extension without pain. Inability of the lumbar spine to move toward full extension results in excessive loading of the thoracic spine.

Walking Push Press From Low Pulley Position

PROGRESSION NAME: Core and Extremity Functional Strength Training

STAGE: Advanced

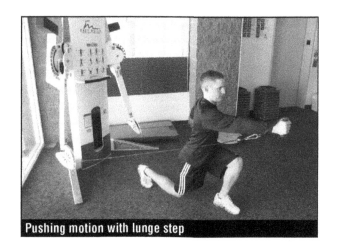

Pushing motion with lunge step

Starting position: Stand, holding pulley handles at shoulder height.

Exercise action: With the descent portion of the lunge, perform bilateral pulley pushing motions or alternately perform unilateral pushing motions.

Primary muscle groups: Spinal extensors, shoulder flexors, scapula upward rotators, hip and knee extensors, abdominal muscles to control rotary motion of lumbar spine

Indications: Strengthens the spine and lower extremity extensors; improves coordination between trunk and lower extremity extensors

Contraindications: Sacroiliac pain; lumbar extension quadrant testing pain; limitation in lumbar extension range of motion

Pearls of performance: This exercise requires a strong spine extensor contraction and the abilty of the lumbar spine to move to end range of extension without pain. Inability of the lumbar spine to move toward full extension results in excessive loading of the thoracic spine. The unilateral pushing motions place additional performance demands on the oblique muscles and the serratus anterior.

Walking Lunge With Medicine Ball Rotations

PROGRESSION NAME: Core and Extremity Functional Strength Training

STAGE: Advanced

Starting position: Stand, holding a medicine ball in front of your body.

Exercise action: With the descent portion of the lunge, rotate the medicine ball toward the right or left side. Upon return to the upright position, bring the medicine ball back to center.

Primary muscle groups: Spinal extensors to counter the flexion and rotary moment over the lumbar spine, shoulder flexors, scapula

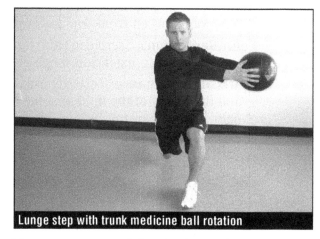

Lunge step with trunk medicine ball rotation

retractors and upward rotators, hip and knee extensors, abdominal muscles to control rotary motion of lumbar spine

Indications: Strengthens the spine and lower extremity extensors; improves coordination between trunk and lower extremity extensors

Contraindications: Sacroiliac pain; lumbar extension quadrant testing pain

Pearls of performance: This exercise requires a strong spine extensor contraction and control by the abdominal obliques. Primary motion of rotation should be through the hips and not through the lumbar spine.

Overhead Medicine Ball Toss

PROGRESSION NAME: Core and Extremity Functional Strength Training

STAGE: Advanced

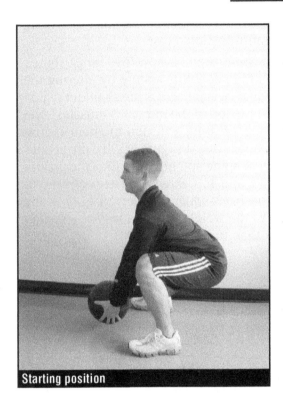
Starting position

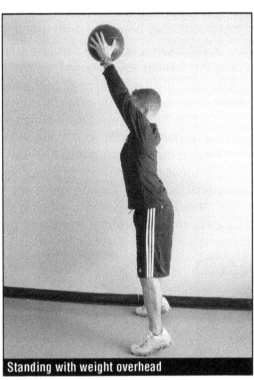
Standing with weight overhead

Starting position: Squat with a medicine ball between your legs.

Exercise action: Push through the heels and accelerate toward standing position, simultaneously bringing the weight upward as if to toss it overhead and behind.

Primary muscle groups: Spinal extensors, shoulder flexors, scapula upward rotators, hip and knee extensors, abdominal muscles to control rotary motion of lumbar spine

Indications: Strengthens the spine and lower extremity extensors; improves coordination between trunk and lower extremity extensors

Contraindications: Lumbar extension quadrant testing pain; degenerative changes of hip joints

Pearls of performance: Monitor the patient for correct form. There should be a coordinated, smooth motion between the shoulder girdle, trunk, and lower extremities. Fatigue or weakness of any one area potentially overloads adjacent areas, making those areas susceptible to injury.

SQUATS

Although the squat is mentioned in chapter 4 of this text, which details lower extremity functional progressions, it is also discussed here because it is an important functional test for the trunk as well. Attention to the principles outlined in this section helps protect the lumbar spine while simultaneously assuring the contribution of the spinal extensors and abdominal mechanism. Most squat injuries to the spine occur because of an uncontrolled rotary force at the lumbar spine, either toward the end of the descent or when the person struggles to come out of the squat position. The other mechanism of injury to the spine occurs when the person does not perform the squat with the muscle activity described here (retracting the scapula, cinching the abdomen, unlocking the hips, and so on) and instead uses the ligamentous tissues rather than strong muscle activity to counterbalance the weight and the motion. This is what the examiner should be carefully analyzing when assessing someone with this important functional test.

The difference between a back squat and a front squat is how load is distributed over the lumbar spine as well as the hip and knee joints simply by altering the position of the bar being held. In the back squat (weight across the shoulder region behind the neck and supported through contraction of the trapezius muscles), the weight line falls anterior to the lumbar spine, creating a flexion moment (figure 5.19a). However, the more the individual leans forward (figure 5.19b), the greater the flexion moment generated over the lumbar spine and hips and thus the greater requirement of the spinal extensor muscles and hip extensors, respectively, to counterbalance the flexion moment. In the front squat the person is typically in a more-upright position, which results in the weight creating less of a flexion moment over the lumbar spine and pelvis than in the back squat.

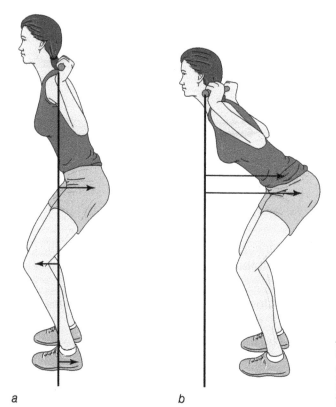

a　　　　　　　　　　*b*

Figure 5.19 Distribution of load over the lumbar spine, hips, and knees with changes in forward lean during a squat.

Back Squat

PROGRESSION NAME: Squats

STAGE: Beginning if no weight is used; intermediate to advanced when weight is used

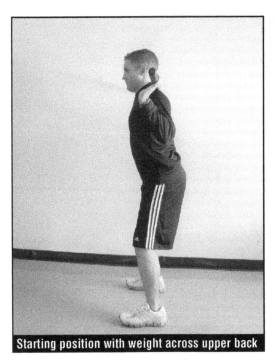

Starting position with weight across upper back

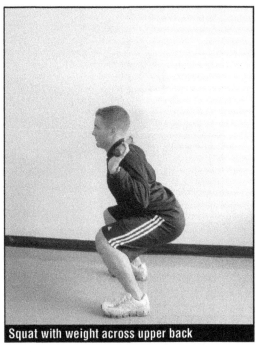

Squat with weight across upper back

Starting position: Begin in standing. If the weight is placed across the upper back, the bar should be supported by a strong contraction of the upper trapezius, not resting on the cervicothoracic junction.

Exercise action: Keep the eyes forward and the head up, and strongly retract the scapulae. These maneuvers result in strong activation of the spinal extensors. Cinch the abdomen (i.e., pull the abdominal wall away from the beltline), which is an excellent way to activate the transversus abdominis. This further stabilizes the lumbar spine. The first movement of a correct squat is to push the buttocks back—in essence, unlocking the hips—rather than simply collapsing into lumbar flexion. The movement should be a precise unlocking of the hip joints (i.e., moving the hips toward a flexed position that actually initiates the descent). Descend straight down and in the sagittal plane, keeping the weight through the heels, both on the descent and during the return to complete upright.

Primary muscle groups: Spinal extensors, abdominal muscles to control rotary motion of lumbar spine, hip and knee extensors

Indications: Strengthens the spine and lower extremity extensors; improves coordination between trunk and lower extremity extensors

Contraindications: Lumbar instability; degenerative changes of the hip joints resulting in loss of hip range of motion

Pearls of performance: It is essential that the first phase of the squat focus on moving the hips toward extension.

Front Squat

PROGRESSION NAME: Squats

STAGE: Beginning when no weight is used; intermediate to advanced when weight is used

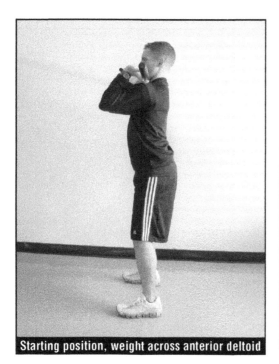

Starting position, weight across anterior deltoid

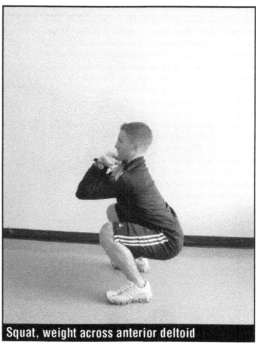

Squat, weight across anterior deltoid

Starting position: Begin in standing. If weight is used, place the bar high on the shoulders across the region of the anterior deltoid.

Exercise action: Keep the eyes forward and the head up, and strongly retract the scapulae. These maneuvers result in strong activation of the spinal extensors. Cinch the abdomen (i.e., pull the abdominal wall away from the beltline), which is an excellent way to activate the transversus abdominis. This further stabilizes the lumbar spine. The first movement of a correct squat is to push the buttocks back—in essence, unlocking the hips—rather than simply collapsing into lumbar flexion. The movement should be a precise unlocking of the hip joints (i.e., moving the hips toward a flexed position that actually initiates the descent). Descend straight down and in the sagittal plane, keeping the weight through the heels, both on the descent and during the return to complete upright.

Primary muscle groups: Spinal extensors, abdominal muscles to control rotary motion of lumbar spine, hip and knee extensors

Indications: Strengthens the spine and lower extremity extensors; improves coordination between trunk and lower extremity extensors

Contraindications: Lumbar instability; degenerative changes of the hip joints resulting in loss of hip range of motion

Pearls of performance: It is essential that the first phase of the squat focus on moving the hips toward extension.

Squat Press

PROGRESSION NAME: Squats

STAGE: Advanced

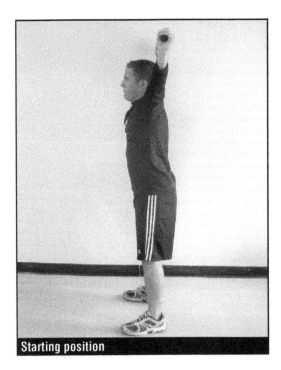

Starting position

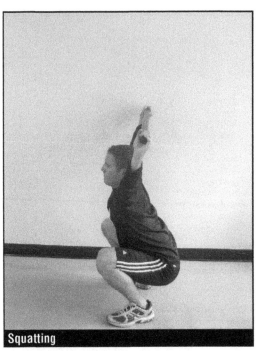

Squatting

Starting position: Begin in standing, with the weight bar pushed completely overhead and held in that position.

Exercise action: While maintaining the bar in an overhead position, descend into a full squat, then return to standing with the weight remaining overhead.

Primary muscle groups: Spine extensors, hip extensors, shoulder girdle elevators

Indications: Strengthens the trunk and lower extremity extensor mechanisms

Contraindications: Limitations in motion of the glenohumeral joint, spine extension, or hip flexion

Pearls of performance: Monitor the patient to ensure correct form. The person must push the weight directly overhead and not allow it to migrate forward. Rotary motion of the spine should be avoided.

Romanian Deadlift (RDL)

PROGRESSION NAME: Squats

STAGE: Intermediate to advanced

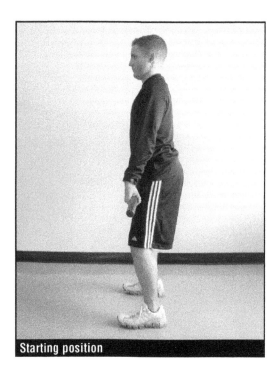
Starting position

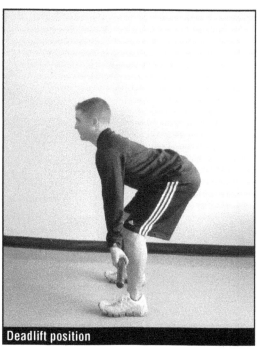
Deadlift position

Starting position: Begin standing, with the head up and looking forward, scapulae retracted, lumbar lordosis maintained, knees slightly bent, and weight held close to the body.

Exercise action: While maintaining scapular retraction and lumbar lordosis, flex the pelvis over the femurs. All motion involves the pelvis moving around the femurs rather than lumbar flexion.

Primary muscle groups: Spine extensors; hip extensors, especially the hamstrings; scapula retractors

Indications: Strengthens the trunk and lower extremity extensor mechanisms

Contraindications: Radicular pain; discogenic pain

Pearls of performance: Monitor the patient to ensure correct form. When the hip extensors are weak, the tendency is to compensate by flexing the lumbar spine. This must be avoided. When bending forward at the hips, the person should feel the stretching sensation in the hamstrings if it is being performed correctly.

PERTURBATION TRAINING

Perturbation training is often used in functional testing of the trunk. Essentially, such testing challenges one's ability to maintain balance. Perturbation is a disturbance of motion, such as when an external force is applied or an unstable surface is used in an attempt to destabilize the athlete. This force can be one that is expected or unexpected during the test. The theory behind using such testing maneuvers is that experiencing pertubations while catching, lifting, or throwing an object can mimic contact events common to sports. Many consider perturbation functional tests an essential progression when training athletes since sports feature unpredictable loading of the human skeleton.

Functional testing and functional progressions implementing this technique often use balance boards or balance discs. The balance boards provide much versatility because different levels can be used, which affects the degree of difficulty. Some boards have a side-to-side range of motion, while others have a full range of motion, increasing the proprioceptive requirements. Balance boards are used for proprioceptive training for elite athletes as well as the general population engaging in rehabilitation exercises. Balance discs are air-filled discs that also provide a variety of training options to assess different skill levels.

Squat Perturbation Training

PROGRESSION NAME: Balance Board Squats

STAGE: Intermediate to advanced

Starting position: Stand on a perturbation apparatus such as a balance disc or balance board. No weight is needed for this exercise, but if you do use weight, keep it very light.

Exercise action: Descend into the squat position and return to standing.

Primary muscle groups: Spine extensors, hip extensors, abdominal muscles

Indications: Strengthens the trunk and lower extremity; improves coordination between trunk and lower extremities; improves reaction times between trunk and lower extremities

Squat on balance disc

Contraindications: Spine instability

Pearls of performance: The patient should start with slow descent training and gradually build speed into the maneuver.

CABLE PULLS

Cable pulls are excellent functional training progressions for the spine and lower extremity extensor mechanism. The value of the cable pull is that it can be modified into high pull, midpull, and low pull actions, thus placing different challenges on the extensor mechanism with a similar exercise stroke. The intent of such activity is to further develop a person's proprioceptive and kinesthetic trunk sense, with the goal of having such training result in rapid reflexive response when needed for sport or other dynamic conditions.

Cable Pull Perturbation Training

PROGRESSION NAME: Balance Board Cable Pulls

STAGE: Intermediate to advanced

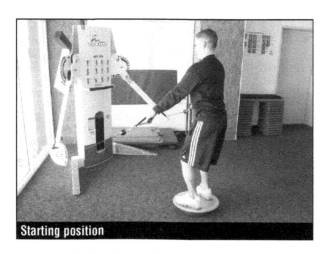
Starting position

Starting position: Stand on a perturbation apparatus such as a balance disc or balance board. Facing the weight stack, hold the cable handles in both hands.

Exercise action: Pull the cables with a shoulder extension and scapular retraction motion.

Primary muscle groups: Scapula retractors, shoulder extensors, spine extensors to counter lumbar extension, abdominal muscles to counter lumbar rotation

Indications: Strengthens the trunk and upper extremity; improves coordination between trunk and upper extremities; improves reaction times between trunk and upper extremities

Contraindications: Spine instability

Pearls of performance: The patient should start with small motions of the shoulder girdle in order to teach trunk control, then progress to greater ranges of motion of the shoulder girdle.

SUMMARY

The trunk presents unique challenges in the development of functional progression programs. This chapter shows that the trunk cannot be viewed in isolation because it serves as the stable yet dynamic base for upper and lower extremity functional progression programs. The sections of this text detailing upper and lower extremity functional progressions illustrate this.

The key to developing functional progression programs that are both safe and effective is to understand the biomechanical vulnerabilities of the lumbopelvic region. To develop scientifically sound programs, the clinician must clearly understand how shear stresses affect the low back and what motions and loading conditions have the potential to adversely affect the apophyseal joints, intervertebral discs, and sacroiliac joints. Finally, this chapter illustrates the anatomical linkages of the shoulder girdle, trunk, and lower extremity musculature. When these linkages are understood, they ultimately serve as the foundation for exercise prescription for training programs, as they are sequenced from simple to complex, non–weight bearing to weight bearing, and static to dynamic.

References

Chapter 1

Barrack RL, Bruckner JD, Kneisl J, Inman WS, Alexander AH. The outcome of nonoperatively treated complete tears of the anterior cruciate ligament in active young adults. *Clin Orthop Relat Res.* 1990;259:192-199.

Buckley SL, Barrack RL, Alexander AH. The natural history of conservatively treated partial anterior cruciate ligament tears. *Am J Sports Med.* 1989;17:221-225.

Carr CM. Sport psychology: Psychologic issues and applications. *Phys Med Rehabil Clin N Am.* 2006;17(3):519-535.

Cook EE, Gray VL, Savinar-Nogue E, Medeiros R. Shoulder antagonistic strength ratios: A comparison between college-level baseball pitchers and nonpitchers. *J Orthop Sports Phys Ther.* 1987;8:451-461.

Cook G, Burton L, Hoogenboom B. Pre-participation screening: The use of fundamental movements as an assessment of function – part 1. *NJSPT.* 2006;1:62-71.

Elmqvist LG, Lorentzon R, Langstrom M, Fugl-Meyer AR. Reconstruction of the anterior cruciate ligament: Long-term effects of different knee angles at primary immobilization and different modes of early training. *Am J Sports Med.* 1988;16:455-462.

Harter RA, Osternig LR, Singer KM, James SL, Larson RL, Jones DC. Long-term evaluation of knee stability and function following surgical reconstruction for anterior cruciate ligament insufficiency. *Am J Sports Med.* 1988;16:434-443.

Indelicato PA, Hermansdorfer J, Huegel M. Nonoperative management of complete tears of the medial collateral ligament of the knee in intercollegiate football players. *Clin Orthop Relat Res.* 1990;256:174-177.

Jokl P, Kaplan N, Stovell P, Keggi K. Nonoperative treatment of severe injuries to the medial and anterior cruciate ligaments of the knee. *J Bone Joint Surg.* 1987;66A:741-744.

Kegerreis S. The construction and implementation of functional progression as a component of athletic rehabilitation. *J Orthop Sports Phys Ther.* 1983;5:14-19.

Kegerreis S, Malone T, McCarroll J. Functional progressions: An aid to athletic rehabilitation. *Phys Sportsmed.* 1984;12:67-71.

Kegerreis S, Wetherald T. The utilization of functional progressions in the rehabilitation of injured wrestlers. *J Athl Train.* 1987;22:32-35.

McMahon LM, Burdett RG, Whitney SL. Effects of muscle group and placement site on reliability of handheld dynamometry strength measurements. *J Orthop Sports Phys Ther.* 1992;15:236-241.

Noyes FR, Torvik PJ, Hyde WB, DeLucas JL. Biomechanics of ligament failure: An analysis of immobilization, exercise, and reconditioning effects in primates. *J Bone Joint Surg.* 1974;56A:1406-1418.

Odensten M, Lysholm J, Gillquist J. The course of partial anterior cruciate ligament ruptures. *Am J Sports Med.* 1985;13:183-186.

Tippet SR, Voight ML. Components of functional progression. In: Tippet SR, Voight ML, eds. *Functional Progressions for Sports Rehabilitation.* Champaign, Ill: Human Kinetics; 1995:3-18.

Wadsworth CT, Krishnan R, Sear M, Harrold J, Nielsen DH. Intrarater reliability of manual muscle testing and handheld dynametric muscle testing. *Phys Ther.* 1987;67:1342-1347.

Walmsley RP, Szybbo C. A comparative study of the torque generated by the shoulder internal and external rotator muscles in different positions and a varying speeds. *J Orthop Sports Phys Ther.* 1987;9:217-227.

Weiss CB, Lundberg M, Hamberg H, DeHaven KE, Gillquist J. Non-operative treatment of meniscal tears. *J Bone Joint Surg.* 1989;71A:811-822.

Wikholw JB, Bohannon RW. Handheld dynamometer measurements: Tester strength makes a difference. *J Orthop Sports Phys Ther.* 1991;13:191-198.

Wyatt MP, Edwards AM. Comparison of quadriceps and hamstring torque values during isokinetic exercise. *J Orthop Sports Phys Ther.* 1981;3:48-56.

Yamamoto SK, Hartman CW, Feagin JA, Kimball G. Functional rehabilitation of the knee: A preliminary study. *Journal of Sports Medicine.* 1975;3:288-291.

Chapter 2

Bolz S, Davies GJ. Leg length differences and correlation with total leg strength. *J Orthop Sports Phys Ther.* 1984;6:123-129.

Bullock-Saxton JE. Local sensation changes and altered hip muscle function following severe ankle sprain. *Phys Ther.* 1994;74(1):17-23.

Bunn J. *Scientific Principles of Coaching.* Englewood Cliffs, NJ: Prentice-Hall; 1972.

Chimielewski TL, Hodges MJ, Horodyski M, Bishop MD, Conrad BP, Tillman SM. Investigation of clinician agreement in evaluating movement quality during unilateral lower extremity functional tasks: A comparison of 2 rating methods. *J Orthop Sports Phys Ther.* 2007;37(3):122-129.

Davies GJ. *A Compendium of Isokinetics in Clinical Usage.* LaCrosse, Wis: S & S; 1992.

Davies GJ, Ellenbecker TS. Scientific and clinical rationale for utilization of a total arm strength rehabilitation program for shoulder and elbow overuse injuries. APTA Orthopaedic Section, Home Study Course. LaCrosse, Wis; 1993.

Ellenbecker TS. *Clinical Examination of the Shoulder.* Philadelphia, Pa: Elsevier Science; 2004.

Elliott B, Fleisig G, Nicholls R, Escamillia R. Technique effects on upper limb loading in the tennis serve. *J Sci Med Sport.* 2003;6(1):76-87.

Elliott B, Marsh T, Blansby B. A three dimensional cinematographic analysis of the tennis serve. *Int J Sport Biomech.* 1986;2:260-271.

Elliott B, Marshall RN, Noffal GJ. Contributions to upper limb segment rotations during the power serve in tennis. *J Appl Biomech.* 1995;11(4):433-442.

Feltner M, Dapena J. Dynamics of the shoulder and elbow joints of the throwing arm during a baseball pitch. *Int J Sport Biomech.* 1986;2:233-259.

Gleim GW, Nicholas JA, Webb JN. Isokinetic evaluation following leg injuries *Phys Sportsmed.* 1978;6:74-82.

Groppel JL. *High Tech Tennis.* 2nd ed. Champaign, Ill: Human Kinetics; 1992.

Hamner DL, Pink MM, Jobe FW. A modification of the relocation test: Arthroscopic findings associated with a positive test. *J Shoulder Elbow Surg.* 2000;9:263-267.

Hanavan EP. A mathematical model of the human body. AMRL-TR-64-102. Wright-Patterson Air Force Base; 1964.

Hardcastle P, Nade S. The significance of the Trendelenburg test. *J Bone Joint Surg Br.* 1985;67:741-746.

Hewett TE, Myer GD, Ford KR, et al. Biomechanical measures of neuromuscular control and valgus loading of the knee predict anterior cruciate ligament injury risk in female athletes: A prospective study. *Am J Sports Med.* 2005;33:492-501.

Kibler WB. Clinical biomechanics of the elbow in tennis: Implications for evaluation and diagnosis. *Med Sci Sports Exerc.* 1994;26(10):1203-1206.

Kibler WB. The role of the scapula in athletic shoulder function. *Am J Sports Med.* 1998;26(2):325-337.

Kibler WB, Press J, Sciascia A. The role of core stability in athletic function. *Sports Med.* 2006;36:189-198.

Marshall RN, Elliott BC. Long-axis rotation: The missing link in proximal-to-distal segmental sequencing. *J Sports Sci.* 2000;18:247-254.

Marshall RN, Noffal GJ, Legnani G. *Simulation of the Tennis Serve: Factors Affecting Elbow Torques Related to Medial Epicondylitis.* Paris: ISB; 1993.

Marshall RN, Wood GA. Movement expectation and simulations: Segment interactions in drop punt kicking. In: Adrian M, Deutsch H, eds. *Biomechanics: The 1984 Olympic Scientific Congress Proceedings.* Eugene, Ore: Microform; 1986:111-118.

Nicholas JA, Strizak AM, Veras G. A study of thigh muscle weakness in different pathological states of the lower extremity. *Am J Sports Med.* 1976;4:241-248.

Piva SR, Fitzgerald K, Irrgang JJ, et al. Reliability of measures of impairments associated with patellofemoral pain syndrome. *BMC Musculoskelet Disord.* 2006;7:33.

Plagenhoef S. 1971. *Patterns of Human Movement.* Englewood Cliffs, NJ: Prentice-Hall.

Priest JD, Braden V, Gerberich SG. An analysis of players with and without pain. *Phys Sportsmed.* 1980;8:81-91.

Priest JD, Nagel DA. Tennis shoulder. *Am J Sports Med.* 1976;4:28-42.

Putnam CA. Sequential motions of the body segments in striking and throwing skills: Descriptions and explanations. *J Biomech.* 1993;26(suppl 1):125-136.

Strizak AM, Gleim GW, Sapega A, Nicholas JA. Hand and forearm strength and its relation to tennis. *Am J Sports Med.* 1983;11(4):234-239.

Tyler TF, Nicholas SJ, Mullaney MJ, McHugh MP. The role of hip muscle function in the treatment of patellofemoral pain syndrome. *Am J Sports Med.* 2006;34(4):630-636.

VanGheluwe B, Hebbelinck M. The kinematics of the service movement in tennis: A three dimensional cinematographic approach. In: Winter DA, Norman RW, eds. *Biomechanics IX-B.* Champaign, Ill: Human Kinetics; 1985:521-526.

Chapter 3

An KN, Hui FC, Morrey BF, Linscheid RL, Chao EY. Muscles across the elbow joint: A biomechanical analysis. *J Biomech.* 1981;14:659-669.

Andrews JR, Alexander EJ. Rotator cuff injury in throwing and racquet sports. *Sports Med Arthrosc.* 1995;3:30.

Andrews JR, Gillogly S. Physical examination of the shoulder in throwing athletes. In: Zarins B, Andrews JR, Carson WG, eds. *Injuries to the Throwing Arm.* Philadelphia, Pa: Saunders; 1985.

Atwater AE. Biomechanics of overarm throwing movements and of throwing injuries. *Exerc Sport Sci Rev.* 1979;7:43-85.

Bagg SD, Forrest WJ. A biomechanical analysis of scapular rotation during arm abduction in the scapular plane. *Arch Phys Med Rehabil.* 1988;238-245.

Bankart ASB. The pathology and treatment of recurrent dislocation of the shoulder joint. *BMJ.* 1938;26:23-29.

Bankart ASB. Recurrent or habitual dislocation of the shoulder joint. *BMJ.* 1923;2:1132-1133.

Basset RW, Browne AO, Morrey BF, An KN. Glenohumeral muscle force and moment mechanics in a position of shoulder instability, *J Biomech.* 1994;23:405-415.

Bennett GE. Elbow and shoulder lesions of baseball players. *Am J Surg.* 1959;98:484-492.

Berryman-Reese N, Bandy WD. *Joint Range of Motion and Muscle Length Testing.* Philadelphia, Pa: Saunders; 2002.

Bitter NL, Clisby EF, Jones MA, Magarey ME, Jaberzadeh S, Sandow MJ. Relative contributions of infraspinatus and deltoid during external rotation in healthy shoulders. *J Shoulder Elbow Surg.* 2007 Sep-Oct;16(5):563-568.

Bourne DA, Choo AM, Regan WD, MacIntyre DL, Oxland TR. Three-dimensional rotation of the scapula during functional movements. *J Shoulder Elbow Surg.* 2007;16:150-162.

Burkhart SS, Morgan CD. The peel-back mechanism: Its role in producing and extending posterior type II SLAP lesions and its effect on SLAP repair rehabilitation. *Arthroscopy.* 1998;14:637-640.

Burkhart SS, Morgan CD, Kibler WB. The disabled throwing shoulder: Spectrum of pathology. Part I: Pathoanatomy and biomechanics. *Arthroscopy.* 2003;19(4):404-420.

Carroll R. Tennis elbow: Incidence in local league players. *Br J Sports Med.* 1981;15:250-255.

Cheng J, Karzel R. Superior labrum anterior posterior lesions of the shoulder:

Operative techniques of management. *Oper Tech in Sports Med.* 1997;5:249-256.

Codman EA. *The Shoulder.* Boston: Privately printed; 1934.

Cyriax JH, Cyriax PJ. *Illustrated Manual of Orthopaedic Medicine.* London: Butterworths; 1983.

Daniels L, Worthingham C. *Muscle Testing: Techniques of Manual Examination.* 4th ed. Philadelphia, Pa: Saunders; 1980.

Dillman CJ. Presentation on the upper extremity in tennis and throwing athletes. United States Tennis Association National Meeting, Tucson, Arizona; March 1991.

Doody SG, Freedman L, Waterland JC. Shoulder movements during abduction in the scapular plane. *Arch Phys Med Rehabil.* 1970;595-604.

Ellenbecker TS. Shoulder internal and external rotation strength and range of motion in highly skilled tennis players. *Isok Exerc Sci.* 1992;2:1-8.

Ellenbecker, TS. Rehabilitation of shoulder and elbow injuries in tennis players. *Clin Sports Med.* 1995;14:87-110.

Ellenbecker TS. *Clinical Examination of the Shoulder.* Philadelphia, Pa: Elsevier Saunders; 2004.

Ellenbecker TS. *Shoulder Rehabilitation: Non-Operative Treatment.* New York, NY: Thieme; 2006.

Ellenbecker TS, Davies GJ. *Closed Kinetic Chain Exercise.* Champaign, Ill: Human Kinetics; 2001.

Ellenbecker TS, Mattalino AJ. Comparison of open and closed kinetic chain upper extremity tests in patients with rotator cuff pathology and glenohumeral joint instability. *J Orthop Sports Phys Ther.* 1997a;25:84

Ellenbecker TS, Mattalino AJ. *The Elbow in Sport.* Champaign, Ill: Human Kinetics; 1997b.

Ellenbecker TS, Roetert EP. Age specific isokinetic glenohumeral internal and external rotation strength in elite junior tennis players. *J Sci Med Sport.* 2003;6(1):63-70.

Ellenbecker TS, Roetert EP, Bailie DS, Davies GJ, Brown SW. Glenohumeral joint total rotation range of motion in elite tennis players and baseball pitchers. *Med Sci Sports Exerc.* 2002;34(12):2052-2056.

Ellenbecker TS, Roetert EP, Piorkowski PA. Shoulder internal and external rotation range of motion of elite junior tennis players: A comparison of two protocols. *J Orthop Sports Phys Ther.* 1993;17(1):65(Abstract).

Ellenbecker TS, Roetert EP, Piorkowski PA, Schulz DA. Glenohumeral joint internal and external rotation range of motion in elite junior tennis players. *J Orthop Sports Phys Ther.* 1996;24(6):336-341.

Elliott B, Marsh T, Blanksby B. A three dimensional cinematographic analysis of the tennis serve. *Int J Sport Biomech.* 1986;2:260-271.

Fleisig GS, Andrews JR, Dillman CJ, Escamilla RF. Kinetics of baseball pitching with implications about injury mechanisms. *Am J Sports Med.* 1995;23:233.

Fleisig GS, Dillman CJ, Andrews JR. Proper mechanics for baseball pitching. *Clin Sports Med.* 1989;1:151-170.

Fleisig GS, Jameson EG, Dillman CJ, Andrews JR. Biomechanics of overhead sports. In: Garrett WE, Kirkendall DT, eds. *Exercise and Sport Science.* Philadelphia, Pa: Lippincott, Williams & Wilkins; 2000:563-584.

Gill TJ, Micheli LJ, Gebhard F, Binder C. Bankart repair for anterior instability of the shoulder. *J Bone Joint Surg.* 1997;79A(6):850-857.

Glousman RE, Barron J, Jobe FW, et al. An electromyographic analysis of the elbow in normal and injured pitchers with medial collateral ligament insufficiency. *Am J Sports Med.* 1992;20:311-317.

Goldbeck TG, Davies GJ. Test-retest reliability of the closed kinetic chain upper extremity stability test: A clinical field test. *J Sport Rehabil.* 2000;9:35-45.

Goldie, I. Epicondylitis lateralis humeri. *Acta Chir Scand Suppl.* 1964;339:1-114.

Golding FC. The shoulder: The forgotten joint. *Br J Radiol.* 1962;35:149-158.

Hang YS, Peng SM. An epidemiological study of upper extremity injury in tennis players with particular reference to tennis elbow. *J Formos Med Assoc.* 1984;83:307-316.

Harryman DT, Sidles JA, Clark MJ, McQuade KK, Gibb TD, Matsen FA. Translation of the humeral head on the glenoid with passive glenohumeral motion. *J Bone Joint Surg.* 1990;72A:1334-1343.

Indelicato PA, Jobe FW, Kerlan RK, Carter VS, Shields CL, Lombardo SJ. Correctable elbow lesions in professional baseball players: A review of 25 cases. *Am J Sports Med.* 1979;7:72-75.

Inman VT, Saunders JB de CM, Abbot LC. Observations on the function of the shoulder joint. *J Bone Joint Surg Am.* 1944;26:1-30.

Itoi E, Kido T, Sano A, Urayama M, Sato K. Which is more useful, the "full can test" or the "empty can test" in detecting the torn supraspinatus tendon? *Am J Sports Med.* 1999;27(1):65-68.

Jobe FW, Kvitne RS. Shoulder pain in the overhand or throwing athlete: The relationship of anterior instability and rotator cuff impingement. *Orthop Rev.* 1989;28(9):963-975.

Jobe FW, Pink M. The athlete's shoulder. *J Hand Ther.* 1994;17(2):107.

Joyce ME, Jelsma RD, Andrews JR. Throwing injuries to the elbow. *Sports Med and Arthrosc.* 1995;3:224-236.

Kamien M. A rational management of tennis elbow. *Sports Med.* 1990;9:173-191.

Karduna AR, Williams GR, Williams JL, Iannotti JP. Kinematics of the glenohumeral joint: Influences of muscular forces, ligamentous restraints, and articular geometry. *J Orthop Res.* 2006;14:986-993.

Kelly BT, Kadrmas WH, Speer KP. The manual muscle examination for rotator cuff strength: An electromyographic investigation. *Am J Sports Med.* 1996;24:581-588.

Kessler RM, Hertling D. *Management of Common Musculoskeletal Disorders: Physical Therapy Principles and Management.* Philadelphia, Pa: Harper & Row; 1983.

Kibler WB. Role of the scapula in the overhead throwing motion. *Contemp Orthop.* 1991;22(5):525-532.

Kibler WB. Evaluation of sports demands as a diagnostic tool in shoulder disorders. In: Matsen FA, Fu F, Hawkins RJ, eds. *The Shoulder: A Balance of Mobility and Stability.* Rosemont, Ill: AAOS; 1993.

Kibler WB. The role of the scapula in athletic shoulder function. *Am J Sports Med.* 1998;26(2):325-337.

Kibler WB, Chandler TJ, Livingston BP, Roetert EP. Shoulder range of motion in elite tennis players. *Am J Sports Med.* 1996;24(3):279-285.

Kitai E, Itay S, Ruder A, et al. An epidemiological study of lateral epicondylitis in amateur male players. *Ann Chir Main.* 1986;5:113-121.

Kraushaar BS, Nirschl RP. Tendinosis of the elbow (tennis elbow). Clinical features and findings of histopathological, immunohistochemical and electron microscopy studies. *J Bone Joint Surg Am.* 1999;81:259-278.

Kvitne KS, Jobe FW, Jobe CM Shoulder instability in the overhead or throwing athlete. *Clin Sports Med.* 1995;14(4):917.

Leadbetter WB. Cell matrix response in tendon injury. *Clin Sports Med.* 1992;11:533-579.

Loudon JK, Jenkins W, Loudon KL. The relationship between static posture and ACL injury in female athletes. *J Orthop Sports Phys Ther.* 1996;24(2):91-97.

Magee DJ. *Orthopaedic Physical Assessment.* 3rd ed. Philadelphia, Pa: Saunders; 1997.

Mallon WJ, Herring CL, Sallay PI, Moorman CT, Crim JR. Use of vertebral levels to measure presumed internal rotation at the shoulder: A radiographic analysis. *J Shoulder Elbow Surg.* 1996;5:299-306.

Matsen FA, Harryman DT, Sidles JA. Mechanics of glenohumeral instability. *Clin Sports Med.* 1991;10:783.

Morgan CD, Burkhart SS, Palmeri M, et al. Type II SLAP lesions: Three subtypes and their relationships to superior instability and rotator cuff tears. *Arthroscopy.* 1998;14:553-565.

Morrey BF. *The Elbow and Its Disorders.* 2nd ed. Philadelphia, Pa: Saunders; 1993.

Nakajima T, Rokumma N, Kazutoshi H, et al. Histologic and biomechanical characteristics of the supraspinatus tendon: Reference to rotator cuff tearing. *J Shoulder Elbow Surg.* 1994;3:79.

Neer CS. Impingement lesions. *Clin Orthop.* 1983;173:70-77.

Nirschl RP. Shoulder tendonitis. In: Pettrone FP, ed. *Upper Extremity Injuries in Athletes. American Academy of Orthopaedic Surgeons Symposium.* Washington, DC: Mosby; 1988.

Nirschl RP. Elbow tendinosis/tennis elbow. *Clin Sports Med.* 1992;11:851-870.

Nirschl RP. Tennis elbow. In: Morrey BF, ed. *The Elbow and Its Disorders.* 2nd ed. Philadelphia, Pa: Saunders; 1993:537-552.

Nirschl R, Sobel J. Conservative treatment of tennis elbow. *Phys Sports Med.* 1981;9:43-54.

Norkin CC, White DJ. *Measurement of Joint Motion: A Guide to Goniometry.* 2nd ed. Philadelphia, Pa: Davis; 1995.

Otis JC, Jiang CC, Wickoewicz TL, Peterson MG, Warren RF, Santner TJ. Changes in moment arms of the rotator cuff and deltoid muscles during abduction and external rotation. *J Bone Joint Surg.* 1994;76A:667-676.

Perthes G. Ueber operationen der habituellen schulterluxation. *Deutsche Ztschr Chir.* 1906;85:199.

Poppen NK, Walker PS. Forces at the glenohumeral joint in abduction. *Clin Orthop.* 1978;135:165-170.

Priest JD, Jones HH, Tichenor CJC, et al. Arm and elbow changes in expert tennis players. *Minn Med.* 1977;60:399-404.

Rathburn JB, MacNab I. The microvascular pattern of the rotator cuff. *J Bone Joint Surg.* 1970;52 (3)-British 540-553.

Roetert EP, Ellenbecker TS. *Complete Conditioning for Tennis.* Champaign, Ill: Human Kinetics; 2007.

Roetert EP, Ellenbecker TS, Brown SW. Shoulder internal and external rotation range of motion in nationally ranked junior tennis players: A longitudinal analysis. *J Strength Cond Res.* 2000;14(2):140-143.

Runge F. Zur genese unt behand lung bes schreibekramp fes. *Berl Kun Wochenschr.* 1873;10:245.

Saha AK. Mechanism of shoulder movements and a plea for the recognition of "zero position" of glenohumeral joint. *Clin Orthop.* 1983;173:3-10.

Slocum DB. Classification of the elbow injuries from baseball pitching. *Am J Sports Med.* 1978;6:62-67.

Snyder SJ, Karzel RP, Del Pizzo W, Ferkel RD, Fiedman MJ. SLAP lesions of the shoulder. *Arthroscopy.* 1990;6:274-279.

Speer KP, Deng X, Borrero S, et al. Biomechanical evaluation of a simulated Bankart lesion. *J Bone Joint Surg.* 1994;76A12:1819-1826.

Uhl TL, Carver TJ, Mattacola CG, Mair SD, Nitz AJ. Shoulder musculature activation during upper extremity weight bearing exercise. *J Orthop Sports Phys Ther.* 2003;33(3):109-117.

United States Tennis Association. Unpublished data.

Walch G, Boileau P, Noel E, Donell ST. Impingement of the deep surface of the supraspinatus tendon on the posterosuperior glenoid rim: An arthroscopic study. *J Shoulder Elbow Surg.* 1992;1:238-245.

Wilk KE, Andrews JR, Arrigo CA, Keirns MA, Erber DJ. The strength characteristics of internal and external rotator muscles in professional baseball pitchers. *Am J Sports Med.* 1993;21:61-66.

Wilk KE, Arrigo CA. Current concepts in the rehabilitation of the athletic shoulder. *J Orthop Sports Phys Ther.* 1993;18:365-378.

Wilk KE, Arrigo CA, Andrews JR. Rehabilitation of the elbow in the throwing athlete. *J Orthop Sports Phys Ther.* 1993;17:305-317

Wilson FD, Andrews JR, Blackburn TA, McCluskey G. Valgus extension overload in the pitching elbow. *Am J Sports Med.* 1983;11(2):83-88.

Wilson JD, Ireland ML, Davis I. Core strength and lower extremity alignment during single leg squats. *Med Sci Sports Exerc.* 2006;35(8):945-952.

Winge S, Jorgensen U, Nielsen AL. Epidemiology of injuries in Danish championship tennis. *Int J Sports Med.* 1989;10:368-371.

Wolf BR, Altchek DW. Elbow problems in elite tennis players. *Tech Shoulder Elbow Surg.* 2003;4(2):55-68.

Wuelker N, Plitz W, Roetman B. Biomechanical data concerning the shoulder impingement syndrome. *Clin Orthop.* 1994;303:242-249.

Yamaguchi K, Riew DK, Galatz LM, Syme JA, Neviaser RJ. Biceps activity during shoulder motion: An electromyographic analysis. *Clin Orthop.* 1997;336:122-129.

Chapter 4

Aagaard P, Simonsen EB, Magnusson SP, Larsson B, Dyhre-Poulsen P. A new concept for isokinetic hamstring:quadriceps muscle strength ratio. *Am J Sports Med.* 1998;26:231-237.

Abernethy PJ, Townsend PR, Rose RM, Radin EL. Chondromalacia patellae a separate clinical entity? *J Bone Joint Surg.* 1978;60B:205-210.

Aglietti P, Insall JN, Cerulli G. Patellar pain in incongruence I: Measurements of incongruence. *Clin Orthop Relat Res.* 1983;176:217-224.

Amis AA, Dawkins GP. Functional anatomy of the anterior cruciate ligament: Fibre bundle actions related to ligament replacements and injuries. *J Bone Joint Surg Br.* 1991;73B:260-267.

Andrews JR, Baker CL, Curl WW, Clancy WG. Surgical repair of acute and chronic lesions of the lateral capsular ligamentous complex of the knee. In: Feagin JA, ed. *The Crucial Ligaments: Diagnosis and Treatment of Ligamentous Injuries About the Knee.* 2nd ed. New York, NY: Churchill Livingstone; 1994:605-622.

Arendt E, Dick R. Knee injury patterns among men and women in collegiate basketball and soccer. *Am J Sports Med.* 1995;23:694-701.

Bahr RM, Krosshaug T. Understanding injury mechanisms: A key component of preventing injuries in sport. *Br J Sports Med.* 2005;39:324-329.

Barber AF, Sutker AN. Iliotibial band syndrome. *Sports Med.* 1992;14:144-148.

Baratta R, Solomonow M, Zhou BH, Letson D, Chiunard R, D'Ambrosia R. Muscular coaactivation: the role of the antagonist musculature in maintaining knee stability. American Journal of Knee Surgery 1988;16:133-22.

Bennell K, Wajswelner H, Lew P, et al. Isokinetic strength testing does not predict hamstrings injury in australian rules footballers. British Journal of Sports Medicine 1998;32:309-14.

Best TM, Kirkendall DT, Almekinders LC, Garrett WE. Basic Science and Injury of Muscle, Tendon and Ligament. In DeLee JC, Drez D, Miller MD eds. *Orthopedic Sports Medicine: Principles and Practices.* Vol. 1. 2nd ed. Philadelphia, PA: Saunders;2003:1-56.

Beynnon BD, Murphy DF, Alosa DM. Predictive factors for lateral ankle sprains: A literature review. *J Athl Train.* 2002;37:376-380.

Bjordal JM, Arnly F, Hannestad B, Strand T. Epidemiology of anterior cruciate ligament injuries in soccer. *Am J Sports Med.* 1997;25:341-345.

Blazina ME, Kerlan RK, Jobe FW, Carter VS, Carlson GJ. Jumper's knee. *Orthop Clin N Am.* 1973;4(3):655-678.

Boden BP, Dean GS, Feagin JA, Garrett WE. Mechanisms of anterior cruciate ligament injury. *Orthopedics.* 2000;23:573-578.

Branch TP, Hunter R, Donath M. Dynamic EMG analysis of anterior cruciate deficient legs with and without bracing during cutting. *Am J Sports Med.* 1989;17:35-41.

Buchanan PA, Vardaxis VG. Sex-related and age-related differences in knee strength of basketball players ages 11-17. *J Athl Train.* 2003;38:231-237.

Burt CW, Overpeck MD. Emergency visits for sports related injuries. *Ann Emerg Med.* 2001;37:301-308.

Chandy TA, Grana WA. Secondary school athletic injury in boys and girls: A three year comparison. *Phys Sportsmed.* 1985;13:106-111.

Childs SG. Pathogenesis of anterior cruciate ligament injury. *Orthop Nurs.* 2002;21:35-40.

Conti SF, Stone DA. Rehabilitation of fractures and sprains of the ankle. In: Sammarco GJ, ed. *Rehabilitation of the Foot and Ankle.* St. Louis, Mo: Mosby; 1995:127-143.

Cook G, Burton L, Hoogenboom B. Pre-participation screening: The use of fundamental movements as an assessment of function, part 1. *N Am J Sports Phys Ther.* 2006a;1:62-71.

Cook G, Burton L, Hoogenboom B. Pre-participation screening: The use of fundamental movements as an assessment of function, part 2. *N Am J Sports Phys Ther.* 2006b;1:132-139.

Cox JS. Patellofemoral problems in runners. *Clin J Sports Med.* 1985;4:699-715.

Cox JS, Cooper PS. Patellofemoral instability. In: Fu FH, Harner CD, Vince KG, eds. *Knee Surgery.* Baltimore, Md: Williams & Wilkins; 1994:953-993.

Croce RV, Pitetti KH, Horvat M, Miller J. Peak torque, average power, and hamstrings/quadriceps ratios in nondisabled adults and adults with mental retardation. *Arch Phys Med Rehabil.* 1996;77:369-372.

Darracott J, Vernon-Roberts B. The bony changes in "chondromalacia patellae." *Rheum Phys Med.* 1971;11:175-179.

DeHaven KE, Collins HR. Diagnosis of internal derangements of the knee. *J Bone Joint Surg.* 1975;57:802-810.

Delahunt E, Monaghan K, Caulfield B. Altered neuromuscular control and ankle joint kinematics during walking in subjects with functional instability of the ankle joint. *Am J Sports Med.* 2006;34:1970-1976.

Dye SF, Boll DH. Radionuclide imaging of the patellofemoral joint in young adults with anterior

Dye SF, Chew MH. The use of scintigraphy to detect increased osseous metabolic activity about the knee. *J Bone Joint Surg Am.* 1993;75:1388-1406.

Ekman EF, Pope T, Martin DF, Walton WC. Magnetic resonance imaging of iliotibial band syndrome. *Am J Sports Med.* 1994;22:851-854.

Ekstrand J, Gillquist J. Soccer injuries and their mechanisms: A prospective study. *Med Sci Sports Exerc.* 1983;15:267-270.

Ekstrand J, Tropp H. The incidence of ankle sprains in soccer. *Foot Ankle* 1990;11(1):41-44.

Engstrom B, Johansson C, Tornkvist H. Soccer injuries among elite female players. *Am J Sports Med.* 1991;19(4):372-375.

Farr J. Patellofemoral articular cartilage treatment. In: Julkerson JP, ed. *Common Patellofemoral Problems.* Rosemont, Ill: American Academy of Orthopedic Surgeons; 2005:85-98.

Ferretti A, Puddu G, Mariani PP, Neri M. Jumper's knee: An epidemiological study of volleyball players. *Phys Sportsmed.* 1984;12:97-103.

Fetto JF, Marshall JL. Medial collateral injuries of the knee: A rationale for treatment. *Clin Orthop* 1978;132:206-218.

Ford KR, Myer GD, Hewett TE. Valgus knee motion during landing in high school female and male basketball players. *Med Sci Sports Exerc.* 2003;34:1745-1750.

Ford KR, Myer GD, Toms HE, Hewett TE. Gender differences in the kinematics of unanticipated cutting in young athletes. *Med Sci Sports Exerc.* 2005;124-129.

Freeman MA, Dwan MR, Hanham IW. The etiology and prevention of functional instability of the foot. *J Bone Joint Surg Br.* 1965;47:678-685.

Fukubayashi T, Torzilli PA, Sherman MF. An in vitro biomechanical evaluation of anterior-posterior motion of the knee. *J Bone Joint Surg Am.* 1982;64A:258-264.

Fulkerson JP, Hungerford DS. Biomechanics of the patellofemoral joint. In: Fulkerson JP, Hungerford DS, eds. *Disorders of the Patellofemoral Joint.* 2nd ed. Baltimore: Williams & Wilkins; 1990:1-39.

Fulkerson JP, Kalenak A, Rosenberg TD, Cox JS. Patellofemoral pain. *American Academy of Orthopedic Surgeons Instructional Course Lectures.* 1992;41:57-71.

Girgis FG, Marshall JL, Monajem ARSA. The cruciate ligaments of the knee joint. *Clin Orthop Relat Res.* 1975;106:216-231.

Giza E, Fuller C, Junge A, Dvorak J. Mechanisms of foot and ankle injuries in soccer. *Am J Sports Med.* 2003;31(4):550-554.

Goodfellow J, Hungerford DS, Zindel M. Patello-femoral joint mechanics and pathology I: Functional anatomy of the patellofemoral joint. *J Bone Joint Surg Br.* 1976;58B:287-290.

Grana WA, Kriegshauser LA. Scientific basis of extensor mechanism disorders. *Clin J Sports Med.* 1985;4:247-257.

Gray H. The bones of the lower limb. In: Goss CM, ed. *Gray's Anatomy.* 114th ed. Philadelphia, Pa: Lea & Febiger; 1973:95-369.

Gray H. The muscles and fasciae. In: Pick TP, Howden R, eds. *The Classic Collector's Edition: Gray's Anatomy.* New York, NY: Bounty; 1978:295-453.

Gray J, Taunton JE, McKenzie DC, Clement DB, McConkey JP, Davidson RG. A survey of injuries to the anterior cruciate ligament of the knee in female basketball players. *Int J Sports Med.* 1985;6(6):314-316.

Grelsamer RP, Klein JR. The biomechanics of the patellofemoral joint. *J Orthop Sports Phys Ther.* 1998;28:286-298.

Hayes CW, Brigido MD, Jamadar DA, Propeck T. Mechanism-based pattern approach of classification of complex injuries of the knee depicted at MR imaging. *Radiographics.* 2000;20:121-134.

Hewett TE, Ford KR, Myer GD. Anterior cruciate ligament injuries in female athletes: Part 2, a meta-analysis of neuromuscular interventions aimed at injury prevention. *Am J Sports Med.* 2006;34:490-498.

Hewett TE, Myer GD, Ford KR. Anterior cruciate ligament injuries in female athletes: Part I, mechanisms and risk factors. *Am J Sports Med.* 2006;34:299-311.

Hewett TE, Myer GD, Ford KR, et al. Biomechanical measures of neuromuscular control and valgus loading of the knee predict anterior cruciate ligament injury risk in female athletes. *Am J Sports Med.* 2005;33(4):492-501.

Hewett TE, Paterno MV, Myer GD. Strategies for enhancing proprioception and neuromuscular control of the knee. *Clin Orthop Relat Res.* 2002;16:69-82.

Hewett TE, Stroupe AL, Nance TA, Noyes FR. Plyometrics training in female athletes: Decreased impact forces and increased hamstring torques. *Am J Sports Med.* 1996;24:765-773.

Heyworth J. Ottawa ankle rules for the injured ankle. *Br J Sports Med.* 2003;37:194.

Hinton RY, Lincoln AE, Almquist JL, Douoguih WA, Sharma KM. Epidemiology of lacrosse injuries in high school-aged girls and boys: A 3-year prospective study. *Am J Sports Med.* 2005;33(9):1305-1414.

Holmes SW, Clancy WG. Clinical classification of patellofemoral pain and dysfunction. *J Sports Phys Ther.* 1998;28:299-306.

Holt KG, Hamill J. Running injuries and treatment: A dynamic approach. In: Sammarco GJ, ed. *Rehabilitation of the Foot and Ankle.* St. Louis, Mo: Mosby; 1995:241-258.

Huberti HH, Hayes WC. Patellofemoral contact pressures: The influence of Q-angle and tendofemoral contact. *J Bone Joint Surg.* 1984;66:715-724.

Hughston JC. Subluxation of the patella. *J Am Acad Orthop Surg.* 1968;50A:1003-1026.

Hungerford DS, Baumgartl F. Biomechanics of the patellofemoral joint. *Clin J Sports Med.* 1979;144:9-15.

Huston LJ, Greenfield M, Wojtys EM. Anterior cruciate ligament injuries in the female athlete: Potential risk factors. *Clin Orthop Relat Res.* 2000;372:50-63.

Hvid I, Andersen LI, Schmidt H. Chondromalacia patellae. *Acta Orthop Scand.* 1981;52:661-666.

Indelicato PA, Linton RC. Knee: Medial ligament injuries. In: DeLee JC, Drez D, Miller MD, eds. *Orthopaedic Sports Medicine Principles and Practices.* 2nd ed. Philadelphia, Pa: Saunders; 2007:1937-1949.

Insall J. Chondromalacia patellae: Patellar malalignment syndrome. *Orthop Clin North Am.* 1979;10(1):117-127.

Insall J. Current concepts review. *J Bone Joint Surg.* 1982;64:147-152.

Insall JN, Falvo KA, Wise DW. Chondromalacia patellae: A prospective study. *J Bone Joint Surg.* 1976;58:1-8.

Isakov E, Mizrahi J, Solzi P, Susak Z, Lotem M. Response of the peroneal muscles to sudden inversion of the ankle during standing. *Int J Sport Biomech.* 1986;22:100-109.

Jacobson BH, Hubbard M, Redus B, et al. An assessment of high school cheerleading: Injury distribution, frequency, and associated factors. *J Orthop Sports Phys Ther.* 2004;34(5):261-265.

Kalund S, Sinkjaer T, Arendt-Nielson L, Simonsen O. Altered timing of hamstring muscle action in anterior cruciate deficient patients. *Am J Sports Med.* 1990;18:245-248.

Karlsson J, Thomeé R, Swärd L. Eleven year follow-up of patello-femoral pain syndrome. *Clin J Sports Med.* 1996;6:22-26.

Kaufer H. Mechanical function of the patella. *J Bone Joint Surg.* 1971;53A:1551-1560.

Krosshaug T, Nakamae A, Boden BP, et al. Mechanisms of anterior cruciate ligament injury in basketball: Video analysis of 39 cases. *Am J Sports Med.* 2007;35:359-367.

Leanderson J, Eriksson E. Proprioception in classical ballet dancers: A prospective study of the influence of an ankle sprain on proprioception in the ankle joint. *Am J Sports Med.* 1996;(24):370-374.

Leetun DTD, Ireland ML, Wilson JD, et al. Core stability measures as risk factors for lower extremity injury in athletes. *Med Sci Sports Exerc.* 2004;36:926-934.

Leslie IJ, Bentley G. Arthroscopy in the diagnosis of chondromalacia patellae. *Ann Rheum Dis.* 1978;37:540-547.

Levy, IM. Posterior meniscal capsuloligamentous complexes of the knee. In: Feagin,JA ed. *The crucial ligaments: diagnosis and treatment of ligamentous injuries about the knee,* 2nd ed. New York: Churchill Livingstone; 1994: 339-349.

Lewis PB, McCarty LP, Kang RW, Cole BJ. Basic science and treatment options for articular cartilage injuries. *J Orthop Sports Phys Ther.* 2006;36(10):717-727.

Lieb FJ, Perry J. Quadriceps function: An anatomical and mechanica study using amputated limbs. *J Bone Joint Surg.* 1968;50A:1535-1548.

Mann RA. Biomechanics of the foot and ankle linkage. In: DeLee JC, Drez D, Miller M, eds. *Orthopaedic Sports Medicine: Principles and Practice.* Philadelphia, Pa: Saunders; 2003:2183-2190.

Maquet PG. Mechanics and osteoarthritis of the patellofemoral joint. *Clin Orthop.* 1979;144:70-73.

McGuine TA, Greene JJ, Best T, et al. Abstract balance as a predictor of ankle injuries in high school basketball players. *Clin J Sports Med.* 2000;10:239-244.

McKay GD, Goldie PA, Payne WR, Oakes BW. Ankle injuries in basketball: Injury rate and risk factors. *Br J Sports Med.* 2001;35:103-108.

McNair PJ, Marshall RN, Matheson JA. Important features associated with acute anterior cruciate ligament injury. *N Z Med J.* 1990;103:537-539.

Merchant AC. Classification of patellofemoral disorders. *Arthroscopy.* 1988;4(4):235-240.

Messina DF, Farney WC, DeLee JC. The incidence of injury in Texas high school basketball: A prospective study among male and female athletes. *Am J Sports Med.* 1999;27(3):294-299.

Moore KL. Lower limb. In: Dalley AF, ed. *Clinically Oriented Anatomy.* 5th ed. Baltimore, Md: Lippincott, Williams & Wilkins; 2005:566-569.

Morgan BE, Oberlander MA. An examination of injuries in major league soccer. The inaugural season. *Am J Sports Med* 2001;29:4:426-30.

Myer GD, Ford KR, Hewett TE. Rationale and clinical techniques for anterior cruciate ligament injury prevention among female athletes. *J Athl Train.* 2004;39:352-364.

Myer GD, Peterno MV, Ford KR, Quatman CE, Hewett TE. Rehabilitation after anterior cruciate ligament reconstruction: Criteria-based progression through the return-to-sport phase. *J Orthop Sports Phys Ther.* 2006;36:385-399.

National Collegiate Athletic Association. NCAA Injury Surveillance System Summary. Indianapolis, Ind: National Collegiate Athletic Association; 2002.

National Federation of State High School Associations. High School Participation Survey. Indianapolis, Ind: National Federation of State High School Associations; 2002.

Noftall F. Knee. In: Gay S, Gery L, eds. *Current Therapy in Sports Medicine.* 3rd ed. St. Louis, Mo: Mosby; 1995: 281-384.

Nogalski MP, Bach BR. Acute anterior cruciate ligament injuries. In: Fu FH, Harner CD, Vince KG, eds. *Knee Surgery.* Baltimore, Md: Williams & Wilkins; 1994:679-730.

Nomura E, Inoue M. Cartilage lesions of the patella in recurrent patellar dislocation. *Am J Sports Med.* 2004;32(1):498-502.

Norkin CC, Levangie PK. The ankle foot complex. In: Norkin CC, Levangie PK, eds. *Joint Structure and Function: A Comprehensive Analysis.* 2nd ed. Philadelphia, Pa: Davis Company; 1992:389.

Olsen OE, Myklebust G, Engebretsen L, Bahr R. Injury mechanism for anterior cruciate ligament injuries in team handball: A systematic video analysis. *Am J Sports Med.* 2004;32:1002-1012.

Pollard CD, Sigward SM, Powers CM. Gender differences in hip joint kinematics and kinetics during side-step cutting maneuver. *Clin J Sports Med.* 2007;17:38-42.

Quatman CE, Ford KR, Myer GD, Hewett TE. Maturation leads to gender differences in landing force and vertical jump. *Am J Sports Med.* 2006;34:806-813.

Rasmussen O, Kromann-Anderson C. Experimental ankle injuries. *Acta Orthop Scand.* 1983;54:356-562.

Rasmussen O, Tovberg-Jensen I. Mobility of the ankle joint. *Acta Orthop Scand.* 1982;53:155-160.

Rasmussen O, Tovberg-Jensen I, Hedeboe J. An analysis of the function of the posterior talofibular ligament. *Int Orthop (SICOT).* 1983;7:41-48.

Rosenberg A, Mikosz RP, Mohler CG. Basic knee biomechanics. In: Scott WN, ed. *The Knee.* St. Louis, Mo: Mosby; 1994:75-94.

Rosenberg A, Mohler CG, Mikosz RP. Gait analysis and its relationship to knee function. In: DeLee JC, Drez D, Miller M, eds. *The Knee.* St. Louis, Mo: Mosby; 1994:95-105.

Rosene JM, Fogarty TD, Mahaffey BL. Isokinetic hamstrings: Quadriceps ratios in intercollegiate athletes. *J Athl Train.* 2001;36:378-383.

Sammarco GJ. Anatomy and physiology. In: Sammarco GJ, ed. *Anatomy of the Foot and Ankle.* St. Louis, Mo: Mosby; 1995:3-23.

Shelbourne KD, Adsit WS. Conservative care of patellofemoral pain. In: Grelsamer RP, McConnell J, eds. *The Patella: A Team Approach.* Gaithersburg, Md: Aspen; 1998:1-14.

Sigward SM, Powers CM. The influence of gender on knee kinematics, kinetics and muscle activation patterns during side-step cutting. *Clin Biomech.* 2006;21:41-48.

Sitler M, Ryan J, Wheeler B, et al. The efficacy of a semirigid ankle stabilizer to reduce acute ankle injuries in basketball. *Am J Sports Med.* 1994;22(4):454-461.

Stauffer RN, Chao EYS, Brewster TC. Force and motion analysis of normal, diseased and prosthetic ankle joints. *Clin Orthop.* 1977;127:189-196.

Steinkamp LA, Dillingham MF, Markel MD, Hill JA, Kaufman KR. Biomechanical considerations in patellofemoral joint rehabilitation. *Am J Sports Med.* 1993;21:438-444.

Teitz CC. Ultrasonography in the knee. *Radiol Clin N Am.* 1988;52:55-62.

Terry GC. The anatomy of the extensor mechanism. *Clin Sports Med.* 1989;8:163-177.

Terry GC, LaPrade RF. The biceps femoris muscle complex at the knee: Its anatomy and injury patterns associated with acute anterolateral-anteromedial rotatory instability. *Am J Sports Med.* 1996;24:2-8.

Tria AJ, Palumbo RC, Alicea JA. Conservative care for the patellofemoral joint. *Orthop Clin N Am.* 1992;23:545-554.

Trojian TH, McKeag DB. Single leg balance test to indentify risk of ankle sprains. *Br J Sports Med.* 2006;40:610-613.

Tropp H, Odenrick P. Postural control in single-limb stance. *J Orthop Res.* 1988;6:833-839.

Tyler TF, McHugh MP, Mirabella MR, Mullaney MJ, Nicholas SJ. Risk factors for noncontact ankle sprains in high school football players: The role of previous ankle sprains and body mass index. *Am J Sports Med.* 2006;34(3):471-475.

Van Dijk CN. Anatomy. In CN van Dijk ed. *On Diagnostic Strategies for Patients with Severe Ankle Sprain.* Amsterdam: Rodopi;1994: 6-50.

Verhagen E, Van der Beek AJ, Bouter LM, Bahr RM, Van Mechelen W. A one season prospective cohort study of volleyball injuries. *Br J Sports Med.* 2004;38:477-481.

Wallace LA, Mangine RE, Malone T. The knee. In: Malone T, McPoil TG, Nitz AJ, eds. *Orthopaedic and Sports Physical Therapy.* 3rd ed. St. Louis, Mo: Mosby; 1997:295-325.

Watts BI, Armstrong B. A randomised controlled trial to determine the effectiveness of double Tubigrip in grade 1 and 2 (mild to moderate) ankle sprains. *Emerg Med J.* 2001;18:46-50.

Wilk KE, Davies GJ, Mangine RE, Malone T. Patellofemoral disorders: A classification system and clinical guidelines for nonoperative rehabilitation. *J Orthop Sports Phys Ther.* 1998;28:307-322.

Chapter 5

Adams MA, Dolan P. Recent advances in lumbar spinal mechanics and their clinical significance. *Clin Biomech.* 1995;10:3-19.

Adams MA, Hutton WC. The effects of posture on the role of the apophyseal joints in resisting intervertebral compression force. *J Bone Joint Surg Br.* 1980;62:358-362.

Akmal M, Kesani A, Anand B, Singh A. Effect of nicotine on spinal disc cells: A cellular mechanism for disc degeneration. *Spine.* 2004;29:568-575.

Barker OJ, Briggs CA, Bogeski G. Tensile transmission across the lumbar fasciae in unembalmed cadavers. *Spine.* 2004;29:129-138.

Beal MC. The sacroiliac problem: Review of anatomy, mechanics, and diagnosis. *J Am Osteopath Assoc.* 1982;81:667-669.

Bergmark A. Stability of the lumbar spine: A study in mechanical engineering. *Acta Orthop Scand.* 1989;230:1-54.

Bogduk N, Engel R. The menisci of the lumbar zygapophyseal joints: A review of their anatomy and clinical significance. *Spine.* 1984;9:454-460.

Bogduk N, Macintosh JE. The applied anatomy of the thoracolumbar fascia. *Spine.* 1984;9:164-170.

Bowan V, Cassidy JD. Macroscopic and microscopic anatomy of the sacroiliac joint from embryonic life until the eighth decade. *Spine.* 1981;6:620-628.

Buckwalter JA. Aging and degeneration of the human intervertebral disc. *Spine.* 1995;20:1307-1314.

Buckwalter JA, Einhorn TA, Simon SR. *Orthopaedic Basic Science: Biology and Biomechanics of the Musculoskeletal System.* Rosemont, Ill: American Academy of Orthopaedic Surgeions; 2000.

Buckwalter JA, Pedrini-Mille A, Pedrini V, et al. Proteoglycans of human infant intervertebral disc: Electron microscopic and biochemical studies. *J Bone Joint Surg Am.* 1985;67:284-294.

Bushell GR, Ghosh P, Taylor TFK, et al. Proteoglycan chemistry of the intervertebral disks. *Clin Orthop.* 1977;129:115-123.

Cholewicki J, McGill S. Mechanical stability of the in vivo spine: Implications for injury and chronic low back pain. *Clin Biomech.* 1996;11:1-15.

DeRosa C, Porterfield JA. *The Sacroiliac Joint.* Berryville, Va: Forum Medicum; 1989.

Fagan A, Moore R, Vernon Roberts B. ISSLS prize winner: The innervations of the intervertebral disc: A quantitative analysis. *Spine.* 2003;28:2570-2576.

Farfan HF. *Mechanical Disorders of the Low Back.* Philadelphia, Pa: Lea & Febiger; 1973.

Farfan HF, Cossette JW, Robertson GH, Wells RV, Kraus H. The effects of torsion on the lumbar intervertebral joint: The role of torsion in the production of disc degeneration. *J Bone Joint Surg.* 1970;52A:468-497.

Gamble JG, Simmons SC, Freedman M. The symphysis pubis. *Clin Orthop Relat Res.* 1986;203:261-272.

Golighty R. Pelvic arthropathy in pregnancy and the puerperium. *Physiotherapy.* 1982;68:216-220.

Gracovetsky S, Farfan HF, Helleur C. The abdominal mechanism. *Spine.* 1985;10:317-324.

Gracovetsky S, Farfan HF, Lamy C. The mechanism of the lumbar spine. *Spine.* 1981;6:249-262.

Gray H. *Anatomy of the Human Body.* Philadelphia, Pa: Lea & Febiger; 2000.

Heylings DJA. Supraspinous and interspinous ligaments of the human spine. *J Anat.* 1978;125:127-131.

Hides JA, Richardson CA, Jull GA. Multifidus muscle recovery is not automatic after resolution of acute, first episode low back pain. *Spine.* 1996;21:2763-2769.

Hodges PW. Is there a role for transversus abdominis in lumbo-pelvic stability? *Man Ther.* 1999; 4:74-86.

Hodges PW, Richardson CA. Inefficient muscular stabilization of the lumbar spine associated with low back pain: A motor control evaluation of transversus abdominis. *Spine.* 1996;21:2640-2650.

Hodges PW, Richardson CA. Contraction of the abdominal muscles associated with movement of the lower limb. *Phys Ther.* 1997a;77:132-144.

Hodges PW, Richardson CA. Feedforward contraction of transversus abdominis is not influenced by direction of arm movement. *Exp Brain Res.* 1997b;114:362-370.

Hungerford B, Gilleard W, Hodges P. Evidence of altered lumbopelvic muscle recruitment in the presence of sacroiliac joint pain. *Spine.* 2003;28:1593-1600.

Kapandji IA. *The Physiology of the Joints.* Vol. 3. Edinburgh: Churchill-Livingstone; 1974.

Kavic N, GrenierS, McGill SM. Determining the stabilizing role of individual torso muscles during rehabilitation exercises. *Spine.* 2004;29(11):1254-1263.

Kippers V, Parker AW. Posture related to electromyographic silence of erectores spinae during trunk flexion. *Spine.* 1984;7:740-745.

Laslett M, Williams M. The reliability of selected pain provocation tests for sacroiliac joint pathology. *Spine.* 1994;19:1243-1249.

Lavignolle B, Vital JM, Senegas J, et al. An approach to the functional anatomy of the sacroiliac joints in vivo. *Anat Clin.* 1983;5:169-176.

Lemperg RK, Arnoldi CC. The significance of intraosseous pressure in normal and diseased states with special reference to the intraosseous engorgement pain syndrome. *Clin Orthop.* 1978;136:143-156.

Luk KDK, Ho HC, Leong JCY. The iliolumbar ligament: A study of its anatomy, development, and clinical significance. *J Bone Joint Surg Br.* 1987;68:197-200.

Macintosh JE, Bogduk N. The morphology of the lumbar erector spinae. *Spine.* 1987;12:658-668.

McCombe PF, Fairbank JCT, Cockersole BC, Punsent PB. Reproducibility of physical signs in low-back pain. *Spine.* 1989;14:908-918.

McDevitt CA. Proteoglycans in the intervertebral disc. In: Ghosh P, ed. *The Biology of the Intervertebral Disc.* Vol. 1. Boca Raton, Fla: CRC Press; 1988:151-170.

McGill SM, Norman RW. The potential of the lumbodorsal fascia forces to generate back extension moments during squat lifts. *J Biomed Eng.* 1988;10:312-318.

Miller JAA, Schultz AB, Andersson GBJ. Load-displacement behavior of sacroiliac joints. *J Orthop Res.* 1987;5:92-101.

Mooney V, Robertson J. The facet syndrome. *Clin Orthop.* 1976;115:149-156.

Moseley GL, Hodges PW, Gandevia SC. Deep and superficial fibers of the lumbar multifidus are differentially active during voluntary arm movements. *Spine.* 2002;27E:29-36.

Niemisto L, Lahtinen-Suopanki T. A randomized trial of combined manipulation, stabilizing exercises, and physician consultation compared to physician consultation alone for chronic low back pain. *Spine.* 2003;28:2185-2191.

O'Neil CW, Kugansky ME, Derby R, et al. Disc stimulation and patterns of referred pain. *Spine.* 2002;27:2776-2781.

Palmoski MJ, Brandt KD. Effects of static and cyclic compressive loading on articular cartilage plugs in vitro. *Arthritis Rheum.* 1980;23:325-334.

Pearcy MJ, Tibrewal SB. Lumbar intervertebral disc and ligament deformations measured in vivo. *Clin Orthop.* 1984;191:281-286.

Porterfield JA, DeRosa C. *Mechanical Low Back Pain: Perspectives in Functional Anatomy.* Philadelphia, Pa: Saunders; 1998.

Porterfield JA, DeRosa CP. The sacroiliac joint. In: Gould JA, ed. *Orthopaedic and Sports Physical Therapy.* 2nd ed. St. Louis, Mo: Mosby-Year Book; 1990:553-573.

Richardson CA, Snijders CJ, Hides, JA et al: The relation between the transversus abdominis muscles, sacroiliac joint mechanics, and low back pain. *Spine.* 2002;27:399-405.

Roberts S, Menage J, Urban PG. Biochemical and structural properties of the cartilage end-plate and its relations to the intervertebral disc. *Spine.* 1989;14:166-174.

Schwarzer AC, Aprill CN, Derby R, Fortin J, Kine G, Bogduk N. Clinical features of patients with pain stemming from the lumbar zygapophyseal joints: Is the lumbar facet syndrome a clinical entity? *Spine.* 1994;19:1132-1137.

Schwarzer AC, Wang S, Bogduk N, McNaught PJ, Laurent R. Prevalence and clinical features of lumbar zygapophyseal joint pain: A study in an Australian population with chronic low back pain. *Ann Rheum Dis.* 1995;54:100-106.

Sturesson B, Selvik G, Uden A. Movements of the sacroiliac joints: A Roentgen stereophotogrammetric analysis. *Spine.* 1989;14:162-165.

Taylor JR. The development and adult structure of the intervertebral disc. *Man Med.* 1990;5:43-47.

Taylor JR, Twomey LT. Vertebral column development and its relation to adult pathology. *Aust J Physiother.* 1985;31:83-88.

Troyanovich SL, Harrison DD, Harrison DE. Motion palpation: it's time to accept the evidence. *J Manipulative Physiol Ther.* 1998;21:568-571.

Tsuji H, Hirano N, Ohshima H, Ishihara H, Terahata N, Motoe T. Structural variation of the anterior and posterior annulus fibrosus in the development of human lumbar intervertebral disc: A risk factor for intervertebral disc rupture. *Spine.* 1993;18:204-210.

Twomey LT, Taylor JR. Age changes in the lumbar articular triad. *Aust J Physiother.* 1985;31:106-112.

Vilensky JA, O'Connor BL, Fortin JD, Merkel GJ, Jimenez AM. Histologic analysis of neural elements in the human sacroiliac joint. *Spine.* 2002;27:1202-1207.

Vleeming A, Pool-Goodzwaard AL, Hammudoghlu D, Stoeckart R, Snidjers CJ, Mens JM. The function of the long dorsal sacroiliac ligaments. *Spine.* 1996;21:556-562.

Vleeming A, Pool-Goudzwaard AL, Stoeckart R, van Wingerden JP, Snidjers CJ. The posterior layer of thoracolumbar fascia: Its function in load transfer from spine to legs. *Spine.* 1995;20:753-758.

Vleeming A, van Wingerden JP, Dijkstra PE, Stoeckhart R, Snijders CJ, Stijnen T. Mobility in the sacroiliac joint in the elderly: A kinematic and radiologic study. *Clin Biomech.* 1992;7:170-176.

Vleeming A, Vries HJ, Mens JM, et al. Possible role of the long dorsal sacroiliac ligament in women with peripartum pelvic pain. *Acta Obstet Gynecol Scand.* 2002;81:430-436.

Weinstein JN, Rauschning W, Resnick D, et al. Part A: Clinical perspectives. In: Frymoyer JW, Gordon SL, eds. *New Perspectives on Low Back Pain.* Park Ridge, Ill: American Academy of Orthopaedic Surgeons; 1989:37-57.

Weiss M, Nagelschmidt M, Struck H. Relaxin and collagen metabolism. *Horm Metab Res.* 1979;11:408-417.

White AA, Panjabi MM. *Clinical Biomechanics of the Spine.* Philadelphia, Pa: Lippincott; 1978.

Yahia LH, Garzon S, Strykowski H, Rivard C-H. Ultrastructure of the human interspinous ligament and ligamentum flavum: A preliminary study. *Spine.* 1990;15:262-268.

Index

Note: The italicized *f* and *t* following page numbers refer to figures and tables, respectively.

A

abdominal muscles
  functional testing of 190-196, 192t
  progressions for 177, 177t, 178t, 179, 192-193, 202-203, 208
  shoulder girdle linkage to 185-186, 189, 196f
  stabilization role 182-186, 182f, 184f, 185f, 186f
Abduction, Prone Horizontal 52
abduction
  in glenohumeral joint strength testing 42-43
  knee injury related to 130, 135
  for rotator cuff 56-60
  in scapular ROM testing 45, 46f
  in total strength concepts 19
  in upper extremity biomechanics 29-31, 36, 40
acceleration 16, 131
acceleration phase, of throwing 34, 34f, 36, 45
acromioclavicular (AC) joint 25-26, 26f, 29, 37
acromioclavicular ligament 25-26, 26f
acromion, impingement and 25, 31-32, 36-37
Active Straight-Leg Raise
  Supine Trunk Curl with 202-203
  as test 136, 137f
Active Trunk Extensions I, II, and III 199-200
activity load. *See* load/loading
adduction
  for rotator cuff 50-56
  in throwing motion 36
  in total strength concepts 19-20
adductor longus muscle 116f
adductor magnus muscle 117, 117f
aerobic/anaerobic base, in progression initiation 9
Aggressive Peroneal Exercise 145
anconeus muscle 28, 28f
angiofibroblastic hyperplasia 40
ankle
  anatomy of
    bone 112, 112f
    ligament 112, 115, 115f, 125
    muscle 120, 120f
  biomechanics of 16, 19, 118, 125
  functional tests of 136
  instability of 125, 127
  sprains of 19, 125, 128, 133-134

annular ligament 26, 26f
annulus fibrosus
  biomechanics of 187-188
  functional anatomy of 168-170, 168f, 170f
  injury to 189-191
anterior chest progressions, modified 92-95
anterior cruciate ligament (ACL)
  anterior vs. posterior bundles of 114, 114f, 123, 123f
  functional anatomy of 110-112, 113f, 114-115, 119f
  injury to 13, 115, 117, 129-130, 134-135, 135f
  in total leg strength 19-20
  in knee biomechanics 123-124, 127, 127f
anterior force couple exercises, for scapula 65-69
anterior superior iliac spine (ASIS), in Q angle 122, 122f
anthropometric girth 14
apophyseal joint 166, 170-171, 187
  injury to 189-190
arm elevation
  biomechanics of 29-32, 37
  for scapula evaluation 42
arm strength, total 18-19
arthrokinematics 28, 32, 121
articular surfaces
  of ankle 125, 127
  of patella 111-112, 111f, 123, 123f
articulations
  as kinetic link 14, 15f, 16, 19, 121
  of lower extremity 110-112, 111f, 113f, 114-115
  of spine 170-173, 186
  of upper extremity 23-26, 24f, 25f, 26f
  of vertebrae 165-167, 165f, 167f, 171
attenuation, of spinal load 170-175, 187-188, 190
  testing for 191-192, 192t

B

back. *See* spine/spinal column
Back Extension, Lumbar 181t
Back Squat 178t
balance 34, 134
Balance Board Squats 213
Ball Catches, Unilateral Quadruped 78
Ball Dribbles
  Floor 87
  Wall 88
Ball Over Edge, Upper Extremity on 83
Ball Slaps, Quadruped 79
Ball Squat 178t

Ball Stabilization, Exercise 82
Ball Toss, Overhead Medicine 207
Bankart lesion, of labrum 39
baseball
  interval throwing program for 102-107
  progressions for 13, 149
  ROM testing for 47, 47t
  strength testing for 43, 43t, 44t
basic progression, as program component 13
basketball 4, 159
Bench Press Narrow Grip 92
bending motion 188-189
Bergmark's model, of core strength 192-193
biceps brachii muscle/tendon
  in shoulder injury 37-40
  stabilization role 28, 28f
biceps femoris tendon 111, 113, 113f, 117-118, 117f, 175
Bilateral Hip and Trunk Extension, Supine 201
Bilateral Leg Lowering, Diagonal 203
Bilateral Row Over Gymnastics Ball 181t
Bilateral Shoulder Extension 69
biomechanics
  of kinetic link system 16-17, 20-21
  of lower extremity 118, 120-128
  of trunk/spine 187-189
  of upper extremity 28-36
Blade Oscillation 91
Blocking Drills, for volleyball 160
Bodyblade, Side-Lying 55-56
body-weight
  distribution during squats 208
  external loading of knee 125-127, 126f
  in strength testing 7, 43, 43t, 44t
bones
  of lower extremity
    ankle 112, 112f
    knee 110-112, 110f, 111f
  progression benefits for 4
  of trunk 164-168
    innominate 164, 167-168, 182
    lumbar vertebrae 164-167, 165f, 166f
    sacrum 164, 167, 167f
  of upper extremity
    elbow 25, 25f
    shoulder 23-25, 24f
Bonnaire's tubercle 167
bony spurs, in elbow 32-33, 33f, 41
BOSU ball platform 82
braces, lower extremity 147
brachialis muscle 28, 28f
brachioradialis muscle 28, 28f
Bridging, Simple 178t
Burn, for volleyball 160

C

Cable Crossover 183, 183f
Cable Pull Perturbation Training 214
Cable Pulls 214
cadence, running, external load in 126
calcaneofibular ligament (CFL) 112, 115, 115f
calcaneus 115, 115f, 118
Calf Raises 147
capitellum 25, 25f
capsular complex, of knee 113-114, 113f, 118-119
capsular ligaments, of shoulder. *See* glenohumeral capsular ligaments
carpal bones 25, 25f
"carrying angle" 25
cartilage
    injury to
        in patellofemoral joint 133, 133t
        in spine 172, 190
    in vertebrae 166, 168-173
cell-matrix response, to tendon injury 40
center of gravity, of body 194
central nervous system (CNS), in trunk/spine movement 163, 188
Chest Fly 93
Chest Pass 75
chest progressions, modified anterior 92-95
chondromalacia
    of elbow 33, 41
    of patellofemoral joint 130-131
Chutes Drill, for football 155
clavicle 23-24, 24f
Closed-Chain Proprioception with Tubing 141-142
closed kinetic chain (CKC) exercises
    for scapula 25, 70-74
    for upper extremity 80-83
closed kinetic chain stability tests
    for lower extremity 124
    for upper extremity 48, 48f
Clubhouse Drill, for volleyball 161
coccyx 164, 167, 167f
cocking phase, of throwing 34-36, 34f
collagen
    in intervertebral discs 168-170, 190
    in thoracolumbar fascia 177
collateral ligaments
    of elbow 26f, 33, 41
    of knee
        biomechanical role 123-124, 123f
        functional anatomy of 110-114, 113f
compensatory movements 14, 30
competition, progression preparation for 5-6
compressive load/force
    constant vs. intermittent, prior to progressions 6
    glenoid concavity and 38
    intervertebral disc countering of 168-170, 188, 190
    lateral patellar 119, 127, 132
    in lumbar spine 164, 166, 168, 171-172, 179, 179f, 186-187, 195
    nerve root irritation with 165, 188-190
    in rotator cuff impingement 37-38

in valgus extension overload of elbow 33f, 34, 41
concentric motion/evaluation 42, 136, 194
connective tissue, of spine 168-170, 168f, 173-174
    injury to 189-191
    periannular 170
conoid ligament 25, 26f
consultation, expert, in functional testing 14
continuous progression, as program component 12-13
coordination development, for core stability 163, 188
coracoacromial ligament 25, 26f, 37
coracobrachialis muscle 27, 27f
coracoid joint 37
core stability. *See also* trunk
    importance of 163, 165, 170, 170f, 174-176, 190
    lower extremity injury risk and 135
    progressions for 13-14, 21
    testing for 191-192, 192t
core strength training 192, 204-207
coronal plane
    lower extremity movements in 109
    of scapular motion 29-30, 45, 46f
    scapular plane vs. 31
court sports, progressions for 148
Crossed Extremity Stability Strengthening 197-198
cruciate ligaments, of knee
    anterior. *See* anterior cruciate ligament (ACL)
        biomechanical role 123-124, 123f
        functional anatomy of 110-115, 113f, 114f
        posterior 110, 112-114, 113f, 119f
        progressions for 13
        in total leg strength 19-20
Curls, Flexion–Extension 84
curl-up, as core stability test 194-195
cutting movements 133-135, 135f
cycling 9, 119

D

Davis' law, of soft tissue healing 4
Deadlift
    Romanian 212
    variations for lumbar overloading 181t
deceleration 16, 129, 132-134
deep squat test 136, 137f
Defensive Ball Drill, for soccer 156
degeneration, of spine 168-169, 171-172, 190
deltoid ligament 112, 125
deltoid muscle 27, 27f, 30f
deltoid–rotator cuff force couple 30-31, 30f
Diagonal Bilateral Leg Lowering 203
dislocations/displacements
    of glenohumeral joint 30, 39
    of patella 110, 116, 131-132
distal joints
    proximal sequencing to, in kinetics 16-17, 188
    of upper extremity
        ROM testing of 45-47

strength testing of 43
distance, as progression guideline 9, 150-151
diving 9
Diving Drill, for soccer 157-158
dorsal root ganglion 165
dorsiflexion, of ankle 125, 127
Drop-Step Drill, for basketball 159
dynamic evaluation
    of lower extremity joint loading 135, 135f
    of scapula 42
    of trunk/spine 192-195, 192t
dynamometer, for strength testing 7, 8f, 42-43, 136

E

eccentric motion
    evaluations of 42, 136
    of spine/hip muscles 186, 188
elbow
    anatomy of
        bone 25, 25f
        ligament 26, 26f
    injury to, total arm strength and 18-19
    as kinetic link 15f, 16-18
    progressions for 84-91
        advanced exercises 87-91
        base exercises 84-87
    ROM testing of 45-47, 46f
    tendinitis of 40
    valgus extension overload of 29, 32-34, 33f, 41
electromyography (EMG)
    of lower extremity function 135, 135f
    of spinal stabilizers 179, 182
electrotherapeutic modalities 6
emotional reactions, to injury 5
empty can test 43
endurance, as progression guideline 9, 163
energy. *See* kinetic energy
epicondylar growth plate, separation of medial 33
epicondylitis, of humerus 40-41
epidural space 167
erector spinae muscles
    functional anatomy of 166, 170, 175
    stabilization role 176, 179, 179f
evaluation, as program component 14-15
eversion movement, of ankle 125
Exercise Ball Stabilization 82
exercises
    movement pattern analysis of 17
    simple vs. complex 5, 9, 109
Extension
    Bilateral Shoulder 69
    Lumbar Back 181t
    Prone 51
    Standing Hip, with selectorized overload 178t
extension
    in lower extremity 121-126, 122f
    lumbar exercises for 180, 181t, 187
    in spine 166, 171-175, 179-180, 180f, 186-189, 208
    in total strength concepts 19, 135-136

Extension Curls, Flexion– 84
Extension Machine, Leg 140
extensor carpi radialis brevis tendon 40
extensor carpi radialis longus tendon 40
extensor carpi radialis muscle 28
extensor carpi ulnaris muscle/tendon 28, 40-41
extensor communis tendon 40
External Rotation
    Oscillation 55
    Prone 56-57
    with Retraction 65
    Side-Lying 50
    Standing 53
    Standing 90/90 57-58
external rotation, in throwing motion 35-36, 40
external rotation/internal rotation (ER/IR) ratio, in strength testing
    for baseball pitchers 43, 44t
    for elite junior tennis players 43, 45t
    of upper extremity 14, 42-43, 45
external rotation test
    of humerus 45-46
    of rotator cuff 14
    of upper extremity 42-43, 44t, 45, 45t
extremities
    arm. See upper extremity
    leg. See lower extremity
    strength training for 163, 197, 204-207
Extremity Stability Strengthening, Crossed 197-198

F
facets
    of patellar articular surfaces 111-112, 111f
    of vertebral bodies 172, 187, 190
        inferior vs. superior 165-167, 165f, 171
fascial system, abdominal 182-183, 182f, 183f
fatigue
    arm, in throwing motion 35
    muscular 12, 14, 19
femoral condyles
    functional anatomy of 110-111, 110f, 114, 117-118
    in knee biomechanics 121-122, 121f, 122f
femoral epicondyles 110, 110f, 114
femoral nerve, in knee 116
femur
    anatomy of 110, 110f, 116, 164
    biomechanics of 121, 121f, 188
fibula, anatomy of 110f, 111-112, 112f
    ligament 113, 113f
field sports, progressions for 149
flexion
    during lateral movements 127-128
    in lower extremity 121, 121f, 123-126
    in total strength concepts 19, 135-136
    in trunk/spine 166, 171-173, 176, 186-187, 189
    in upper extremity 29, 31
Flexion–Extension Curls 84

flexion–extension cycles, spine injury and 166
flexor carpi radialis muscle/tendon 28, 41
flexor carpi ulnaris muscle/tendon 28, 41
Flips 90
"flip sign" 43
Floor Ball Dribbles 87
Flys, Prone 98
follow-through phase, of throwing 34, 34f, 36, 40
foot
    ankle muscle attachments to 120, 120f
    biomechanics of 125, 128, 128f
    contact in throwing 35
football 10, 154-155
foot flat phase, of gait 125, 126f, 128
foot strike phase, of lateral movement 127-128, 127f, 128f
force 4
    in kinetic link system 15f, 16
    knee biomechanics and 111, 123-124
        during running 125-126, 126f
    in labrum injury 39-40
    lower extremity injury related to 129, 131-132, 134
    spine dynamics and 167-170, 170f, 179, 179f, 186, 189
        attenuation of 170-175, 187-188, 190-191
    of tennis serve 17, 17t
force-couple concept
    anterior, in scapula 65-69
    in upper extremity 29-31, 30f
forearm, kinetics of 16-17, 19
Forearm Pronation and Supination 86-87
Forward Lunge 144
fractures, of spine 166, 166f, 187, 190
    compression 164
    microfracture 171, 189
Free Weight, Walking Push Press with 205
frontal plane
    lower extremity movements in 110-111, 113
    lumbar spine and 171, 180, 182, 189
    scapular plane vs. 31
functional movement patterns 15-18, 15f
    of ankle 118, 125
    kinetic analysis of 17
    of knee 125-128
        during gait 125, 126f
        during lateral movement 127-128, 127f, 128f
        during running 125-127, 126f
    of lower extremity 125-128, 147
    of trunk/spine 168, 170-173, 188, 208
    of upper extremity 47-49
Functional Movement Screen (FMS) 8, 9f
    of lower extremity 136, 137f
    of upper extremity 47-49
functional progression programs
    application examples of 11-12, 20
    benefits of 4-6
    clinical guidelines for 6-8
    definition of 3
    goals of 3, 6, 112
    initiation guidelines for 5, 8-10

introduction, 3-4, 10-12
    key components of 12-15
    kinetic link principle of 14-20
    for lower extremity 109, 147, 161
        basic strength exercises vs. 138-147, 214
        sport-specific 147-161
    for postpartum female 173
    regional exercises for 21, 23, 109, 163-164
    for trunk 163-164, 195, 215
        core exercises 192-193, 195, 197-208
        overlap with testing 193-194
        perturbation training 213-214
        squat exercises 208-212
    for upper extremity 23, 49
        anatomy-specific 50-79, 84-99
        closed kinetic chain exercises 80-83
        sport-specific 100-108
functional tests/testing
    of lower extremity 13-14, 14f
        clinical measures in 134-136
        isokinetic 135
        neuromuscular 134-135
        screening measures in 136, 137f
    as progression guideline 12-13
    for range of motion 13-14
    for strength. See strength tests/testing
    of trunk/spine 164, 192t, 195-196
        overlap with training 193-194
    of upper extremity 14, 41-49
        clinical measures in 41-47
        screening measures in 47-49

G
gait cycle/pattern
    ankle biomechanics during 125
    knee biomechanics in 118, 124, 131
    phases and duration of 125, 126f
    progression benefits for 11, 147
galvanic stimulation, high-volt 6
gastrocnemius muscle
    functional anatomy of 110, 113, 118, 118f
    functional testing of 136, 137f
gender, lower extremity injury and 129-130, 134-135, 135f
Gerdy's tubercle 118
glenohumeral capsular ligaments 25, 26f
    in labrum injury 38-39
glenohumeral joint
    anatomy of 25, 26f, 27-28
    arthrokinematics of 28, 32
    biomechanics of 16-17, 30
    instability of 30-31, 37-39
    rehabilitative stresses to 25
    ROM testing of 45-47, 46f
    scapular plane evaluation of 31
    strength testing of 42-43
    in throwing motion 34-36
glenoid fossa
    antetilting of 30, 35
    functional anatomy of 24-25, 24f
    in glenohumeral kinematics 32, 38-39
glenoid labrum 38
    injury to 31, 36, 38-40
gliding, in knee 121, 121f

gluteal nerve, in knee 118
gluteus maximus 117*f*, 128, 175-176
gluteus medius 13-14, 117*f*, 118, 128
Gluteus Medius Exercise, Side-Lying 138-139
glycosaminoglycans, sulfated, in intervertebral discs 169
goalies, soccer 157-159
golf 107-108
goniometer, for ROM testing 45, 46*f*
gracilis muscle 117*f*, 119
gravitational force, in spine 171, 174, 186, 195
gym-based exercises, for shoulder 31
gymnastics 9, 9*f*, 152-153
Gymnastics Ball, Bilateral Row Over 181*t*

H
hamstrings 19, 127, 136
    functional anatomy of 117-118, 117*f*
hamstring to quadriceps (H/Q) ratio 136
hand, kinetics of 17
head and neck position, in trunk progressions 164, 209-212
healing-time constraints, progression and 3-4, 6
heel off phase, of gait 125, 126*f*
heel strike phase, of gait 124-125, 126*f*, 127-128
High-Knees Drill, for football 154
Hip and Trunk Extension
    Supine Bilateral 201
    Supine Unilateral 201-202
hip drop 13-14, 14*f*
Hip Extension, Standing, with selectorized overload 178*t*
hips
    anatomy of 167-168, 175
    biomechanics of 118-119, 127, 182, 188
        during running 125-126, 184, 184*f*
    functional tests for 13-14, 135-136
    as kinetic link 15*f*, 16-17, 19-20
    progressions for 13, 208
Hit and Recover, for volleyball 161
Hit-the-Target Drill, for soccer 159
homeostasis theory, of tissue 131
humeral head
    forced migration of 30-31, 39
    functional anatomy of 24-25, 24*f*
    in glenohumeral kinematics 32
    in throwing motion 36, 38
humerus
    anatomy of 23-25, 24*f*, 27
    epicondylitis of 40-41
    in glenohumeral kinematics 32
    as kinetic link 16-17
    ROM testing of 45-46
hurdle step test 136, 137*f*
hyperangulation, in throwing motion 36
hyperextension, of knee 124

I
iliolumbar ligaments 173*f*, 174
iliopatellar band 119, 132

iliopsoas muscle 117*f*, 128, 179, 181-182
iliotibial (IT) band 117*f*, 118-119, 119*f*, 132
ilium
    force transfer role 167, 172-174, 187
    in knee anatomy 116*f*, 118
impingement
    in knee 117
    in rotator cuff 36-38
    in spine 180
    in upper extremity 25-27, 31-32, 41
impingement test 14
inflammation
    of iliotibial band 132
    of nerve roots 189
    of spinal joints 172, 189
    tendon injury and 40
infraspinatus muscle 27, 27*f*, 30*f*
infraspinatus tendon 37-38
injuries
    to ankle 19, 125, 128, 133-134
    contact vs. noncontact 129-130, 134
    to elbow 18-19, 33, 40-41
    emotional reactions to 5
    to glenoid labrum 31, 36, 38-40
    healing factors of 6
    to knee
        anterior cruciate ligament 129-130, 135, 135*f*
        medial collateral ligament 130
        patellofemoral joint 130-133
    lower extremity mechanisms of 115, 129-135
    overuse 25, 28, 31, 33, 38-41, 45, 132
    rehabilitation of, progressions for 3
    reinjury risk with 5, 9
    to rotator cuff 37-38
    to spine 164-168, 166*f*, 171-172, 189-191, 208
    total arm strength and 18-19
    trunk mechanisms of 187
    upper extremity mechanisms of 36-41
in-line lunge test 136, 137*f*
innominate bone 164, 167-168, 182
instantaneous center of rotation (ICR), of scapulothoracic joint 29
intercondylar notch, of femur 110-111, 121
Internal Rotation
    Plyos at 90° Abduction 63
    Standing 54
    Standing 90/90 58-59
internal rotation
    long-axis, in kinetics 16-17
    in throwing motion 36
internal rotation test
    of humerus 45-46
    of rotator cuff 14
    of upper extremity 42-43, 44*t*, 45, 45*t*
International Cartilage Repair Society (ICRS), chondral injury classification 133, 133*t*
interosseus ligament 174, 175*f*
interspinous ligaments 166-167, 173*f*, 174
interval golf program 107-108
interval tennis program 100-102

interval throwing program, for baseball 102-107
    Little League 106-107
    phase I 102-104
    phase II 105
intervertebral disc
    biomechanics of 187-188
    functional anatomy of 168-170, 168*f*, 173, 181
    injury to 189-190
    vertebral body interface with 165, 168, 172, 186-187
intervertebral foramen 165, 165*f*, 189-190
inversion movement, of ankle 125, 127
ischial tuberosity 175
isokinetic testing, for strength 7, 7*f*
    in baseball pitchers 43, 43*t*, 44*t*
    in elite junior tennis players 43, 44*t*, 45*t*
    of lower extremity 136
    of rotator cuff 14

J
jogging 9
joint reaction force, of patellofemoral joint 124
joints. *See* articulations
jumper's knee 132
jumping
    ankle sprain related to 133-134
    EMG studies of 135, 135*f*
    functional programs for 109, 135, 152-153
    leg strength for 19-20
jump-landing task 109, 135, 152

K
kicking, kinetics of 16
kinesthetic awareness 8, 128, 195, 214
kinetic chain exercises
    for scapula 25, 70-74
    for upper extremity 80-83
kinetic chain principle 14-20
kinetic chain stability tests. *See* closed kinetic chain stability tests
kinetic energy 15*f*, 16
    of tennis serve 17, 17*t*
kinetic link 16
kinetic link principle 14-20
    biomechanical demonstrations of 16-17, 17*t*, 20-21
    introduction to 14-16, 15*f*
    total arm strength concept in 18-19
    total leg strength concept in 19-20
kinetic link system 15-16, 15*f*
    nonoptimal use of 17-18, 18*f*
knee
    anatomy of
        bone 110-112, 110*f*, 111*f*
        capsular complex 113-114, 113*f*, 118-119
        ligament 110, 112-115, 113*f*, 114*f*
        muscle compartment 110, 115-119, 116*f*, 117*f*, 118*f*, 119*f*, 120*f*, 127
    biomechanics of 7*f*, 118, 121-125

arthrokinematic principles of 121, 121*f*

dynamic 123-125

functional movement patterns in 125-128, 126*f*, 127*f*

ligaments in 123-124, 127, 127*f*

patellofemoral joint in 122-125, 123*f*

Q angle in 116, 122, 122*f*

screw-home mechanism in 121-122, 122*f*

functional tests of 13-14, 136

as kinetic link 16, 19-20

pain in 19-20, 119, 124, 126-127, 130-132

progression importance for 11, 208

stability of

anatomical factors 110-112, 115, 117-118

biomechanical factors 121, 122*f*, 123-124

L

labrum. *See* glenoid labrum

lamellae, of vertebrae 168-170

laminae, of vertebral bodies 165, 165*f*, 167

lateral collateral ligament (LCL) 110-114, 113*f*, 118

lateral complex, of ankle 125, 134

lateralis muscle 112

lateral malleolus 112, 115, 120

lateral meniscus 113, 113*f*, 119, 119*f*

lateral movement

knee movement patterns during 119, 125-128, 127*f*, 128*f*, 132

in spine 127, 173, 180

lateral raphe 176

latissimus dorsi muscle 28, 176-177, 177*t*

Latissimus Pull-Down 177*t*

Lat Pull in Front 96

Lawn Mower 67-68

Leg Extension Machine 140

leg length discrepancy 19

Leg Lowering, Diagonal Bilateral 203

Leg Press 145, 178*t*

Leg Raises

Active Straight-

Supine Trunk Curl with 202-203

as test 136, 137*f*

Calf 147

Quadriceps Straight-Leg 139

leg strength, total 19-20

levator scapulae muscle 27, 27*f*

lever arm 188, 192

for lumbar extension 179-180, 179*f*, 180*f*

ligamenta flava 173*f*, 174

ligaments

of lower extremity

ankle 112, 115, 115*f*, 125

knee 112-115, 113*f*, 114*f*, 123

of pubic symphysis 173

of spine 166-167, 170, 173-175, 173*f*, 175*f*, 208

of upper extremity

elbow 26, 26*f*

shoulder 25-26, 26*f*

Little League baseball, interval throwing program for 106-107

Little League elbow 33

load/loading

compressive. *See* compressive load/force

lower extremity absorption of 119, 124-125

during lateral movements 127-128, 127*f*, 128*f*

during running 125-127, 126*f*

testing for 134-135, 135*f*

nonoptimal kinetics and 17-18, 18*f*

for progression initiation 4, 10, 195

in scapula evaluation 42, 42*f*

spine dynamics with 163, 166-170, 186, 190, 195, 208

attenuation of 170-173, 187-191

in valgus elbow extension 29, 32-34, 33*f*

load-to-failure rate, of ankle ligaments 112

longitudinal ligaments, anterior vs. posterior 173*f*, 174

lordosis, lumbar 168, 171, 174

loss of control, muscular 12

low back pain

causes of 170-171, 173

exercise prescriptions for 180, 181*t*, 191

functional exam of 189, 191

peripartum 175

lower extremity 109-161

anatomy of 109-115

biomechanics of 118, 120-128

clinical exercise progressions for 138-147

functional progression programs for 109, 147, 161

basic strength exercises vs. 138-147, 214

sport-specific 147-161

functional testing of 13-14, 14*f*, 134-137

injury to 115, 129-135

as kinetic link 15*f*, 16

muscular stabilization of 115-120

Low Pulley Position, Walking Push Press from 206

Lumbar Back Extension 181*t*

Lumbar Range of Motion, Quadruped 197

lumbar spine

anatomy of

bone 164-167, 165*f*, 166*f*, 170

muscle 175-182, 176*f*, 185, 185*f*

extensor overload exercises for 180, 181*t*

force/load dynamics of 167-168, 172, 187, 208

functional movements in 186-188, 195, 208

functional testing of 164, 190-196, 192*t*

lordosis of 168, 171, 174

zygapophyseal joints of 170-172

lumbopelvic region

anatomy of 164, 167-168, 170-175, 175*f*

functional testing of 164, 190-196, 192*t*

muscular stabilization of 181-182

progressions for 164, 195, 197, 208

lumbosacral angle 167, 167*f*

Lunge

Forward 144

in-line, as test 136, 137*f*

Walking 204

M

malleolus 112, 115, 120

mechanical engineering model, of core strength 192-193

mechanoreceptors 127, 170, 173

medial collateral ligament (MCL)

functional anatomy of 110, 112-114, 113*f*

injury to 130

in knee biomechanics 123-124, 123*f*

medial ligament, of ankle 125

medial malleolus 112

medial meniscus 113, 113*f*, 117, 119, 119*f*

Medicine Ball Balance 74

Medicine Ball Toss, Overhead 207

meniscus

anatomy of 113, 113*f*, 117, 119, 119*f*

in knee biomechanics 121, 122*f*

progressions for 13

metacarpophalangeal (MCP) joints 19

metatarsals 120

midstance phase, of gait 125, 126*f*

mid-support phase, of lateral movement 127, 127*f*

midswing phase, of gait 125, 126*f*

Military Press Modification 94

Mirror Dodge Drill, for football 155

mobility tests, for lumbopelvic region 191-192, 192*t*

Monster Walk, Step-Up 72

motion disturbance, in functional trunk tests 213

motion velocity, neuromotoric control over 195

motor learning, for core stability 163

multifidus muscle

functional anatomy of 166, 170, 176

stabilization role 179-180, 180*f*

multiplanar motions, of trunk 189

muscle contraction, in core stability tests 194-195

muscles

of abdomen. *See* abdominal muscles

agonist-antagonist concept of 7, 29

axiohumeral 28

fatigue of 12, 14, 19

functional testing of 12, 14

of lower extremity

ankle 120, 120*f*

knee 110, 115-119, 116*f*, 117*f*, 118*f*, 119*f*, 120*f*

reflex inhibition of 6

scapulohumeral 27-29, 27*f*

of shoulder girdle 164

of spine 165-166, 168, 170

lumbar 175-182, 176*f*

optimal positioning function of 188

muscles (*continued*)
  of spine (*continued*)
    pathomechanical tests for 191-193, 192*t*
    squat positions and 208
    strains of 190
  strength of. *See* strength tests/testing
  in total leg strength 19
  of upper extremity
    elbow 28, 28*f*
    scapula 26-28, 27*f*
muscular stabilization
  dynamic
    of knee 123-124
    of trunk 189
    of lower extremity 115-120
      ankle joint 120, 120*f*
      knee quadrants 115-119, 123-124
      during lateral movements 127-128
    of scapula. *See* scapular stabilization
  static, of knee 123-124
  of trunk 174-186, 176*f*
  of upper extremity 26-28
    primary 27-28, 27*f*
    superficial 28, 28*f*
musculoskeletal surface, kinetics of 16

N
Neer's stages, of rotator cuff impingement 37
nerve root compression, in spine 165, 188-190
nerves
  in ankle 120
  in knee 116-119
  in spine 163, 165, 170-171, 179-180
neuromuscular control
  over motion velocity 195
  testing lower extremity for 134-135
  trunk role in 163-164, 188, 193
90/90 External Rotation, Standing 57-58
90/90 Plyo Reverse Catches 61-62
90/90 Prone Plyos 60
nociceptors, in spine 170, 172
notches
  of femur, intercondylar 110-111, 121
  of vertebral bodies, inferior vs. superior 165, 165*f*
nucleus pulposus
  biomechanics of 187-188
  functional anatomy of 168-170, 168*f*, 170*f*
  injury to 189
nutrient foramina 164, 165*f*, 169-170

O
objective tests, as program component 13-14
oblique muscles, abdominal 176-177, 182*f*, 183-187, 184*f*, 186*f*
observation, clinical, in functional testing 14
obturator nerve, in knee 119
olecranon, in valgus extension overload 33, 33*f*, 41

Olympic clean and jerk 193-194
One-arm Row 177*t*
one-leg squat test 13-14
one-leg stability test 13, 49
open kinetic chain exercises, for scapula 25, 70-74
Oscillation
  Blade 91
  External Rotation 55
  scapular plane 73
osteochondritis dissecans, of elbow 34
osteophytes, in elbow 32-33, 33*f*, 41
Outerbridge Scale, Modified, of chondral injury 133, 133*t*
Overhead Medicine Ball Toss 207
Overhead Pull-Over 177*t*
overload
  for core stability tests 193
  selectorized, for hip extension 178*t*
  of spinal articular cartilage 172
  tensile, in rotator cuff impingement 37-38
  valgus extension, of elbow 29, 32-34, 33*f*, 41
overuse injuries. *See* repetitive stress injuries

P
pain
  in knee 119, 124, 126-127, 130-132
  in leg 189
  patellofemoral syndrome of 19-20, 127-128, 132
  as program guideline 6, 12, 14, 147
  referred 189-190
  in spine 163, 170-171, 173, 175, 188-190
pars interarticularis 166, 166*f*, 187, 190
Partner Drill, for football 155
patella
  anatomy of 110, 110*f*, 111-112, 111*f*, 119
  force vs. stress encountered by 124
  instability of 110, 116, 131-132
  in Q angle 122
patellar ligament 113*f*, 119*f*
patellar tendon 128, 132
  functional anatomy of 111, 116-117, 116*f*
patellar tracking, lateral, with joint compression 119, 127, 132
patellofemoral (PF) joint
  anatomy of 110
  biomechanics of 118, 122-123
    dynamic 124-125
    during running 125-127
  contact points of 123, 123*f*
  painful dysfunction of 19-20, 127-128, 130-132
    with malalignment 131-132
    without malalignment 131-132
patellofemoral ligaments 112, 113*f*, 119, 120*f*
patellofemoral syndrome 19-20, 127-128, 132
patellotibial ligaments 119
pathomechanical tests, of lumbopelvic region 191-193, 192*t*, 195

pectoralis major muscle 28, 182*f*, 183-184
pectoralis minor muscle 28
pedicles, of vertebral bodies 165, 165*f*, 190
pelvis
  anatomy of 167-168, 170, 172-173
  in bending motion 188
  functional tests of 14, 187, 191-192, 192*t*
  muscular stabilization of 118-119, 132, 180-183, 186, 188
  in running motion 184*f*, 185, 185*f*
  in throwing motion 35
performance enhancement 5, 16-17, 109
Peroneal Exercise, Aggressive 145
peroneal nerve, in knee 118
peronei brevis ligament 112, 120, 120*f*
peronei longus ligament 112, 120, 120*f*
Perturbation Training, in functional trunk tests 188, 213
  Cable Pull 214
  Squat 213
pes anserinus 114, 117, 119
physical evaluation
  of low back pain 191-192, 192*t*
  preseason 13
physiological benefits, of functional progression 4-5
piano key sign 26
Pilates 194
pitching
  interval throwing program for
    flat-ground 104
    Little League 106-107
    off the mound 105
  ROM testing for 47, 47*t*
  strength testing for 43, 43*t*, 44*t*
Planks
  Prone 179, 198
  Side 199
plantar flexion, of ankle 125-127, 134
plyometric exercises, for rotator cuff 60-64
Plyos
  90/90 Prone 60
  90/90 Reverse Catches 61-62
  Internal Rotation at 90° Abduction 63
  Wall 77
Pointer, Triped to 81
popliteal ligament, oblique 113*f*
popliteal nerve, in ankle 120
popliteus muscle/tendon 110, 119*f*
posterior cruciate ligament (PCL) 110, 112-114, 113*f*, 119*f*
Posterior Tibialis Exercise 146
postpartum female, functional progressions for 173
Post-Up Hook Shot, for basketball 159
posture
  of ACL-deficient athlete 127
  standing. *See* standing position
pregnancy 173
Press
  Leg 145, 178*t*
  Squat 211
preswing phase, of lateral movement 127, 127*f*

preventive programs, for lower extremity injury 109, 129, 135
processes, of vertebral bodies
    posterior 165, 165*f*
    spinous 165*f*, 166-167, 176, 179
    transverse 165*f*, 166, 181
pronation
    of foot and ankle 125-126, 128
    of forearm
        for elbow and wrist progression 86-87
        in kinetics 16-17, 19
pronator quadratus muscle 28
pronator teres muscle 28
pronator teres tendon 41
Prone Extension 51
Prone External Rotation 56-57
Prone Flys 98
Prone Horizontal Abduction 52
Prone Plank 179, 198
Prone Plyos, 90/90 60
prone position, for lumbopelvic exam 192*t*, 195
proprioception 3, 8, 194
    lower extremity activities for 109, 128, 134, 147
    trunk exercises for 194-195, 213-214
    upper extremity activities for 141-142
proprioceptive neuromuscular facilitation (PNF) 136, 170, 173
proteoglycans, in intervertebral discs 169-170, 172
protraction, in upper extremity 30, 183-184, 183*f*
provocation tests
    in lumbopelvic exam 191-192, 192*t*
    for rotator cuff strength 43
    in scapula evaluation 42, 42*f*
proximal to distal sequencing, in kinetic link system 16-17, 188
psoas major muscle 117*f*, 128, 179, 181-182
psychological benefits, of functional progression 5-6
pubic symphysis 167-168, 170, 173, 185
Pull-Down, Latissimus 177*t*
Pulley Position, Walking Push Press from Low 206
Pull in Front, Lat 96
Pull-Over, Overhead 177*t*
Pulls, Cable 214
push-up, as functional test 47-48, 48*f*
    for trunk stability 136, 137*f*

Q
quadratus lumborum ligament 174
quadratus lumborum muscle 180
quadriceps angle (Q angle), of knee 116, 122, 122*f*
    patellofemoral force and 127-128
quadriceps muscle/tendon
    biomechanical role 19, 123-124, 127-128
    functional anatomy of 111, 116-117, 116*f*
    functional testing of 136
    strengthening of 11, 13, 19

Quadriceps Straight-Leg Raise 139
Quadruped Ball Catches, Unilateral 78
Quadruped Ball Slaps 79
Quadruped Lumbar Range of Motion 197
Quadruped Rhythmic Stabilization 80
Quartet Squats 143

R
radial collateral ligament 26, 26*f*
Radial Ulnar Deviation 85
radiculopathy, spinal 165, 188-190
radiocapitellar joint, in valgus extension overload 34
radius 19, 25-26, 25*f*
range of motion (ROM)
    anatomy-specific. *See* biomechanics
    ER/IR ratio and. *See* external rotation/ internal rotation (ER/IR) ratio
    objective measures of 13-14
    as progression guideline 7, 11-12
    total rotation, in glenohumeral joint 46-47, 47*t*
rectus abdominis muscles 182*f*, 183, 184*f*
rectus femoris muscle 116, 116*f*
repetitive stress injuries
    to lower extremity 132
    to upper extremity 25, 28, 31, 33, 38-41, 45
respiration phases, in core stability tests 194-195
retinacula, of knee 112-113, 116, 119, 120*f*
retraction, in upper extremity 30
Retraction, External Rotation with 65
return-to-sport programs
    functional progression concept in 3-6
    lower extremity testing and 136, 137*f*
    spinal pain and 188
    for upper extremity 100-108
Reverse Catches, 90/90 Plyo 61-62
rhomboid muscles 27, 27*f*, 185, 186*f*
Rhythmic Stabilization
    Quadruped to Triped 80
    Supine 66-67
Robbery 68
rolling
    in glenohumeral joint 32
    in knee 121, 121*f*
Romanian Deadlift (RDL) 212
rotary stability test, for lower extremity 136, 137*f*
rotation
    in ankle biomechanics 125
    external. *See* external rotation
    internal. *See* internal rotation
    in kinetic link system 16-17
    in knee biomechanics 121, 122*f*, 127, 130
    in spine/trunk biomechanics 168, 171-173, 180, 186-190, 208
    in throwing motion 35-36
    in upper extremity
        biomechanics of 29-32, 183
        testing for 14, 42-47, 44*t*, 45*t*, 46*f*
rotator cuff
    force couple concept of 30-31, 30*f*

impingement of 31, 36-38
injury to 25, 37-38
muscles of 27-28, 27*f*
progressions for 50-64
    abducted position 56-60
    adducted position 50-56
    plyometric 60-64
    specific exercises 11-13
strength testing of 14, 42-43
in throwing motion 36
Row 70
    One-arm 177*t*
    Seated Variation 99, 177*t*
    Unilateral Bent-Over 97
rowing 9
Row Over Gymnastics Ball, Bilateral 181*t*
running
    knee loading during 125-127, 126*f*
    knee pain with 119
    pelvis motion during 184*f*, 185, 185*f*
    progressions for 9-10, 13
        distance 150-151
ruptures. *See* tears

S
sacral hiatus 167
sacroiliac (SI) joint
    anatomy of 167-168, 170, 172
    biomechanics of 172-173, 182, 187, 195
sacroiliac ligaments 174-175, 175*f*
sacrospinous ligament 175
sacrotuberous ligament 175
sacrum
    anatomy of 164, 167, 167*f*
    biomechanics of 172, 187-188
sagittal plane
    lower extremity movements in 109-111, 113, 121
    of scapular motion 29-30
    scapular plane vs. 31
    spine movements in 171, 179, 182, 186-189, 195
Scaption 0 to 90° 95
scapula
    anatomy of 23-24, 24*f*, 27, 164, 185
    biomechanics of 16, 19, 27, 29-30
    functional evaluation of 41-42, 42*f*
    progressions for 11-13. *See also* scapular stabilization
    strength testing of 42-43
    in throwing motion 36
scapular plane
    functional anatomy of 24-25, 24*f*
    kinetic chain movement patterns in 25
    in upper extremity biomechanics 28-29, 31
Scapular Plane Oscillation 73
scapular stabilization
    evaluation of 42-43
    primary muscles for 27, 27*f*
    progressions for 65-79
        kinetic chain exercises 70-74
        plyometric exercises 75-79
        trapezius–serratus anterior force couple exercises 65-69

scapular stabilization (*continued*)
    ROM testing of 45-46, 46*f*
scapulothoracic motion 29, 35, 164, 200, 202
sciatic nerve, in knee 117-118
scientific principles, of functional progression 3-4, 8
screw-home mechanism, in knee biomechanics 121, 122*f*
Seated Row Variation 99, 177*t*
semimembranosus muscle 117, 117*f*
semitendinosus muscle 117, 117*f*
sequence/sequencing
    improper timing of 17-18, 18*f*
    in kinetic link system 15*f*, 16-17, 18*f*, 188
serratus anterior muscle
    in scapular exercises 65-69
    stabilization role 27, 27*f*, 29-30, 183-185, 186*f*
Serratus Press 66
Serratus Punch 66
serving. *See* tennis serve
shear force/stress
    in labrum injury 39
    in lumbar spine 169-172, 179, 179*f*, 184, 187, 195
shoulder
    anatomy of
        bone 23-25, 24*f*
        ligament 25-26, 26*f*
    injury to, total arm strength and 18
    as kinetic link 15*f*, 16-18
    mobility testing of 137*f*
    progressions for 11-12, 92-95
    strength training for 31, 50-60
Shoulder Extension, Bilateral 69
shoulder girdle
    abdominal mechanism linkage to 185-186, 189, 196*f*
    anatomy of
        bone 23-25, 24*f*
        muscle 164, 182*f*, 183-184
Side-Lying Bodyblade 55-56
Side-Lying External Rotation 50
Side-Lying Gluteus Medius Exercise 138-139
side-lying position, for lumbar spine tests 195
Side Plank 199
side-step maneuver
    EMG studies of 135, 135*f*
    knee movement patterns during 125, 127-128, 127*f*, 128*f*
signs and symptoms, monitoring of 12
Simple Bridging 178*t*
sitting position
    knee biomechanics in 124
    for lumbopelvic exam 192*t*
skill guidelines, for progression initiation 5, 9-10, 195
sliding, in glenohumeral joint 32
Snaps 89
soccer 156-159

softball 149
soft tissue
    progression benefits for 4
    of spine. *See* connective tissue
soleus muscle 136, 137*f*
specific adaptations to imposed demands (SAID) 3-4
speed. *See also* velocity
    external lower extremity load with 127-128, 136
    in kinetic link system 16-17
    in progression initiation 9
spinal nerve 165
Spin Drill, for football 154
spine/spinal column
    anatomy of
        bone 164-168, 165*f*, 166*f*, 167*f*
        connective tissue 168-170, 168*f*, 170*f*
        joint 170-173
        ligament 166-167, 170, 173-175, 173*f*, 175*f*, 208
        muscle 165-166, 168, 170, 208
        nerve 163, 165, 170-171, 179-180
    biomechanics of 15*f*, 16, 187-189
        with lateral movement 127, 173, 180
    functional testing of 164, 190-196, 192*t*
    injury to 164-166, 166*f*, 168, 171-172, 189-191, 208
    pain in 163, 170-171, 173, 175, 188-190
    progression programs for 163-164, 195, 215
        core exercises 195, 197-208
        modified for upper 96-99
        perturbation training 213-214
        squat exercises 208-212
spondylolisthesis 166, 166*f*, 187, 190
spondylolysis 166, 166*f*
sport performance
    enhancement of 5, 16-17, 109
    movement pattern analysis of 17
sport rehabilitation. *See also* functional progression programs
    functional progression concept in 3
    for lower extremity 109, 147, 161
    for trunk 163-164, 195, 215
    for upper extremity 23, 49
sport-specific progression 13
    for lower extremity rehabilitation 147-161
    for upper extremity rehabilitation 100-108
sprains, of ankle 19, 125, 128, 133-134
sprinting 9
Square Drill, for football 154
Squat Perturbation Training 213
Squats
    Back 178*t*, 209
    Balance Board 213
    Ball 178*t*
    deep, as test 136, 137*f*
    Front 210
    for lumbar overloading 181*t*, 208
    Perturbation Training 213
    Press 211

Quartet 143
Romanian Deadlift 212
squatting, knee biomechanics in 124-125
Stability Strengthening, Crossed Extremity 197-198
stability tests
    closed kinetic chain 48, 48*f*, 124
    for lumbopelvic region 191-192, 192*t*
    one-leg 13, 49
    rotary, for lower extremity 136, 137*f*
    for scapula 42-43, 45-46, 46*f*
stair ambulation, knee biomechanics in 124
stance, in throwing motion 35
stance phase, of gait 125, 126*f*, 127
Standing 90/90 External Rotation 57-58
Standing 90/90 Internal Rotation 58-59
Standing External Rotation 53
Standing Hip Extension, with selectorized overload 178*t*
Standing Internal Rotation 54
standing position
    lumbar weight-bearing and 168, 172, 175-176, 184
    for lumbopelvic exam 192*t*
    for scapula evaluation 41-42
static evaluation, of scapula 41-42
Statue of Liberty 59-60
step, hurdle, as test 136, 137*f*
Step-Downs 144
step-down sign 26
step-down test 14
Step-Up Monster Walk 72
Step-Ups 71
Straight-Leg Raise
    Active
        Supine Trunk Curl with 202-203
        as test 136, 137*f*
    Quadriceps 139
strains, of spinal muscles 190
strength
    as program guideline 7, 8*f*
    total, in kinetic link system 18-19
strength tests/testing
    isokinetic. *See* isokinetic testing
    of lower extremity 136
    manual 7, 43
    objective measures in 13-14, 42
    of upper extremity 7, 8*f*, 14, 42-45, 43*t*, 44*t*, 45*t*
strength training
    basic exercises for 138-147, 214
    core 192, 204-207
    for extremities 163, 197, 204-207
    for shoulder 31, 50-60
    for thoracolumbar fascia 177, 178*f*
stress(es) 4
    manual, in lumbopelvic tests 191
    nonoptimal kinetics and 17-18, 18*f*
    of patellofemoral joint 124, 126-128
stride, running, external load in 126
stride angle, in throwing motion 35
subacromial space 37
subchondral bone, in spine 169, 171, 189-190
subjective tests, of strength 7

subluxation relocation test 14
subluxations. *See* dislocations/displacements
subpedicular recess 165, 165*f*
subscapularis muscle 27, 27*f*
subtalar joint 118, 125, 127
summation of speed principle 16
superior labrum anterior posterior (SLAP) lesions 39-40
Supination, Forearm 86-87
supination
    of foot and ankle 125, 128
    of forearm 19
Supine Bilateral Hip and Trunk Extension 201
supine position, for lumbopelvic exam 192*t*, 195
Supine Rhythmic Stabilization 66-67
Supine Trunk Curl 202
    with Active Straight-Leg Raise 202-203
Supine Unilateral Hip and Trunk Extension 201-202
supraspinatus muscle 27, 27*f*, 30*f*, 43
supraspinatus tendon 37-38
supraspinous ligaments 167, 173*f*, 174
swelling 6, 12
swimming 9
swing phase, of gait 125, 126*f*
synovial joint
    of knee 111-112, 114
    of vertebral facets 166, 171-172

T
talocrural joint. *See* ankle
talofibular ligaments, anterior vs. posterior 112, 115, 115*f*, 125
talus 112, 112*f*, 115, 125
tape/taping, of lower extremity 147
tears
    of labrum 39
    of rotator cuff 37-38
tendinitis 40, 132
tendons
    cell-matrix response to injuries 40
    injury to
        in elbow 18-19, 40-41
        in knee 132
    of lower extremity 111, 116-117, 116*f*, 128, 132
    of upper extremity 28, 28*f*, 37-40
tennis
    return-to-sport progressions for 100-102
    ROM testing for 45-47, 47*t*
    strength testing for 43, 44*t*, 45*t*
    total arm strength and 18-19
tennis elbow 18-19, 40-41
tennis serve
    kinetics of 16-18, 17*t*
    pre-serve progressions for 101-102
    valgus extension overload with 32-34, 33*f*, 41
tensile load/force
    intervertebral disc countering of 168-170, 170*f*
    in rotator cuff impingement 37-38

in trunk biomechanics 175-176, 187
tensor fasciae latae 116*f*, 118
teres major muscle 27, 27*f*, 30*f*
teres minor muscle 27, 27*f*, 30*f*
terminal extension, in knee biomechanics 121, 122*f*
thoracic wall, in upper extremity biomechanics 30, 42
thoracolumbar fascia (TLF)
    biomechanics of 176, 180, 184
    functional anatomy of 166, 175-176, 176*f*
    strength exercises for 177, 178*f*
throwing
    arm strength for 7, 14, 43, 45
    impingement with 37-38
    interval program for 102-107
        Little League 106-107
        phase I 102-104
        phase II 105
    kinetics of 16-17, 189
    labrum injury from 40
    overhead
        biomechanics of 34-36, 34*f*
        impingement with 37-38
    phases of 34, 34*f*
    progressions for 9, 11-13
    valgus extension overload with 32-34, 33*f*, 41
tibia
    anatomy of 110*f*, 111-112, 112*f*
        ligament 113, 113*f*, 119
    in knee biomechanics 121, 121*f*, 127
tibial eminence 111
Tibialis Exercise, Posterior 146
tibial nerve, in knee 118
tibial plateau 110*f*, 111, 121, 121*f*
tibial tuberosity 111, 121-122
tibiofemoral joint
    anatomy of 111, 113, 113*f*, 119
    biomechanics of 121, 122*f*, 127
tibiofibular ligament, posterior 113*f*
time, in distance running progressions 151
timing, in kinetic link system 17-18, 18*f*
tissue healing
    cell-matrix response with 3, 6, 40
    homeostasis theory of 131
    as program guideline 3-4, 6
toe off phase, of gait 125, 126*f*
tolerance
    in functional movement screening 6, 8
    as program guideline 12-13
torque
    in knee abduction, ACL injury and 19
    of tennis serve 17-18
    in trunk/spine 187-188
torque-to-body-weight ratio, in strength testing 7
    for baseball pitchers 43, 43*t*
    for elite junior tennis players 43, 44*t*
torsional force/load
    in labrum injury 40
    in lumbar spine 169, 171, 180, 187, 195
    in patellar dislocation 132

in sacroiliac joint 172-173, 182, 187, 195
torso. *See* trunk
total arm strength (TAS) 18-19
total leg strength (TLS) 19-20
total rotation range of motion, in glenohumeral joint 46-47, 47*t*
translation
    of anterior tibia 124, 127
    of humeral head 30-31, 39
    obligate, in upper extremity 29, 32
    in throwing motion 35
    of vertebral segments 173, 182, 189
transverse plane
    lower extremity movements in 121
    of scapular motion 29-30
transversus abdominis muscle 176, 179, 182-186, 182*f*, 184*f*, 185*f*
trapezius muscle
    in scapular exercises 65-69
    stabilization role 27, 27*f*, 29-30
trapezoid ligament 25, 26*f*
Trendelenburg sign 13-14, 14*f*
Triangle Drill, for soccer 156
triceps brachii muscle 28, 28*f*
Triped Rhythmic Stabilization 80
Triped to Pointer 81
trochlea
    functional anatomy of
        in lower extremity 110-111, 122-124
        in upper extremity 25, 25*f*
    patellar dislocation and 131-132
trunk 163-215
    activity performance role 163-164
    anatomy of 164-175
    biomechanics of 187-189
        with lateral movement 127, 173, 180
    functional progression programs for 163-164, 195, 215
        core exercises 195, 197-208
        perturbation training 213-214
        squat exercises 208-212
    functional testing of 164, 190-196, 192*t*
    injury to 189-190
    as kinetic link 15*f*, 16-17, 19
    muscular stabilization of 26, 163, 175-186
    in throwing motion 36
Trunk Curl, Supine 202
    with Active Straight-Leg Raise 202-203
Trunk Extensions
    Active I, II, and III 199-200
    Supine Bilateral Hip and 201
    Supine Unilateral Hip and 201-202
trunk stability push-up test 136, 137*f*
Tubing, Closed-Chain Proprioception with 141-142

U
ulna 19, 25-26, 25*f*
ulnar collateral ligaments 26, 26*f*, 33, 41
ulnohumeral joint 25, 25*f*
underloading, of spinal articular cartilage 172
Unilateral Bent-Over Row 97

Unilateral Hip and Trunk Extension, Supine 201-202
Unilateral Quadruped Ball Catches 78
upper back exercises 96-99
upper extremity 23-108
    anatomy of 23-26
    biomechanics of 28-36
    functional progression programs for 23, 49-108
        anatomy-specific 50-79, 84-99
        closed kinetic chain exercises 80-83
        sport-specific 100-108
    functional testing of 14, 41-49
    impingement in 25-27, 31-32, 41
    injury to 36-41
    as kinetic link 15f, 16
    muscular stabilization of 26-28, 27f, 28f
    ROM testing in 45-47, 46f
    strength testing of 7, 8f, 14
Upper Extremity BOSU 82
Upper Extremity on Ball Over Edge 83

V
valgus collapse, in ACL injury 129-130
valgus extension overload, of elbow 29, 32-34, 33f, 41
valgus stress
    ACL biomechanics and 19, 123-124, 135
    knee injury related to 129-130
    in tennis serve 18
    upper extremity anatomy and 26, 29

varus stress 28, 124
vascular channels, in intervertebral discs 169, 172, 189-190
vastus intermedialis muscle 116, 116f
vastus lateralis muscle 116, 116f, 119
vastus medialis muscle 112, 116-117, 116f, 119
vastus medialis oblique (VMO) muscle 116-117, 116f
velocity. *See also* speed
    high, patellofemoral stress with 128
    joint angular, in kinetics 16
    motion, neuromotoric control over 195
    of tennis serve, segmental contribution to 17, 17t
vertebrae
    lumbar 164-167, 165f, 166f
    sacral 164, 167, 167f
vertebral bodies 164-168, 165f, 166f
vertebral body–intervertebral disc interface 165, 168, 172, 186-187
video analysis
    of ACL injury 129
    in functional testing 14
visual analog scale (VAS), for pain assessment 12
volleyball 160-161

W
Walking Lunge 204
Walking Push Press
    with Free Weight 205
    from Low Pulley Position 206

Wall Ball Dribbles 88
Wall Plyos 77
water component, of intervertebral discs 169-170
weight bearing
    lower extremity injury related to 131, 134
    lower extremity mechanics of 119, 123, 125
    lumbar spine and 168-172, 174-175
    in progression initiation 9, 195
weight shift, in progression initiation 9
Windshield Wiper 64
windup phase, of throwing 34, 34f
winging, of scapula 42, 42f
Wolff's law, of soft tissue healing 4
Wood Chops 76
work-to-body-weight ratio, in strength testing
    for baseball pitchers 43, 43t
    for elite junior tennis players 43, 44t
wrestling 9-10, 148
wrist
    as kinetic link 15f, 16-17, 19
    progressions for 84-91
        advanced exercises 87-91
        base exercises 84-87

Y
yoga 194

Z
zygapophyseal joints, in spine 166, 171-172

About the Authors

Todd S. Ellenbecker, DPT, CSCS, is clinic director for Physiotherapy Associates Scottsdale Sports Clinic in Scottsdale, Arizona, and the national director for Clinical Research Physiotherapy Associates. He has been a physical therapist for more than 35 years, specializing in orthopedic and sports physical therapy. He is also a certified strength and conditioning specialist.

Ellenbecker is the primary author of more than 20 peer-reviewed research publications in orthopedic and sport physical therapy, and he is the primary author of more than 10 books in these fields. He serves as director of Sports Medicine ATP Tour (Association of Tennis Professionals) and chairman of the United States Tennis Association Sport Science Committee. He is a member of the American Physical Therapy Association (APTA), the American College of Sports Medicine (ACSM), and the Society for Tennis Medicine and Science.

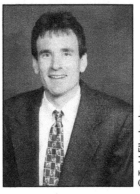

© Todd Ellenbecker

In 2007 Ellenbecker received the Ron Peyton Award for sport physical therapy, and in 2008 he earned the International Tennis Hall of Fame Education Merit Award.

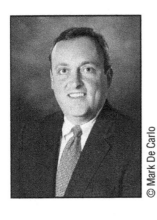

© Mark De Carlo

Mark S. De Carlo, PT, MHA, SCS, ATC, is vice president of clinical services for Methodist Sport Medicine/ The Orthopaedic Specialists in Indianapolis. He has more than 23 years of clinical experience with high school, college, and professional athletes and has more than 40 published articles and book chapters to his credit. A certified athletic trainer and board-certified sports clinical specialist, De Carlo is president of the Sports Physical Therapy Section for the APTA and current board member of the International Federation of Sports Physical Therapy.

Carl DeRosa, PT, PhD, FAPTA, is professor of physical therapy at Northern Arizona university and co-owner of DeRosa Physcial Therapy in Flagstaff, Arizona. Dr. DeRosa completed his physical therapy education at the Mayo Clinic and earned his master's and doctoral degrees in human anatomy. His scholarly interests over the past 25 years have been focused on the anatomy and mechanics of the human spine and shoulder girdle with particular emphasis on their relationship to orthopedics, sport, and rehabilitation sciences. He has co-authored

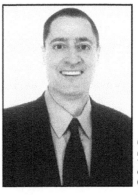

© Carl DeRosa

several textbooks, textbook chapters, journal articles, and two series for home study. In addition to research and invited presentations throughout the United States, Dr. DeRosa has presented his work at numerous national and international conferences, including the International Federation of Manual Therapists' World Congress on Low Back and Pelvic Pain. In recognition of his contributions to the profession of physcial therapy, Dr. DeRosa was awarded the Lucy Clair Service Award and, in addition, was selected by the APTA Board of Directors as a Maley Lecturer. He is a Catherine Worthingham Fellow of the APTA.